Genetics and the Unsettled Past

Rutgers Studies in Race and Ethnicity

Controversies in race and ethnicity cannot be fully understood through a single analytical lens or disciplinary approach. Such issues require sustained, collaborative analysis—drawing on insights from law to history, from sociology to literature, from labor studies to anthropology, from political science to health-related scholarship, and from biology to cultural studies. Focusing primarily on edited volumes, the series aims to bring multiple theories, methods, and approaches to bear on how racial and ethnic politics, identity, culture, structures, and social relations function in the modern world. Through innovative critical commentary and sustained policy engagement, this series encourages scholarship aimed at expanding and deepening the study of these issues in the United States and around the globe. Organized by the Rutgers Center for Race and Ethnicity, the series is an outgrowth of the breadth, depth, and strength of the field at the University and is committed to new collaborative scholarship that bridges boundaries. Readers will find a deep and expansive understanding of the intricate and often unrecognized ways in which race and ethnicity shapes and is shaped by modern societies.

Series Editors: Keith Wailoo, Karen M. O'Neill, Mia Bay, and Lisa Miller

Keith Wailoo, Karen M. O'Neill, Jeffrey Dowd, and Roland Anglin, eds., *Katrina's Imprint: Race and Vulnerability in America*

Keith Wailoo, Alondra Nelson, and Catherine Lee, eds., *Genetics and the Unsettled Past: The Collision of DNA, Race, and History*

Genetics and the Unsettled Past

The Collision of DNA, Race, and History

EDITED BY

KEITH WAILOO
ALONDRA NELSON
CATHERINE LEE

RUTGERS UNIVERSITY PRESS

NEW BRUNSWICK, NEW JERSEY, AND LONDON

LIBRARY OF CONGRESS CATALOGING-IN-PUBLICATION DATA

Genetics and the unsettled past : the collision of DNA, race, and history / edited by Keith Wailoo, Alondra Nelson, and Catherine Lee.

    p. cm. — (Rutgers studies in race and ethnicity)

Includes bibliographical references and index.

ISBN 978–0–8135–5254–5 (hardcover : alk. paper) — ISBN 978–0–8135–5255–2 (pbk. : alk. paper) — ISBN 978–0–8135–5336–8 (e-book)

    1. Human population genetics.   2. Genomics.   3. Gene mapping.   4. Genetic markers.   5. Race.   6. Ethnicity.   I. Wailoo, Keith.   II. Nelson, Alondra. III. Lee, Catherine.

GN289.G463   2012

611′.0181663—dc23

2011023491

A British Cataloging-in-Publication record for this book is available from the British Library.

Visit our Web site: rutgerspress.rutgers.edu

Manufactured in the United States of America

CONTENTS

PART THREE
Stories Told in Blood

Conclusions: The Unsettled Past

ACKNOWLEDGMENTS

Drawn together by a common interest in race, history, and science, the editors of this volume—Keith Wailoo, Alondra Nelson, and Catherine Lee—along with Mia Bay, organized a conference on "Race, DNA, and History" in late 2007. Submissions for the conference came in from scholars across many disciplines, indicating the ways in which questions concerning the genetic view of race stretched across fields in the humanities, social sciences, the sciences, and the professions. The essays in this collection were among the most compelling essays in the conference, and a subsequent meeting of the authors transformed the often disparate questions of race, genes, and history across law, medicine, culture, and society into one multidimensional conversation. This book is the product of those rich conversations tracking the unfolding problems of genes and identity. We must first thank Mia Bay for her contributions toward the conceptualization and organization of the conference. Helpful as well were the contributions of Eviatar Zerubavel, Nadia Abu El-Haj, Julie Livingston, Stephen Pemberton, Ann Jurecic, and Sumit Guha. The logistical challenges of the conferences and planning the volume were deftly handled by Mia Kissil, the senior program coordinator at Rutgers Center for Race and Ethnicity. We could not have held the conference nor put together this volume without the financial support of the Center for Race and Ethnicity and Rutgers University more generally. The center also provided sustained commentary, insight, and organizational energy of the graduate research assistants over many years who offered incisive comments and administrative support. They are: Jill Campaiola, Elizabeth Reich, Simone Delerme, Sonja Thomas, Anantha Sudhakar, Jeffrey Dowd, Dora Vargha, Bridget Gurtler, Fatimah Williams-Castro, Melissa Stein, Stephanie Jones-Rogers, Fred Hanna, Isra Ali, Nadia Brown, Dana Brown, and finally, Shakti Jaising, who offered extraordinary editorial insight at multiple stages of this project. We are also grateful for the helpful evaluations of two anonymous reviewers for their critical questions and trenchant comments. We also wish to thank the Russell Sage Foundation, the James S. McDonnell Foundation (Centennial Fellowship in the History of Science), Yale University, Columbia University, Rutgers University, colleagues in the Rutgers History Department and Sociology Department, and the Institute for Health, Health Care Policy, and Aging Research for many years of support for the multidisciplinary research at the heart of this study. Finally, we must thank our tireless and patient editor at the Rutgers University Press, Leslie Mitchner, for her extraordinary engagement and insight on this important project.

Genetics and the Unsettled Past

Introduction

Genetic Claims and the Unsettled Past

KEITH WAILOO, ALONDRA NELSON, AND CATHERINE LEE

As the American geneticist, anthropologist, and television presenter Spencer Wells boldly claims in his 2003 PBS documentary *The Journey of Man*, the study of genetic variation in people around the globe opens an unparalleled view into the past. One drop of blood or a few cells swabbed from the inside of the cheek, he insists, not only unveils mankind's origins in Africa, but also reveals the pathways along which human beings traveled into Europe, Asia, and North and South America.

It is a compelling narrative of the body as a microcosm of the past. And, in another bold move that marries science to business, Wells and others like him have commercialized this vision—successfully translating laboratory insights from population genetics into an international collaborative science endeavor, the Genographic Project, in which individual consumers purchase DNA test kits that yield personal genetic results *and* scientific data toward the further elucidation of "the ultimate human history . . . written in our genes."[1] Wells's recent venture is but one instance of the countless ways that this new era of genetic analysis has expanded far beyond the arena of origin stories and popular science over the last few years—connecting individuals and groups to imagined ancestors.

These recent developments in genetic analysis have been employed to uncover, not only individual ancestry, but also group heritage. Genetic markers—referring to tiny sections where miniscule variations on the chromosomes are evident from person to person, tiny data points standing out against the otherwise vast uniformity across all humanity—have come to be regarded as scientific portals to the past. Analysis of these markers is increasingly employed to investigate and adjudicate issues of social membership and kinship; rewrite history and collective memory; arbitrate legal claims and human rights controversies; and open new thinking about health and wellbeing.[2] Not surprisingly, these latest applications have attracted much attention, and at times generated intense public controversy.

1

In 2010 alone, the debates and assertions arising over genetic analysis were almost as numerous as the genetic practices themselves. In April, the Havasupai Indians, who reside within the Grand Canyon, won their fight with academic geneticists over the analyses of their members' genes and history, which the tribe had never sanctioned. In May of this same year, Walgreens announced that it was reconsidering its plan to sell Pathway Genomics's do-it-yourself at-home DNA kit that infers genetic predisposition for several diseases after the FDA ordered testing companies to "prove the validity of such products."[3] In July, DNA analysis was credited with leading to the arrest of a suspect in the twenty-five-year-old so-called "Grim Sleeper" serial murders in Los Angeles. In September, as news outlets announced that the genome of an Irish man had been fully sequenced for the first time under the headline "The Irish Are Different—Genetically." That same month, a court in Iceland debated the validity of DNA findings regarding the claims of a young Filipino woman that her daughter was the child of deceased chess champion Bobby Fischer.[4] This diverse array of cases highlights how DNA has become central to the claims and counterclaims of many stakeholders—from university researchers to ethnic communities, from consumers to entrepreneurial companies to district attorneys, and from mothers to citizens of a nation.

Coding Race

As the "Irish genome" case suggests, one central element in the new genetics has been the remaking of individual and collective identity and the rethinking of the meaning of race and ethnicity.[5] The implications are not merely rhetorical. As Henry Greely has noted, "with enough data, population geneticists can estimate how closely related different populations of humans are to each other. . . . [But] genetically based historical information could have modern political implications."[6] As Greely anticipated, DNA analysis—much-sought in order to resolve questions of ancestry, community, and justice, among other matters—has become a potent political touchstone as well as a social, legal, and historical one.

Genetics today has become a standard for shaping how we think about our collective past; at the same time, this politics of genetics has real effects in the present, for example, by impinging concretely upon the rights of groups within a nation-state or redefining the very boundaries of kinship and nationality. In addition, these genetic claims can shape how future rights and responsibilities tied to these relationships are articulated. The mere hint that genetic markers are distributed in different frequencies across populations has led some people to quickly treat such variation as a proxy for racial and ethnic differences, lending renewed authority to biological conceptions of human difference and providing fodder for national debates over belonging, self-definition, and political power.[7] Although many scholars have long agreed that race is a social phenomenon rather than a biological fact, these recent developments in DNA analysis have blurred this distinction.[8] In these and many other ways, the rise of this singularly potent science has transformed scholarly and popular opinion about the "nature" of race.

Since the early-twentieth century, genetics scientists have had a rocky relationship with the politics of race and nationality. The flowering of modern genetics—after the rediscovery of Mendel's work on inheritance of traits—brought with it bold and specious claims about how biology and heredity defined race and racial possibilities. By the mid-twentieth century, in response to these overblown claims most scientists insisted that races in the classic sense do not exist.[9] They regarded the supposedly fundamental human divisions conceived by their nineteenth century predecessors—such as Caucasian, Mongoloid or Asian, and Negroid—as problematic, because these categories were based on superficial differences only. But in recent decades, genetic science has changed its tune. To be sure, many geneticists would insist that in revisiting race they are not endorsing old racial thinking, but only creating more fine-grained statistical groupings of gene frequencies and populations which, by chance and science, overlap considerably with older racial categories.[10] Yet their analyses of genes across human populations have provoked a resurgence in race thinking—and fostered efforts, not only to locate race in biology, but also to connect people today to their own scientific ancestors. In these ways, genetics has returned to its own controversial past, using gene-level differences across groups, enormous similarities, and a relative handful of variations across genomes as a template for reconfiguring groups and for building new notions of racial difference for a new era.

Given the field's contentious history, it should not surprise us that each new assertion about genetic or biological group identity becomes a collision point—a nexus of often heated discussion about evidence, science, and political authority. Press headlines that readily draw conclusions about ancestry and behavior, intelligence, or drug metabolism suggest that the social conceptualization of race may be losing ground in the era of genetics or they might be seen as illustrating the point that some "[s]cientists never did give up on [its] biological meaning," as sociologist Jenny Reardon proposed.[11] Furthermore, a number of geneticists and biological anthropologists—as well as sociologists and political scientists—have begun making bold claims based on variations of seemingly distinctive gene markers across populations, ranging from contentions about racial predisposition to cancer to the genetic transmission of political orientation.[12] Analyzing these flashpoints and tensions over the claims and credibility of genetic science are among this book's central concerns, for they have dramatic implications for the American discourses about race and biological difference, and pose potentially far-reaching implications in media and policy settings.

Genetics today has become a novel yet thorny enterprise—a set of laboratory practices packaged as commodities that are undergirded by far-reaching intellectual, scientific, and technical assumptions about human difference. This book seeks to chart the development of how these assumptions about human difference are often bundled—sometimes unwittingly—into diverse genetic endeavors. In some instances, genetics and DNA analysis are being deployed as new technological advances to address old, longstanding questions about identity and history. In other instances, we are witnessing the emergence of new questions and claims about the meaning of human difference and relations of shared or broken history based on the premise that genetics can offer answers and remedies. Our aim is not to specify precisely when genetics provides access to the truth and when it does not. Although our essays have much to say about the credibility of genetic evidence in law, medicine, politics, and consumer culture, we seek primarily to describe and analyze those social contexts and political settings. In so doing, we explore how the authority of genetic evidence about race and history are linked to the social, political, and cultural utility of racialization.

As the essays in this volume make clear, genetic science does not exist apart from its context and uses; nor can its claims be fully understood apart from these contexts and uses. What is particularly notable is the way in which the genetic ventures examined in the pages ahead are enacting "racial projects,"[13] in which race (including whiteness, and also to some extent, ethnicity) is being reconstituted, and in which notions of race and the past offer both liberating possibilities (for example, a feeling of belonging to the nation, release from false imprisonment, the promise of better health, social healing) and also confinement (for example, racial reification and the biological essentialization of the family and groups). Herein lies one paradox of genetics and the unsettled past: in relying upon genetic analysis to resolve historical mysteries or clear the way for restitution and healing, we are at the same time manipulating and transforming already politicized notions of race and the past, and implicitly making claims about the social, political, and personal significance of biological human difference. Throughout this volume we also ask how ancestry testing has transformed our notions of kinship, placing *en famille* those individuals whose association is based on genetic markers and pushing aside notions of family that are based on social norms, interaction, or cultural codes. To what extent is genetically fashioned genealogy overtaking other, long practiced ways of rendering the family and, in turn, the community and the nation?

At the end of the day, we argue, only a multidisciplinary approach can illuminate this collision of DNA, race, and history, and help us to identify and expose the cultural, ethical, social, and philosophical challenges and possibilities posed by genetics. Understanding and dissecting the implications of DNA in multiple realms is a complex undertaking, for its uses span across the realms of politics, the courtroom, the laboratory, the clinic, and the media.[14] The pages ahead therefore bring together scholars from history, sociology, anthropology, molecular biology, law, medicine, cultural studies, ethnic studies, and other fields to examine the emerging, and often contested, connections among race, genetics, and history. In these chapters, readers find discussions of the historical use of DNA (and claims made about DNA) in biomedicine, in genealogy, in the law, in epidemiology, and in the complex processes of memory, reparation and nation building. These diverse essays also put forward commentaries and critiques of the uses and mis-uses of genetic race analyses within particular social settings and across cultural and national boundaries.

Genes, Kinship, and Historical Revisionism

Bold claims have become commonplace in the selling of genes as historical tools. In his influential best-selling work, *The Seven Daughters of Eve*, Bryan Sykes, the geneticist and founder of the genetic genealogy company Oxford Ancestors, provocatively proposes that the advent of the genetics era may mark the end of historical inquiry as we know it (see Marianne Sommer's detailed discussion of Sykes's enterprises in chapter 13).

> Within the DNA is written not only our histories as individuals, but the whole history of the human race. With the aid of recent advances in genetic technology, this history is now being revealed. We are at last able to begin to decipher the messages from the past. Our DNA does not fade like an ancient parchment; it does not rust in the ground like the sword of a warrior long dead. It is not eroded by wind or rain, nor reduced to ruin by fire and earthquake.[15]

In this volume, we explore whether we have indeed entered a new stage of histor-ical understanding dominated by genetics and bereft of culture as Sykes suggests. If this is true, what are the implications of this new rendering of the past for how we understand race in various domains? Genetics may well be transforming the very way we define history, but it is also clear that the evidence and concepts guiding this genetic/historical revisionism must be examined closely before the nature and limits of that transformation can be fully assessed.

All efforts to connect to the past are bound to be fraught with supposition and speculation, and troubled by problems of credibility of evidence. In the annals of history, new evidence and novel methods of analysis come and go, provoking the very type of question of history, revisionism, and memory that are raised by genetic analysis. Of course, what makes the genetic revision of race and history so compelling is its intimate implications for individuals, its widespread marketing and popularity, its close connection to a set of commercial products, and the promise it offers to unlock past mysteries.

The new genetic data have quickly produced theories of human difference and kinship, even as they have provoked debate about the nature of the data col-lection and DNA analysis, about how and whether the resulting genetic evidence truly relates to social categories of identity, and about whether the evidence indeed offers a portal into the past. Despite such uncertainties, the analysis of sequences of genes—when compared across large data sets gathered in patchwork fashion around the globe—is being used to provide insights about the past and relationships among people in cases where there may be little other connection.

In some cases, this analysis comes into conflict with existing knowledge—most notably when geneticists proclaim to Native Americans, for example, that they are not originally American but (like others) merely earlier immigrants from Europe. In the process, DNA analysis is also re-creating how we know the past and even how we now define the social world.

THE OPENING PART (entitled "History, Race, and the Genome Era") features three essays by Keith Wailoo, Alondra Nelson, and Catherine Lee that describe the stakes and limits of DNA analysis—for individuals grappling with the personal questions of race, identity, and the past; for groups and stakeholders in different national settings who use this information in adjudicating conflicts and in pursuit of reconciliation and social justice; and for the fraught political enterprises of nation-building around ideas of biological difference. Wailoo's essay offers a personal look at the stakes for one individual pondering multiple lineages and historical connections to the past. Nelson's illuminates the stakes for social groups and nations, viewing genetics in the broader politics of group struggles for justice and reconciliation. And Lee's explores the implicit role of gender in this genetic turn and its implications for familial and nation-building claims. These essays see these realms—the personal, the social, and the political—as among the most important for understanding the stakes of DNA analysis today.

A second part (entitled "Decoding the Genomic Age") takes us into the science of genetic analysis, revealing precisely how genetic material is collected and analyzed, turned into detailed claims about race and identity, and how such knowledge is reworked in settings from laboratories to courtrooms and in the new entrepreneurial practices of genetic genealogy. Abram Gabriel provides an academic biologist's perspective (in contrast to that of a commercial biologist) on the advent and limits of genetic evidence about difference, and a critique of the curious rise of personalized genomics companies, with their far-reaching claims about connecting people to their ethnic roots. Scientists' efforts to construct and categorize populations have an extensive history, and Lundy Braun and Evelyn Hammonds offer historical reflection on the longstanding dilemma of racial classification and its challenging implications for gene theories of race today. Peter Chow-White situates the fascination with genetics in the broader context of the technical possibility and cultural allure of manipulating large databases. What emerges here is a portrait of the complexity and contingency of genetic classification—the ways in which these new developments relate to the long history of racial bio-typologies; limitations in how DNA scientists make claims about history using specific techniques (from Ancestry Informative Mapping (AIMS) to forensic DNA phenotyping); how geneticists strategically bracket off and answer objections to their claims; how the manipulation of large-scale databases shape these new ideas about identity; and how novel forms of genetic identity are made in the process. Also in this part, the authors ask how we should decode this genomic age, by looking closely at how genetic evidence and racial theories are developed, interpreted, and manipulated in three realms: the courts and policing, the clinic, and the laboratory. In two separate essays, legal scholar Jonathan Kahn and anthropologist/ethicist Pamela Sankar examine American legal practice as it merges forensic DNA with race thinking. Sociologists of science Ramya Rajagopalan and Joan Fujimura examine how particular techniques (such as admixture mapping) depend upon social definitions of race which are then reified in the science. Medical anthropologist Sandra Soo-Jin Lee examines the new field of pharmacogenomics, the notion of medicine tailored to individual and group identity, and the political economy of difference upon which the enterprise is founded.

A third part (entitled "Stories Told in Blood") turns to an analysis of the poignant, if flawed, social narratives about DNA, blood, and racial identity that are woven by genealogists, political actors, and others in the present and used strategically in order to recount the past and lay claims on the present and future. This section describes how DNA is being used to rewrite notions of race, kinship, and nation, and how such genetic renderings are employed in the pursuit of reparations, justice, nation building, and reconciliation. In a study of genetic genealogy in Quebec, cultural anthropologist Nina Kohli-Laven points to the influence of French Canadian identity politics on biological renderings of the past. Bioscience scholar Amy Hinterberger relates the unfolding debate over genetic ancestry in Canada to the nation's multicultural policy regarding "visible minorities" and "Aboriginal" people; with this broad context in mind, historian of science Marianne Sommer analyzes the limits of anthropological genetics as applied history. Literary scholar Priscilla Wald unravels how these narratives of technological innovation and identity have long been embedded in commercial, colonial, and political claims and interests. In these essays, then, we see how anthropologists, sociologists, historians, and literary scholars track the expanding impact of genetics for how we understand history. What becomes evident is the way in which the past is contested and how the fraught knowledge of genetics is deployed in service of contemporary political and social goals of cultural inclusion, political exclusion, and mediating social relationships.

The three final essays in this part add further richness to our understanding of the racially tinged claims, counterclaims, and stakes at the heart of these kinship-genetics-history disputes. Jennifer Hamilton, an anthropologist and legal studies scholar, explores genetic ancestry tracing and the legal status of the "genetic ancestor" in the context of recent court cases. Sociologist Michelle M. Jacob examines the use, politics, and limits of genetic analysis in Native American claims regarding land, belonging, and identity. Turning to post-apartheid South Africa, historian Jay Aronson illuminates the forensic DNA profiling of the remains of disappeared black political activists from the apartheid era as part of the politics of reconciliation and repair in that fraught national context. Here, as throughout the volume, we examine the political, scientific, and social implications of calling upon genetic analysis (in Quebec, the United States, South Africa, England, and elsewhere) to perform a kind of racially charged cultural work—to repair and recast the past; to settle claims; to establish the parameters of kinship, belonging, and national identity; to validate proper and rightful claims; and to reshape identity in the present and possibly the future.

Any study of genetic analyses' multiple implications for race and history demands a wide methodological and geographic sweep, multiple voices, and diverse approaches to science and its meaning. As such, some of the essays in this volume look closely at legalistic reasoning and argumentation in the court; others examine closely the nuances of biological analysis; yet others scrutinize cultural and literary representations of genes and identity; and others explore personal meanings or political speech or sociological dimensions of genetics. The diversity of approaches highlights, in its own fashion, the complex ways in which this enterprise is attempting to rewrite normative views of kinship, identity, memory, ancestral rights, national identity, and social justice. Moving us inside this new enterprise, and also beyond old debates about whether race is biological or social in nature, we emphasize the importance of understanding the expansive "social life of DNA" particularly in relation to societies' already fraught and complex narratives of race and history.[16]

DNA analysis in our time is not merely about predicting a future that is supposedly written in our genes, warning us, for example, about our predisposition to disease. The practice also makes fundamental, if problematic, claims about the present and the distant past—and as such, the claims, credibility, and applications of the genetic sciences must be examined closely and in multiple venues. It would be a mistake for those involved with this enterprise—at the clinical, legal, or scientific level—to ignore these ethical, legal, and epistemological questions swirling around the field. Yet in the concluding part (entitled "The Unsettled Past"), sociologist Reanne Frank examines the disturbing tendency of genetics advocates and entrepreneurs to mischaracterize critiques as stemming from ignorance of the enterprise, fear of the truth, or political correctness. The scientific and social challenge, however, is not so simple. As a final essay by Keith Wailoo, Alondra Nelson, and Catherine Lee makes clear, there are questions of evidence and credibility that sit at the heart of genetic claims about history and race, and precisely because of their sweeping implications in politics, law, and society, they must be investigated carefully. With the maturity, commercialization, and rapid expansion of the genetic sciences (particularly into the realm of the so-called racial past), the time is long behind us when geneticists could ignore the cultural world in which their work is applied or ignore the influence of cultural politics on their science. As we see it, the past is one of the principal arenas where this new story of genetic knowledge is being told and where genetic authority is being developed. The essays that follow, then, take us into the center of this conflicted terrain to reveal how historical ideas are refashioned and unsettled through the lens of DNA, to see how genetic claims about race and difference are concocted, and to observe how the distant, otherwise unreachable past has become the site for debate and conflict in the present. From this vantage point, we can observe that the collision of DNA, race, and history is as much about remapping the unsettled past as it is about shaping the unsettled present and imagining the future stretching out before us.

NOTES

1. Adam Geller, "Consumers Turn to Their DNA for Answers," *Boston Globe* (March 28, 2006) www.boston.com/business/personalfinance/articles/2006/03/28/consumers_turn_to_their_dna_for_answers/ [Accessed March 19, 2010].

2. The literature in the field of race and genetics has grown exponentially in recent decades, growing alongside controversies over the meaning of markers and biological indices of difference. Notable works include, Catherine Lee, "'Race' and 'Ethnicity' in Biomedical Research: How Do Scientists Construct and Explain Difference in Health?" *Social Science and Medicine* 68 (2009): 1183–1190; Alondra Nelson, "Bio Science: Genetic Genealogy Testing and the Pursuit of African Ancestry," *Social Studies of Science* 38 (October 2008): 759–783; Adele E. Clarke, Janet Shim, Sara Shostak, and Alondra Nelson, "Biomedicalizing Genetic Health, Diseases and Identities," in Handbook of Genetics and Society: Mapping the New Genomic Era, ed. Paul Atkinson, Peter Glasner, and Margaret Lock (London: Routledge, 2009); Deborah Bolnick, Duana Fullwiley, Troy Duster, Richard Cooper, Joan H. Fujimura, Jonathan Kahn, Jay S. Kaufman, Jonathan Marks, Ann Morning, Alondra Nelson et al., "The Business and Science of Ancestry Testing," *Science* 318 (2007): 399–400; Keith Wailoo and Stephen Pemberton, *The Troubled Dream of Genetic Medicine: Ethnicity and Innovation in Tay-Sachs, Cystic Fibrosis, and Sickle Cell Disease* (Baltimore: Johns Hopkins University Press, 2007); Keith Wailoo, *Dying in the City of the Blues: Sickle Cell Anemia and the Politics of Race and Health* (Chapel Hill: University of North Carolina Press, 2001); Ian Whitmarsh and David S. Jones, *What's the Use of Race?: Modern Governance and the Biology of Difference* (Cambridge, MA: MIT Press, 2010); Jenny Reardon, *Race to the Finish: Identity and Governance in an Age of Genomics* (Princeton, NJ: Princeton University Press, 2005). On the cultural, political, and ideological allure of modern genetics in American society, see Dorothy Nelkin and M. Susan Lindee, *The DNA Mystique: The Genes as a Cultural Icon* (Ann Arbor: University of Michigan Press, 2004); Richard Lewontin, *Biology as Ideology: The Doctrine of DNA* (New York: Harper, 1993); Troy Duster, *Backdoor to Eugenics* (New York: Routledge, 1990); Daniel J. Kevles, *In the Name of Eugenics: Genetics and the Uses of Human Heredity* (Berkeley: University of California Press, 1985).

3. David Brown, "FDA Challenges Companies over DNA Tests Sold to Customers," *Washington Post* (June 11, 2010) www.washingtonpost.com/wp-dyn/content/article/2010/06/11/AR2010061106097.html [Accessed August 2010].

4. "When Two Tribes Go to War," *Nature* 430 (July 2004): 500–502; Amy Harmon, "Indian Tribe Wins Fight to Limit Research of Its DNA," *New York Times* (April 21, 2010); Jennifer Epstein, "DNA Test Replaces Summer Reading Project at UC-Berkeley," *USA Today* (May 18, 2010); Rosemary Black, "Freshmen at UC Berkeley Can Find Out Alcohol Tolerance from DNA Test," *New York Daily News* (May 22, 2010); Rachel Gross, "A Few Wrinkles in UC Berkeley's Plan to Test Freshmen's Genes," *New York Times* (May 24, 2010); Robert Sanders, "UC Berkeley Alters DNA Testing Program," UC Berkeley Press Release (August 12, 2010) berkeley.edu/news/media/releases/2010/08/12_dna_change.shtml [Accessed August 2010]; "At-Home Genetic Test Kit Hits FDA Wall," *ABC News* (May 13, 2010); Daniel B. Wood, "'Grim Sleeper' Case Raises Privacy Concerns over Use of DNA," *Christian Science Monitor* (July 8, 2010); Maura Dolan, Joel Rubin, and Mitchell Landsberg, "DNA Leads to Arrest in Grim Sleeper Killings," *Los Angeles Times* (July 8, 2010); Dylan Loeb McClain, "Fischer's Paternity Test Released," *New York Times* (September 9, 2010); Rachel Panizzo,

"The Irish Are Different—Genetically," *BioNews* (Published by the Progress Educational Trust), (September 13, 2010).

5. Barbara A. Koenig, Sandra Soo-Jin Lee, and Sarah S. Richardson, eds., *Revisiting Race in a Genomic Age* (New Brunswick, NJ: Rutgers University Press, 2008); Evelyn Hammonds and Rebecca Herzig, eds., *The Nature of Difference: Sciences of Race in the United States from Jefferson to Genomics* (Cambridge, MA: MIT Press, 2009).

6. Henry T. Greely, "Legal, Ethical, and Social Issues in Human Genome Research," *Annual Review of Anthropology* 27 (1998): 478.

7. For a recent scientific perspective, see Neil Risch, Estaban Burchard, Elad Ziv, and H. Tang, "Categorization of Humans in Biomedical Research: Genes, Race, and Disease," *Genome Biology* 3 (July 2002), genomebiology.com/2002/3/7/comment/2007.

    For social science perspectives on these debates, see Nadia Abu El-Haj, "The Genetic Reinscription of Race," *Annual Review of Anthropology* 36 (2007): 283–300; and Troy Duster, "Race and Reification in Science," *Science* 307 (February 18, 2005): 1050–1051.

8. See, for example, one manifestation of this tension in Ruth Hubbard, "Constructs of Genetic Difference: Race and Sex," and in David L. Hull, "Species, Races, and Genders: Differences Are Not Deviations," both from *Genes and Human Self-Knowledge: Historical and Philosophical Reflections on Modern Genetics*, ed. Robert Weir, Susan C. Lawrence, and Evan Fales (Iowa City: University of Iowa Press, 1994).

9. See, for example, the influential paper by Richard Lewontin, "The Apportionment of Human Diversity," *Evolutionary Biology* 6 (1972): 381–398. Here the evolutionary biologist and geneticist argued that "human races and populations are remarkably similar to each other, with the largest part by far of human variation being accounted for by the differences between individuals. Human racial classification is of no social value . . . no justification can be offered for its continuance" (397).

10. Risch et al., "Categorization of Humans in Biomedical Research."

11. Jenny Reardon, "Decoding Race and Human Difference in a Genomic Age," *differences: A Journal of Feminist Cultural Studies* 15 (2004): 38–65.

12. See, for example, John R. Alford, Carolyn L. Funk, and John R. Hibbing, "Are Political Orientations Genetically Transmitted?" *American Political Science Review* 99 (2005): 153–167.

13. Michael Omi and Howard Winant, *Racial Formation in the U.S.: From the 1960s to the 1990s*, 2nd ed. (New York: Routledge, 1994), 56.

14. In using this approach, we follow in the footsteps of Koenig, Lee, and Richardson, whose recent edited volume *Revisiting Race in a Genomic Age* also considered the themes of race and genetics from an multidisciplinary perspective. In this volume, we also extend the discussions inaugurated in that important anthology by looking closely at the socio-political circulation of genetic analysis, especially its mediation in debates about history and ancestry.

15. Bryan Sykes, *The Seven Daughters of Eve* (New York: Norton, 2002), 1.

16. Alondra Nelson, "The Social Life of DNA," *Chronicle of Higher Education* (September 3, 2010), B10.

PART ONE

History, Race, and the Genome Era

1

Who Am I?

Genes and the Problem of Historical Identity

KEITH WAILOO

A fundamental conundrum at the heart of the new genetics is the question "Who am I?" Despite what we may believe about ourselves—based on our family lore, our photographs, our documented past, or the recollections and memorabilia of our ancestors—genetics makes possible bold claims about self and family that may be at odds with these long-relied-upon artifacts of identity. When seeking historical guidance as to who we are, we can look backward in multiple ways—the matrilineal line, the patrilineal line (along which names are often, but not always, transferred), some combination of family lines (the mother's father's family line, for example), or in ways totally outside the biological family. Genetic science has emerged from the laboratory and clinic in recent years to add new complexity to this already complex process, and to revise our self knowledge.

No longer promising only that "new breakthroughs can cure diseases and save lives," genetic technologies have entered the courtroom, the genealogy business, and popular culture, posing profound challenges to older ways of knowing ourselves.[1] For Americans like me, who look back across an ocean for links to ancestry and the past and who pine for answers about heritage, the possibilities inherent in the new genetics have been exciting. With a cheek swab, a thousand dollars or less, and a sophisticated analysis, comparing my genes to those in the company's database, which have been gathered from several populations around the world, the mystery of my roots can be unlocked.

Over the past decade or so, popular media—for example, multiple covers of *Time* magazine—have suggested that DNA's insights are far reaching. DNA, some speculate, may define our religiosity and our compulsion to "seek a higher power"; "infidelity," too, "may be in our genes"; an "I.Q. gene" just might explain our intellectual capacity; and a "gay gene" might explain our sexual orientation.[2] Whatever I believed about myself—my behaviors and predilections or other features of who I am—can be opened via genetic analysis. Or, so we are relentlessly told.

Spencer Wells's 2002 National Geographic documentary, *Journey of Man: A Genetic Odyssey*, begins with an audacious assertion—that the blood coursing through my veins is "the greatest history book ever written." Such narratives of genetic insight and omniscience have taken a new turn—with the rise of genetic genealogy now also claiming to reopen one's past and to divulge new realities about my family heritage or about the true lineage of a community. The argument at the heart of this captivating made-for-TV drama was simple and shocking: that none of us can truly know who we are without genetic analysis. We might speculate and dream, but the blood and genes would reveal the truth. The power of Wells's program stems from skillfully borrowed science fiction tropes—in this case, a merging of the time machine/time travel theme of H. G. Wells (no relation) with the marvelous 1966 into-the-body motif of the film *Fantastic Voyage*, in which a miniaturized team of scientists venture into a man's body in order to destroy a blood clot and save his life. As Spencer Wells travels the world, collecting blood and comparing its patterns to the vast database of already-collected samples, he stages a new fantastic voyage—an odyssey, not only into the body, but back in time, weaving a compelling set of stories about how each of us is connected to one another, how we all have migrated out of Africa, and yet how we have come to be so different today.

Before geneticists began to visit the past in this fashion, each of us had well-established and complex, often conflicted, ways of knowing ourselves, of pointing to a past, and of situating ourselves in the present. The fierceness with which we hold onto these older beliefs about ourselves explains, in part, the skepticism that confronts genetic revisionists. In what follows, my argument is simple: Rather than seeing a fundamental tension between genetic knowledge and other non-genetic ways of answering the question "Who am I?" there is rather a curious way in which genetic knowledge gains plausibility, not through any inherent power of science, but by reinforcing already-existing cultural and political forms of imagining self and the past in films, popular media, public commemoration, family lore, nationalistic display, and so on. Yet, all efforts to connect to the past are bound to be speculative, fraught with supposition, and troubled by problems of evidence. Indeed, selective editing and interpretation is just as prevalent in the fashioning of historical identity using genetic analysis as it is in the use of other evidence, from family photos to genealogical archives. To put it another way, whatever the data we draw upon to answer the question who am I (whether photographs, family trees, birth certificates, or genetic analysis), we engage in a willful paring down of multiple lines of descent, choosing between mothers and fathers in crafting the story of one's self. Genetic analysis, then, like other forms of historical memory, is as much about making meaning in the present as it is about the past. Hence it is as deeply mired in the politics of identity as are these other forms.

LET ME OFFER A PERSONAL CASE in point on the complexities surrounding "who I am." Since I was eight years old, my identity has been that of a migrant—an immigrant from South America, and (by sixteen) a naturalized American citizen.

Despite appearing to be phenotypically and culturally African American, the fact of my coming into this identity has been something I know about myself, but something that is not obvious to most people. Where I emigrated from is less relevant here than the fact that it was to the United States that I emigrated. My "coming to America" immigration narrative still figures in the stories I choose to tell my children about who I am. Because of my age when this journey took place, the transition to America was traumatic and memorable—more so than if I had been a five- or two-year old with few vibrant recollections. I can still recall forty years later the way my accent (even though I was an English speaker) marked me off in elementary classes. I can recall having to explain where it was that I had arrived from. Even as time passed and I learned to speak like an American (merging different intonations from my New York City surroundings), I knew I was from somewhere else even if others did not—or chose to forget. But at some point, people ceased asking, because I had learned a new way of talking. My parents, by contrast, still retain the "old world" lingo—marking them distinctly as from "somewhere else." For many new Americans who come from "somewhere else," that old place is marked by one's parent's ways of speaking, by one's memories, and by one's family. Like many Americans, I have relatives who remain "back home," linking me to one version of who I am. For me, this form of identity is still powerful and resonant—strong enough for me to want to pass the knowledge on to my children and to keep it alive, so that they know where they are from. Before genetics and even after the rise of genetic genealogy, this remains one of the powerful ways in which I know, perform, and understand who I am.

Geneticists might argue that this is a fable, a myth I tell myself because, in truth, my people were only passing through South America on our way to the United States. In the ultimate truth of genetics, no one can truly, historically be from South America because South Americans—even indigenous people—are migrants and new world beings. In history as told through genetic analysis, there must be a deeper historical story. Against this backdrop, the language of genetics makes a bold claim—that this knowledge that I have carried for decades about who I am, could be richer and deeper. It could also be plain wrong. Why stop in the old country? Why not go further back or travel in different directions to build a more expansive sense of myself, especially by reflecting on ancestors I have never met and who lived thousands of years ago?

Genetic analysis promises to take me back even further. How should one think of this option? And are these opportunities offered by genetic genealogy truly radical departures from the pathways previously available to me? My strong sense is that the difference is not as great as one might think. Indeed, the genetic options available to us are filled with all of the same interpretive complexities associated with the conventional sources—the photographs, family lore, and documents—that we commonly use to decide who we are. As it happens, all ways of answering the question, "Who am I?" contain false narratives based on incomplete samples, and they are false in surprisingly consistent ways.

Starting Points and Stopping Points

When I am asked where I'm from, first I pause to decode what the questioner is asking and to decide where to begin. Does he mean where was I born? Where I grew up? Or does the questioner mean the name of the country, the state, or the region of my birth and early years? How specific should I be? I usually choose to speak about the country of my birth—a small country with a British colonial past and a diverse population defined by the in-migration of South Asians, Africans, and Europeans during the century-plus of British imperial rule. Based on what I know about my grandparents and great-grandparents, I can point to an obvious African heritage. I also point to a South Asian ancestry which, although a small percentage of my family tree, is still attached to me by way of my name—privileging my patrilineal descent, as is the custom where I come from. Usually, I skip the details unless asked for them and point to the country of my birth. Doing so appeals to my sense of self; it "feels right" in most situations. Yet, I know that I have relatives (on one side) who make different choices—pointing for example more insistently to South Asia. I have always believed that the important feature of the country of my birth is that it provides these multiple avenues for anyone confronted with the question, "Who are you?"

By contrast, what are the starting points and stopping points of genetic analysis? In order to place myself in the most distant past, the world of genetic genealogy must create that past. It is a past largely defined by genetic material gathered from contemporary individuals around the globe—material contained in vast archives and databases against which snips and sections of any particular person's genes can be compared. As Peter Chow-White explains in another essay in this volume, these data sources (composed by each company or compiler from populations they have selected as representative genetic populations) have become a biomedical and informational paradigm around which new ideas of race and identity are generated. Since the human genomes in these databases (each genome with 3,000,000,000 base pairs, spread across our 23 chromosomes) are 99.9 percent similar to one another, the starting point of genetic differences analysis is the 0.1 percent (or 3 million base pairs) where the variations and differences are notable. In most studies, as in one 2004 report in *Nature Genetics*, an even smaller selection of the 0.1 percent provides the raw material for locating the sources of our differences. Analyzing just over 100 selected markers in small population samples from sub-Saharan Africa, Western Europe, and East Asia, the authors (a collaboration between a genetics department, a pediatrics unit, and a pharmaceutical company) observed that many studies "confirmed that there is a relationship between patterns of genetic variation and geographical ancestry, with a high degree of accuracy and reliability, using a relatively modest number of multilocus genotypes, individuals can indeed be allocated to groups that represent broad geographical regions."[3] The power to situate individuals in the past and, in particular, places, based on genes, however, was more limited for certain people and regions, because of the data itself and because of the complexities of certain populations. As the authors observed, for example, "the sampling of individuals from many parts of the world (such as sub-Saharan Africa, India, North and South America) has been extremely limited, even though genetic diversity in some of these regions (such as Africa or India) seems to be higher than in many parts of the world." This very diversity of population raises a set of conceptual problems at the heart of the new genetics/ancestry business: what sources of data are best equipped to link us to the past we seek to create; what populations exist in the genetic databases and how does this shape what past will be found; and if we are "all from Africa" originally, as genetic genealogy insists, then what should be the end-point of my quest for an ancestral home? As most historians know, these questions about sources and limitations of evidence are not specific to genetic data; rather, they are inherent to the use of any data linking past to present identity.

Choosing a Lineage

When I speak about who I am, I have the option of choosing among a range of lineages. I can speak about my mother's side of the family or my father's. Beyond that, I can recall the story of my father's father life as an East Indian child of immigrants to the South American continent, or I can speak of my father's mother's mixture of African and Native American roots, or I can point to my mother's own four grandparents all with their own cultural lineages. I have physical markers on my own body linking me, in highly selective ways, to each of these lines. My skin color links presumably to one line, an inherited oddity on the little fingers of my hands is clearly inherited from my mother's mother and has been passed to my daughter, and so on. One cannot, then, speak of a single ancestral lineage—but of many lineages (four grandparents, eight great-grandparents, sixteen for the next generation, and thirty-two after that). The lineage chart is a tree pointing back in multiple directions, ever expanding into the past and comprising the individual in the present. Choosing which one of these lineages to speak about is often a situationally shaped social act.

Genetic testing offers specific yet highly limited entry into this complex past. As the authors of the 2004 *Nature Genetics* article noted, "much of the genetic data available on many populations is limited to genotypes of the mitochondrial genome and the non-recombining portion of the Y chromosome."[4] The first type of genetic data points backward along one line (the paternal or father's father's father's line), offering insight into that portion of the genome passed down along that hereditary pathway. The second type of genetic data points backward along another line (the mother's mother's mother's line), offering insight into that portion, and analysis of its frequency elsewhere in the world. These two types of testing provide one way of situating oneself in the past—but only if one is concerned about the matrilineal past or the patrilineal past. In my own family, the collective memory, evidence, and lore point patrilineally to India (whence my surname) and matrilineally to somewhere in England or Europe (owing to my mother's mother's mother's mother's place of origin). Ironically, these two forms of testing would not place me where the bulk of my own family history and phenotypic appearance would place me, a self-identified first-generation African American—in Africa. To boil down my complex DNA another way, a third type of analysis might be useful. Called Ancestry Informative Marker (AIM) testing, it offers a general statistical comparison of one's markers with those gathered in company databases from populations around the world. AIM testing (each company has its own database) purports to tell me statistically what percentages of supposedly pure old-world identities I embody. These forms of testing were used in the popular American television show "Faces of America," in which Professor Henry Louis Gates Jr. (and founder of AfricanDNA.com) has the genome of famous Americans tested before presenting them with a dubious pie chart representing their ethnic makeup. The Mexican American actress Eva Longoria is told that she is 70 percent European, 27 percent Asian, and 3 percent African; and when she is told that this percentage makes her genetically similar to the Parisian-born American cellist of Chinese parents Yo-Yo Ma, her bemused response ("He's Mexican?") captures the impossible tension between genetic claims and personal modes of identification.[5]

Genetic analysis raises the same question that I raise for myself: Do I privilege my mother's mother's lineage or my father's mother's line (while playing down the significance of other ancestors) in telling the story of who I am? As the essays in Part One of this volume illustrate, the high-tech memory-making of DNA analysis contains the same kinds of uncertainties one finds in many other forms of historical reconstruction. The true difference is that mitochondrial DNA ancestry and Y-chromosome ancestry leave these ambiguities about one's true self unstated and unarticulated.[6] Genetic analysis, as we also learn in chapters ahead, blurs the question of starting points and end points of analysis, preventing me from seeing South America clearly and locating that continent as my point of origin, or from understanding the more complex story of who I am—that is, how many still genetically-invisible strands of my family dispersed over time from several regions and countries that are as yet unmapped genetically, how this process unfolded in highly specific ways and how these many ancestors combined to make me who I am.

Any one of us has multiple pathways for building a strong historical sense of self. Genetic analysis offers its own multiple pathways for self-knowledge. In some ways, the social logic of ancestry is not so different from the logic of genetic ancestry, for both depend on selective data that require us to make deliberate human choices in reconstituting the past. Both also depend upon complicated social machinery that makes the past available to us in the present. Finally, both depend upon assemblages of arbitrary databases, mixed with suppositions and memories. The essays in this volume take us, then, into the world of how genetic knowledge is selectively made. They also allow us to examine the question, "How different is this new form of analysis from more conventional ways of knowing who I am?"

NOTES

1. "Genetics: The Future Is Now," *Time* magazine cover (January, 17, 1994).

2. "The God Gene," *Time* magazine cover (October 25, 2004); "Infidelity: It May Be in Our Genes," *Time* magazine cover (August 15, 1994); "The I.Q. Gene," *Time* magazine (September 13, 1999).

3. Michael Bamshad, Stephen Wooding, Benjamin A. Salisbury, and J. Claiborne Stephens, "Deconstructing the Relationship between Genetics and Race," *Nature Genetics* 5 (August 2004): 601.

4. Ibid.

5. Alessandra Stanley, "Genealogy for a Nation of Immigrants," *New York Times* (February 9, 2010) tv.nytimes.com/2010/02/10/arts/television/10faces.html?_r=1.

6. Troy Duster, "Deep Roots and Tangled Branches," *Chronicle of Higher Education* (February 3, 2006): B13.

2

◇◇◇

Reconciliation Projects

From Kinship to Justice

ALONDRA NELSON

Among the many possibilities presented by the decoding of the human genome has been the expansion of the types and availability of genetic analysis. These techniques are now ubiquitous. They are employed in biomedical settings—for instance, to examine an individual's genetic predisposition to disease. They have driven developments in forensic investigation, such as the so-called "DNA finger-printing" techniques.[1] These postgenomic transformations have also spurred the conception of a range of goods and services that make genetic technologies broadly available for public consumption. Indeed, these direct-to-consumer (DTC) genetic tests that claim to infer racial and ethnic identity, genealogical affiliation, and health potential are among the most visible manifestations of the genomics era. For example, the pervasiveness of DTC genetic ancestry testing, is evident in the media's powerful depictions of the unearthing of personal pasts, ranging from journalist Amy Harmon's Pulitzer Prize–winning articles for the *New York Times* to Harvard University professor Henry Louis Gates Jr.'s television franchise of celebrity-focused genealogy documentaries.

Information derived from genetic science is now widespread at a range of social sites. Through this circulation, the "logics" of DNA analysis—that is, the centrality of "the prism of hereditability,"[2] the privileging of molecular scale, the use of statistical methods and probabilistic algorithms alongside bio-banks and genetic databases, and so forth—move across and beyond their characteristic domains of biomedicine and forensic science into practices of self-fashioning, kin-keeping, and family formation, among others. Tracking this broader social transmission of the logics and techniques of genetic science—*the social life of DNA*—we can apprehend how genetics is increasingly relied upon to answer fundamental questions, not only about human identity, but also about national and political community, social justice, and collective memory.[3]

In one particular and striking trend in recent years, genetic information is being applied in what I term *reconciliation projects*—endeavors aimed at ameliorating the injurious repercussions of the past. Reconciliation projects are efforts to repair the damage caused by fractious social and political struggles—efforts that are being undertaken in many arenas, including courts of law, laboratories, social justice organizations, and museums. The concept, reconciliation projects, of course connotes the idea of reparative justice that underlies late twentieth-century truth and reconciliation commissions such as those that took place in post-apartheid South Africa, in post-civil-rights-era Greensboro, North Carolina, and, in post-junta Argentina of the early 1980s, following the fall of the military authoritarian state that had brutally "disappeared" its critics.[4] For the purposes of this essay, and with the social life of DNA in mind, the phrase furthermore points to the constitutive role played by genetic analysis in endeavors to "mak[e] whole what has been smashed," to paraphrase the title of sociologist John Torpey's recent comparative study of "reparation politics."[5] Genetics has become a medium through which the "unsettled past" is reconciled, be it through commemoration of historical events or making expiation for past injury.

Extending Torpey's reparation metaphor once more, DNA testing may also be relied upon to "make whole" both formerly opposed parties or formerly unified ones, rejoining broken ties within a community, nation-state, or diaspora. The information yielded from genetic genealogy testing, such as that conducted by African Ancestry and other companies, has been employed in attempts "reunite" individuals, for example, by offering the prospect of membership in both kin groups and national communities. A case in point is the Leon H. Sullivan Foundation, a nonprofit organization with roots in the U.S. civil rights movement. This organization endorses the use of genetic ancestry testing and DNA affiliation as a medium of African American involvement in entrepreneurship and philanthropy on the African continent.

Employing genetic information in another way, other subjects, citizens, or social groups increasingly engage in DNA testing, not to forge cross-national connections, but in the hope of repairing injury and rectifying injustices committed by states, institutions, or other entities. The Innocence Project, a U.S. initiative "dedicated to exonerating wrongfully convicted people through DNA testing and reforming the criminal justice system," is one such example.[6] In Argentina, DNA analysis has been used to examine the remains discovered in mass graves and determine the identities of persons suspected to have been abducted by agents of a repressive seven-year military dictatorship that began in 1976. More recently, now-adult children suspected to have been taken from their "disappeared" mothers and placed in adoptive families are now being compelled by the Argentinean government to undergo genetic testing, whether or not the adoptees desire this information.[7] Genetics is in these ways being put to the use of mending what has been "smashed."

DNA techniques and genetic evidence are now sought to fill perceived voids (and settle disputes) in many social landscapes, as the essays by Jay Aronson, Jennifer Hamilton, and Michele Jacobs describe and analyze. Aronson, for example, directs us to the "convergence of DNA and history in the context of post-apartheid South Africa." He assays how "forensic DNA profiling" is used in order to attend to an issue that could not be fully addressed by the country's Truth and Reconciliation Commission—the more than two thousand "missing and disappeared (primarily black)" anti-apartheid activists who were abducted and murdered by agents of the state. Forensic DNA analysis, as in the Argentinean example, is used to perform what we might understand as a social autopsy, with the aim of producing post-mortem information that can help reconcile South African society across the color line by restoring to families—and to the nation-state—the bodies of activists who gave of their lives in the fight for racial justice and equality.

As these and other examples in this volume illustrate, the courtroom has been one critically important realm in which the power of genetic information to validate ancestral claims has been deployed, tested, and challenged. Hamilton's contribution, by contrast, examines how genetic analysis is being used to discover and codify unknown or unacknowledged genealogy with the hope of securing legal recognition and, in turn, rights and recompense. She illustrates this process with a close reading of two U.S. legal cases in which genetic ancestry tracing has been used as an evidentiary tool—a suit in which the plaintiffs seek reparations for slavery and a suit filed by the Freedman or "Black Indians" of Oklahoma, who seek to reaffirm their full tribal membership in Native communities. These suits suggest how the legal construction of what Hamilton describes as the "genetic ancestor" is strategically exercised by the plaintiffs "as a way to configure [themselves] as legitimate, legally cognizable subjects, who can make claims to rights and benefits under the law."

Thus one tension that sits at the heart of the modern collision of DNA, race, and history is this: the employment of genetic ancestry testing or other forms of DNA analysis does not guarantee resolution of historical controversies or claims. For some members of oppressed groups, genetic science, moreover, may be deemed both an undesirable arbitrator and unreliable narrator of the past. As Jacob argues in her essay about the Kennewick Man controversy from a Native American perspective, "genetic-based" ideas about ancestry may place at risk the "land-based identities" of indigenous peoples. For these communities, DNA analysis does not offer the horizon of justice, but is rather a threat to their worldview, it is a medium through which both their "homeland and legal status" come under "assault." A genetic framing of history, ethnicity, and the past in this case presents a barrier to mutual understanding; Jacob's analysis asserts how one Native American group renders its history and limns how this same community must necessarily contend with different ways of knowing the past as a facet of socialization and cultural transmission.

The Selling of Direct-to-Consumer Reconciliation

In order to better understand the relationship of DNA and reconciliation projects, it is instructive to look closely at the role that the company African Ancestry has played in such endeavors in the United States. Given the schismatic force of racial slavery, colonialism, and imperialism—and the enduring effects of this fracturing—it is unsurprising that efforts toward reunion and repair have also been longstanding in African-descended communities. Late nineteenth- and early twentieth-century ventures by Martin R. Delany and Marcus Garvey to return enslaved Africans to the African continent, Queen Mother Audley Moore's slavery reparations activism, and Alex Haley's popularization of root-seeking in the 1970s, among other endeavors, readily come to mind. The historical events that propelled the African diaspora, in ensuing decades, inspired varied social and cultural attempts at reconciliation—most notably, documentation of the slave trade and its impact, and the quest of some African Americans for justice and reparations through DNA testing.

Among the most recent (and certainly the most technologically facilitated) of these reconciliation enterprises is the DTC (direct-to-consumer) genetic ancestry testing business and its burgeoning use by diasporic blacks intent on inferring African descent. The use of DTC genetics by blacks in the United States and else-where represents a small, but active, segment of the larger commercial genetic genealogy terrain. Established in the last decade, genetic ancestry testing contin-ues to grow in popularity and is now a multimillion-dollar industry. These testing services have a particular attraction for those people of African descent for whom, for multiple reasons, it may be especially difficult to track their family history beyond one or two generations.

Since the introduction of widely available genetic ancestry testing about a decade ago, it has been increasingly called upon to repair the injury and injustice that some understand to be inherent in the African diaspora. These initiatives are apparent in identity politics and self-fashioning, in how the memory of racial slavery has been institutionalized, and in reparations politics. Genetic analysis has been adopted to cement affiliations among members of a transnational network of blacks; to redeem and restore the contemporary, stigmatized African American family by reuniting it with a past, idyllic "African" one; to inscribe the "official memory" of slavery; and to adjudicate historical wounding, among other issues.

The line between genetics' role in public memory and its role as a business has become increasingly blurred in these DTC enterprises. The prominence of African-diaspora reconciliation projects becomes readily apparent if one tracks the phenomenal trajectory of the genetic ancestry tracing company AfricanAncestry.com and of its co-founder, geneticist Rick Kittles. African Ances-try, Inc., a Washington, D.C.-based company, purveys what is arguably the most popular brand of genetic genealogy testing among U.S. blacks.[8] Founded in early 2003 by University of Illinois at Chicago human geneticist Kittles and his business partner Gina Paige, African Ancestry matches customers to nation-states and ethnic groups on the African continent. Kittles honed the skills and techniques that would facilitate the formation of his African Ancestry company as a doctoral student in genetics at George Washington University. At this time, he was concurrently working as a junior researcher on the team of scientists tasked with investigating the remains of several hundred free and enslaved blacks found in lower Manhattan in the 1990s (this site is now the African Burial Ground Memorial of the U.S. National Parks Service). The researchers employed a then relatively novel process, in which DNA from the deceased individuals was compared to a database containing genetic samples from contemporary Africans, with the aim of inferring the ethnic origins of these colonial-era American blacks. Kittles left the team before the project was completed. His decision to convert these research techniques, with partner Paige, into a commercial enterprise caused a rift amongst the researchers and also created some public controversy among his fellow scientists. Consumers, however, clamored for the company's services. This commercialization of genetics—a theme taken up in the essays ahead—challenges us to think broadly about the nature, meaning, and circulation of genetic claims.

This is how African Ancestry (and most other DTC genetic genealogy testing) works: After a root-seeker has paid a fee (typically from $99 to $500, depending on the company used and the particular service purchased), the company mails test kits to customers that contain the implements necessary to secure a DNA sample. The customer returns the sample to the company by mail. It is amplified and sequenced, and then compared to African Ancestry's proprietary DNA bio-bank— the African Lineage Database (ALD), which is said to contain more than 25,000 DNA samples from over thirty countries and 200 ethnic groups on the African continent. After several weeks, a customer will receive a results package.[9]

Over the last several years, the services of Kittles and Paige's African Ancestry company have come to play a central role not only in the lives of individual consumers, but also in broader reconciliation projects. Present for some time in the criminal justice context, DNA is now moving more squarely into the courts and engaging genetics with other legal arguments and processes. Recently, genetic genealogy testing migrated to the domain of civil law when results of this kind of analysis was introduced as evidence in a well-known U.S. class-action suit for reparations for slavery, *Farmer-Paellmann v. FleetBoston Financial Corp. et al.*[10] This case is discussed by Hamilton in this volume. Here I rehearse some of Hamilton's discussion and draw from my own research in order to locate it within the broader circulation of what I term "reconciliation projects" and, more particularly, to establish what can be revealed through tracing one genetic ancestry testing company's role in these socio-political endeavors.

Acts of Reparation

From the "forty acres and a mule" promised to emancipated blacks after the Civil War to contemporary reparations social movements, U.S. history is punctuated with instances in which bondsmen and bondswomen and their descendents have endeavored to gain restitution for the forced, unpaid labor of slavery. Despite such efforts, prospects for such recompense have never been promising. During Reconstruction, few emancipated blacks received either land or livestock. In the mid-twentieth century, black radical Queen Mother Audley E. Moore, the granddaughter of slaves, made several attempts to secure reparations for blacks. In 1959, she presented to the United Nations a petition that charged that genocide had been perpetrated against black Americans and demanded reparations in the form of land and economic resources. Moore made a similar request in a 1962 meeting with President John F. Kennedy. In this same year, she also founded the Committee for Reparations for Descendants of U.S. Slaves, an entity that works for social repair and economic restitution.[11] But neither Queen Mother Moore's lobbying nor grassroots organizing resulted in any significant movement toward reparations before her death in the 1990s. More recently, Representative John Conyers has introduced bill H.R. 40, the Commission to Study Reparation Proposals for African Americans Act, every year since 1989. In more than twenty attempts, the bill has never made it out of committee.

Attorney Deadria Farmer-Paellmann was well aware of these fits and starts toward the goal of slavery reparations when she decided to take another tack, moving from legislation and lobbying to litigation. In 2002, she became the lead plaintiff in *Farmer-Paellmann v. FleetBoston*, a class action suit coalesced from several individual cases, in which corporations were sued by the descendents of slaves for the return of lost wages and, consequently, lost wealth. In March 2002, Farmer-Paellman's attorney Edward Fagan, who had successfully obtained a settlement of $2 billion from Swiss banks on behalf of Holocaust victims, filed a complaint and demand for a jury trial in a New York federal Court on behalf of his client and "all other persons similarly situated," against FleetBoston Financial Corporation, Aetna, and CSX.[12] The plaintiffs sought a national apology to the descendants of slaves and financial reparations from these corporations in the form of large trust funds that would be used for social welfare programs to improve housing, education, and health care.

The case was heard in late 2003 by the United States District Court for the Northern District of Illinois. It was discharged in January 2004, when the court granted the corporate defendants' motion requesting a dismissal of the case. District Judge Charles R. Norgle's decision of dismissal was based on several grounds—though primarily he found the plaintiffs' case lacking in the area of the legal doctrine of "standing."[13] In his ruling, the judge asserted that the plaintiff class did not have a precise, or even a proximate, connection to former slaves, and thus the plaintiffs could not sue for injury as their descendents. Norgle noted that "[the] Plaintiffs cannot establish a personal injury sufficient to confer standing by *merely alleging* some genealogical relationship to African-Americans held in slavery over one-hundred, two-hundred, or three hundred-years ago."[14] With this line of reasoning, the court contested the plaintiff class's claim of "hereditary or genetic standing," to use the words of legal scholar Eric J. Miller.[15] Put another way, the court rejected the assumption of a "familial relationship between the ancestor victim and the descendant plaintiff."[16]

The plaintiffs sought to persuade the court of their "hereditary injury"[17] and to counter Judge Norgle's assertion that they "merely alleged" a genealogical relationship to enslaved men and women with scientific evidence of genetic inheritance. In March of 2004, Farmer-Paellmann and the seven other plaintiffs filed a second, narrower reparations case against just three companies, FleetBoston, Lloyd's of London, and R. J. Reynolds, that they claimed had "aid[ed] and abet[ted] the commission of genocide" by providing insurance and financing for slavers. In this suit, the plaintiffs responded to the court's argument that they lacked standing to bring the slavery reparations case with genetic genealogy results—provided free of charge by African Ancestry—that linked each of them to an ethnic group and/or nation-state on the continent of Africa.[18] Genetic ancestry test results that associated Farmer-Paellmann with the Mende people of Sierra Leone, another plaintiff in the group to Niger, and a third to the Gambia, among other contemporary locations on the African continent, were submitted as an evidential retort to the standing doctrine. The DNA data, the plaintiffs argued, confirmed their hereditary connection to enslaved Africans brought to the United States and thus was also evidence of their legal legitimacy as aggrieved parties.

In March 2005, in a lengthy decision, Judge Norgle dismissed the plaintiffs' second case—once again primarily on the basis of standing. The judge maintained that the genetic genealogy tests did not sufficiently establish a relationship between deceased slaves and the signatories to the class action suit. He wrote that "there may well be no perfect method of determining exactly who is a descendent of a slave and thus a member of the group entitled to receive reparations." Continuing this line of argument, the judge noted the strengths and weaknesses of genetic genealogy as hereditary evidence, compared to other indices of "race," ethnicity, kinship, and nationality:

> Genealogical research "often fails to provide significant information about a person's ancestry." "The blood, or 'one drop,' test (whereby anyone with any trace of African ancestry is deemed part of the group entitled to receive reparations) "fails to differentiate between descendants of US slaves and those of other nationalities with African heritage . . ." Genetic mapping, or *DNA testing, is more promising than the above two methods, but "alone is insufficient to provide a decisive link to a homeland."*[19]

Invoking both the problem of the incomplete archive and the pernicious logic of hypodescent, Norgle concluded, in keeping with legal doctrine, that the only suitable means to establish "a decisive link to a homeland" was DNA evidence that could show an uninterrupted, definitive line of ancestry from an exploited former slave to an aggrieved present-day descendent or descendents *and simultaneously*, a direct line of capital gained (and lost) from accused corporation to expropriated laborers and their offspring. Genetic genealogy test results, the court surmised, neither supplied the plaintiffs with genetic standing nor substantiated their hereditary injury.

From Genetic Kinship to Social Justice?

With reconciliation projects, the insights of genetic science are applied to the discovery or confirmation of ancestry in the hopes of securing social inclusion, including rights and reparation. But to what extent can DNA identification be efficacious for African diasporic and/or racial reconciliation? What might be the consequences of the genetic mediation of African diasporic cultural politics that have historically involved social movement tactics and civil rights organizations?

To be sure, the reconciliation projects described in this volume suggest that it may not be possible to settle political controversies and correct historical misdeeds on strictly technical grounds. As Aronson demonstrates, the reconciliation sought by the activists' families may remain elusive despite the turn to genetics because while "biological recognition" may be accomplished, the "social recognition" and "historical recognition" that are sought and are at stake may remain unattainable.

In the case of the reparations suit, there is the problem of "genetic standing" manifested as a gap between how the court and the plaintiffs respectively interpret relatedness. Tort law requires the succession of capital, matrilineage, and patrilineage to constitute what Hamilton calls "legal cognizance." The reparations plaintiffs, on the other hand, introduced genetic genealogy tests into the litigation not only to demonstrate "hereditary injury" but also to highlight the "social death" that was inherent to the chattel slavery system.[20] "The injury that we're focusing on," Farmer-Paellmann proclaimed in an interview,

> is the loss of our, the destruction of our ethnic and national groups. African-Americans today do not know who we are. That is a human right, to know who you are. . . . There are now DNA tests available where we can determine the precise ethnic and national groups we come from in Africa, so we're able to trace ourselves back to the slave trade and determine who underwrote those slave trading expeditions, which nations, which companies supplied whatever resources necessary to brutally enslave my ancestors.[21]

Farmer-Paellmann and the other plaintiffs believe that they have found in genetic genealogy testing a vehicle of racial repair both within and beyond the courtroom. Yet, as with Aronson's analysis, legal cognizance is not fully achieved, because of the incommensurability between how the civil court, on the one hand, and the plaintiffs, one the other, differently perceive ancestry. This fundamental political and epistemological incommensurability leads one strongly toward the conclusion that social repair may not be attainable by means of genetic analysis.

Following this line of reasoning, one could conclude that genetic genealogy testing is of little value as a true medium of reconciliation. However, even if the plaintiffs ultimately lose the reparations litigation, they may gain ground in other ways. Legal scholar James Davey explains, for instance, that the reparations case could be considered a form of legal "sparring" used by counsel in *Farmer-Paellmann v. FleetBoston* "in order to gain access to the Supreme Court, where the novel nature of the issue might force a change in judicial attitudes to the doctrine of standing."[22] Davey also offers that the lawsuit "is a form of 'quasi-public' litigation."[23] With such an understanding, he continues, although "the nature of the litigation remains adversarial. . . . The role of the litigant is therefore, in part, to raise awareness of the issues beyond the confines of the courtroom, in wider social, legal and political fora."[24] In this task, Farmer Paellmann and her allies will likely succeed. And, more to Davey's point, this litigation in the court of popular opinion will be occurring in the context of the increased ubiquity of DNA, with the legal gatekeepers and the public alike being more exposed to the influence of genetics in numerous aspects of their lives.

In 1998, before genetic testing became widely available to the public, this analysis was used to test the hypothesis that President Thomas Jefferson fathered children with an enslaved woman owned by him, Sally Hemings.[25] Historian Annette Gordon-Reed exhaustively researched the controversy over the paternity of bondswoman Hemings's children and the nature of her relationship with the founding father and slave-owner Jefferson.[26] Gordon-Reed demonstrates that archival evidence that might typically be used to by historians to resolve this issue was ignored or selectively interpreted. What lies at the heart of Gordon-Reed's claim is the problem of fact and evidence, and more specifically, the capacity of certain forms of evidence to prove histories that have been disavowed and denied, in particular, the ultimately unknowable (but, certainly provable) details of the peculiar institution. Genetic analysis was deemed capable of resolving centuries-old and deeply entrenched disputes and debates about racial slavery in the United States. But as Mia Bay and others have shown, the results of the genetic testing that established Jefferson's possible paternity of one of Hemings's children has not accomplished reconciliation among his descendents and those of Hemings.[27]

Clearly, the issues, controversies, and questions we pose to science about race and the unsettled past can never find resolution in the science itself. A troubling reality for these reconciliation projects is the fact that the purposes to which DNA is put are, in the words of Alvin Weinberg, "trans-scientific."[28] For Weinberg, some questions posed to science—typically metaphysical questions or moral ones—cannot be answered or resolved by science. The illegibility of genetic testing as proof of ancestry in civil suits and historiography—despite its use in other courts and for other operations of state power, such as the reunification of immigrant families (as described in work in progress by sociologist Catherine Lee), suggests the trans-scientific.

As the essays in this volume demonstrate, the stakes of genetic genealogy testing and of the broader issues of race and history in genetics are largely trans-scientific. The issues, controversies, and mysteries we pose to science about race and the unsettled past may never find resolution. Those instances in which genetic science fails to fully resolve concerns suggests that what is sought is not biogenetic facts as proof of injury or vectors of repair, but rather reconciliation in its fullest sense. The repair that is sought cannot necessarily be found in genetic science solely. Aronson's work reveals that "complexity and ambiguity" remained, even after DNA technologies helped to identify deceased activists, because social recognition was not fully accomplished even as biological recognition was. The families of deceased anti-apartheid activists also seek recognition of the sacrifice that their loved ones made for a better South Africa. In this sense, DNA can offer an avenue toward recognition, but cannot stand in for reconciliation: voice, acknowledgment, mourning, forgiveness, and healing. These reconciliation efforts also raise interesting and fraught contradictions: they threaten to reify race in the pursuit of repair for injury; they suggest how justice pursuits can be uneasily intertwined with commercial enterprises; they may substitute genetic data for the just outcomes that are sought, and, indeed, they demonstrate well that facts may not, in and of themselves, secure justice.

Reconciliation projects are becoming commonplace. It is by tracking genetic analysis from its conditions of possibility into some of its unexpected applications that the profound and expansive manner in which DNA now shapes social arenas and engenders social norms comes into relief. Even if they lack formal, legal efficacy, the very phenomenon of reconciliation projects tells us something about the proliferation and social utility of genetics beyond the hospital, the science bench and the criminal court room, and sheds light upon *the social life of DNA*.

NOTES

1. Mildred Cho and Pamela Sankar, "Forensic Genetics and Ethical, Legal, and Social Implications Beyond the Clinic," *Nature Genetics* 36 (2004): S8–S12.

2. Troy Duster, *Backdoor to Eugenics*, 2nd ed. (New York: Routledge, 2003), 21–38.

3. Alondra Nelson, "The Social Life of DNA," *Chronicle of Higher Education* (August 29, 2010), chronicle.com/article/The-Social-Life-of-DNA/124138/ [Accessed August 29, 2010].

4. The Greensboro Truth and Reconciliation Commission, www.greensborotrc.org/. On the National Commission on the Disappearance of Persons in Argentina, see Emilio Fermin Mignone, Cynthia L. Estlund, and Samuel Issacharoff, "Dictatorship on Trial: Prosecution of Human Rights Violations in Argentina," *Yale Journal of International Law* 10 (1984): 118–150.

5. John Torpey, *Making Whole What Has Been Smashed: On Reparations Politics* (Cambridge, MA: Harvard University Press, 2006).

6. Innocence Project website, www.innocenceproject.org/ [accessed February 10, 2010]. See also, Edward F. Connors, ed., *Convicted by Juries, Exonerated by Science: Case Studies in the Use of DNA Evidence to Establish Innocence after Trial* (New York: National Institute of Justice, Institute for Law and Justice, 1996).

7. Rory Carroll, "Argentina's Authorities Order DNA Tests in Search of Stolen Babies of Dirty War," *The Guardian* (UK), (December 30, 2009). www.guardian.co.uk/world/2009/dec/30/argentina-dna-tests-babies-disappeared; Associated Press, "Argentina Forces DNA Tests in 'Dirty War' Cases," (November 20, 2009), www.msnbc.msn.com/id/34071255/ns/world_news-americas/.

8. This popularity stems in large part because africanancestry.com supplies its customers with "matches" to ethnic groups and nation-states on the African continent, rather than simply haplotype groups or percentages of racial ancestry that are less easily imported

into self-fashioning. See Nelson, "Bio Science: Genetic Ancestry Tracing and the Pursuit of African Ancestry," *Social Studies of Science* 38 (2008): 759–783.

9. African Ancestry reports that approximately 25 to 30 percent of male root-seekers using its PatriClan (Y-chromosome) test will not match any of the paternal lines in the African Lineage Database (ALD). In such instances, the customer may be advised to have his sample matched against a "European database." See Greg Langley, "Genealogy and Genomes: DNA Technology Helping People Learn More About Who They Are and Where They Come From," *Baton Rouge Advocate* (July 20, 2003). A page about the PatriClan (Y-chromosome) test on African Ancestry's website states: "We find African ancestry for approximately 65% of the paternal lineages we test. The remaining 35% of the lineages we test typically indicate European ancestry. If our tests indicate that you are not of African descent, we will identify your continent of origin." "Discover the Paternal Roots of Your Family Tree," africanancestry.com/patriclan.html [accessed July 1, 2010]. Because the ALD (African Lineage Database) is extensive, but not exhaustive, there is some chance that matching "African" genetic markers are not yet included.

10. "Judge Drops Suit Seeking Reparations, Slave Descendents Vow to Appeal," *Chicago Tribune*, (January 27, 2004).

11. queenmothermore.org/reparations.htm [accessed April 13, 2009].

12. "Judge Drops Suit Seeking Reparations, Slave Descendents Vow to Appeal," *Chicago Tribune* (January 27, 2004).

13. On standing in reparations suits, see Eric J. Miller, "Representing the Race: Standing to Sue in Reparations Lawsuits," *Harvard BlackLetter Law Journal* 20 (2004): 91–114.

14. "Judge Rejects Slavery Reparations Lawsuit," *Chicago Sun-Times* (January 27, 2004) (emphasis added).

15. Miller, "Representing the Race," 93.

16. Ibid.

17. Ibid., 94.

18. Farmer-Paellmann's fervor for genetic genealogy testing led her several years ago to establish the Organization of Tribal Unity, a "not-for-profit organization established to create a network of those who have restored their African ethnic and national identities through DNA testing." In 2006, the OTU initiated an online petition to nominate geneticist Rick Kittles (co-founder of the African Ancestry company genetic genealogy tests, which had been submitted in the Farmer-Paellmann reparations suit) for the Nobel Prize. The petition read: "We, the undersigned, propose that Dr. Rick Kittles be nominated for the Nobel Prize for his profound contribution to the field of genetic research. Dr. Kittles, a 40-year-old geneticist descended from enslaved Africans, has earned this honor and recognition for his original DNA research and analysis that is repairing the effects of 450 years of slavery[-]related ethnic cleansing committed against people of African descent. His unique method compares genetic sequences to restore ethnic and national identity—two of the most fundamental human attributes. Prior to Dr. Kittles' groundbreaking work, this information was inaccessible to millions of descendants of enslaved Africans. For using science to 'unlock the door of no return,' Dr. Kittles deserves the greatest honors and recognition the world has to offer. We propose and support his nomination for the Nobel Prize."

19. Justice Charles R. Norgle, "Opinion and Order," In re African-American Slave Descendants Litigation, United States District Court, N.D. Illinois, Eastern Division, July 6, 2005, 20. (emphasis added)

20. Orlando Patterson, *Slavery and Social Death: A Comparative Study* (Cambridge, MA: Harvard University Press, 1985).

21. DF-P interview with the Australian Broadcasting Corporation, "The World Today," March 30, 2004.

22. James Davey, "From 'Jim Crow' to 'John Doe': Reparations, Corporate Liability, and the Limits of Private Law," in *Ethics, Law, and Society* (Vol. 3), ed. Jennifer Gunning and Soren Holm (Burlington, VT: Ashgate, 2007), 199.

23. Ibid. Here Davey is drawing on the work of Paige A. Fogarty, "Speculating a Strategy: Suing Insurance Companies to Obtain Legislative Reparations for Slavery," 9 *Connecticut Insurance Law Journal* 9.211 (2003): 224–241.

24. Ibid.

25. Eugene A. Foster, Mark A. Jobling, P. G. Taylor et al., "Jefferson Fathered Slave's Last Child," *Nature* 396 (5 November 1998): 27–28.

26. Annette Gordon-Reed, *Thomas Jefferson and Sally Hemings: An American Controversy* (Charlottesville: University of Virginia Press, 1997).

27. Mia Bay, "In Search of Sally Hemings in the Post-DNA Era," *Reviews in American History* 34 (December 2006): 407–426.

28. A "father" of the nuclear age, Weinberg deployed the idea of "trans-science" to forestall criticism of potentially dangerous research and to draw a line between politics and "pure science" (as he put it). As a scholar working in the social studies of science and contra Weinberg, I take it as a given that science and its applications are inherently social (and thus also political) phenomena. But I nevertheless find Weinberg's insight to be of use in a new era in which genetic science is being asked to resolve myriad issues.

3

The Unspoken Significance of
Gender in Constructing Kinship,
Race, and Nation

CATHERINE LEE

In 2007, the *New York Times* reported the fourteen-year effort of Isaac Owusu to be reunited with the four sons he left behind in Ghana. After becoming a citizen in 2002, Owusu petitioned to have his sons join him in the United States, a right afforded to him as a citizen. When given the opportunity to prove his familial claims by taking a DNA test, Owusu confidently swabbed the inside of his cheek. Test results quickly dashed his hopes for reuniting with his children when government officials notified him that the test could verify paternity for his oldest son only. With these test results, Owusu learned that his deceased wife may have been unfaithful and that his three younger sons were not biologically his. The government permitted the admission of his oldest son to the United States, but the other three were denied entry. The only recourse Owusu had was to petition for the younger boys' entry as his stepsons. Awaiting the government's decision, he had chosen to withhold the information generated by the DNA test from his sons, explaining that he could not tell them they were fatherless when they were already motherless. Although he called himself their "daddy" as he wept, genetic tests rendered null and false the affective ties of familial bond between father and son that Owusu unequivocally knew for nearly two decades (Swarns 2007).

The Owusu case illustrates powerfully the ways in which DNA analysis has become a critically important tool in the definition of family and in the administration of national identity. As the U.S. government considers moving toward the use of DNA testing for proving eligibility for immigration, the practice has the potential to drastically affect the implementation of immigration policy as well as the meaning of family and familial ties.[1] Despite the highly personal nature of his experience with genetic testing, Owusu's claim to retain his role as "daddy" underscores four general points illustrated by essays throughout this volume, which range from individual, to group, to population genetics.

First, as the case makes clear, genetic analysis does not always provide unwavering answers to how people are related, and certainly not to how they understand their attachments to one another. Owusu's test results did not nullify his feelings of affection and filial responsibility for the boys who were not his *biological* sons, although they altered the legal parameters of their relationship. Many of the examples discussed in essays in this volume also attest to this point by showing how the construction of populations or groups used in genetics research obscures the complex and contested ways in which familial ties, racial difference, or ancestry is understood and mobilized. Genetics is thus not only *an* answer to questions of nation, race, or kinship and belonging, but also a *way* of answering or even framing questions of how collective ties ought to be formulated, evaluated, and understood for purposes of connecting individuals across time and space.

The Owusu case illustrates a second point, that there exists an evolving tension between the supposed absolute nature of genetic tests versus the seemingly contingent nature of personal accounts. Seen through the lens of genetic analysis, the stories we repeatedly tell about ourselves and our origins—passed down from one generation to the next—are deemed to be less real than the results of a buccal swab test. Of course, nationalism scholars have long shown that such ancestral storytelling is part of the mythologizing of nations, and this continues to be true in the era of genetic analysis. The putative claims of nativists and nationalists and of business entrepreneurs marketing genetic ancestry testing are entrenched in various and overlapping measures of fact and fiction. In replacing personal, familial, or national narratives with DNA analysis, some scientists, government officials, business entrepreneurs, and consumers of ancestral testing have failed to recognize that genes tell stories as well, which are rooted in equivocal and challengeable claims.

Third, Owusu's experience highlights how these issues of determining collective ties have become matters of widespread legal, administrative, and social contest, as migration increases and as institutional actors assert greater authority to adjudicate kinship claims. In this context, DNA test results have meaning and are consequential to the extent that they provide an avenue for exercising a right, privilege, or demand, such as family reunification provisions in American immigration policy. As such, genetic testing becomes the terrain upon which issues of inequality and access to scarce or contested resources unfold.

A fourth important point that is raised by Owusu's story is the role of gender in molding the boundaries and meanings of family, race, or nation. The issue has been paradoxically absent from discussions of genetics and kinship. Gender—the system of meanings that shape actions and expectations about roles and behavior for men and women—is critical to how notions of family, race or ethnicity, genetic identity, nation, and state are connected in four important ways. First, gender frames the questions that individual family members, government officials, or nationalists may demand that genetics answer, since gender helps structure the relations we have with one another, a larger ethnic or racial group, the nation, or the state. Second, gendered rules govern intimate relations, such as marriage and reproduction, as well as more formal ones related to migration and settlement.

Third, these relations shape the development of physical materials, including populations, genome banks, and even DNA and cell lines, which delineate the boundaries, for example, of legal or legitimate families, racial formation, and the nation-state. These physical materials provide the basis upon which genetic, familial, racial, and national claims are made. Finally, gender molds the symbolic meaning of these materials and the significance of the relations from which they arise. Thus, gendered ideals and claims lie at the heart of how individual family members, nationalists, or geneticists collect, interpret, and narrate such materials for familial, racial, and nationalist questions and claims, although these actors often hide, ignore, or deny these processes. Therefore, gender is crucial for how we construct kinship in its various forms and for how it structures cultural and political projects. In the rest of this chapter I examine the significance of gender in these endeavors.

Gendered Questions and Claims

The absence of Owusu's sons' mother in the case raises several questions that both Owusu and the U.S. government believed DNA analysis could answer. Gender shaped the relationship Owusu had with his wife, guiding decisions such as migration and child rearing. Questions about sexuality, reproductive choice, and paternal responsibility arise from gendered expectations about men and women. Because Owusu's boys are "motherless," the mother's claim to her sexual history are absent, along with critical bits of information that could ostensibly determine where the kids belong, including to which nation. If the mother were still alive, the issue of whether Owusu would make an effort to bring them to the United States would perhaps be uncertain as well. Without her presence, genetics is used to provide answers to the questions of where the sons belong and to whom. Yet the prism of gender guides how Owusu and the government should interpret "facts" such as DNA, and this meaning is not self-evident. Instead, the apparent contradiction to the decades-long affection Owusu knew and felt forces a reinterpretation of his familial ties in the absence of the mother.

The use of biometric tests for evaluating the veracity of ties is not new, especially in the administration of American immigration policy. For example, American immigration officials at various points throughout the twentieth century relied on blood analysis and other biometric measurements for assessing familial claims made by would-be Chinese immigrants as well as other excludable groups of immigrants (Lau 2006). The contest over Chinese immigrants' rightful claims to enter the United States as the biological children—often sons—of native-born citizens included applicants that immigration officials derisively called "paper sons" in order to highlight the presumably forged nature of documents on which these familial claims were based. This was part of a history of immigrant exclusion, especially of women, which led to great gender imbalances and resulted in the formation of bachelor societies and the denial of Chinese family formation and settlement (Lee 2010). This fact illustrates the point that genetics stands as part of a long history of our efforts to determine what is "real" and "true" about our relations, and that such efforts intertwine with gendered processes such as immigration.

Owusu's "motherless" children and Chinese "paper sons" exemplify the gendered ways in which nation-building practices operate. Nationalists and immigration officials seek to answer the question of who truly belongs, not just to the family, but to the nation as well. As such, immigration control and border gatekeeping are about the construction and maintenance of a national identity. The contests over this process include the testing of familial claims and measures that dictate which immigrant women have the right to settle physically and give birth to the next generation. The recent debates over "anchor babies"—babies born to foreign born, particularly undocumented, immigrants in the United States—and demands for changes to the constitutional protection of birthright citizenship further demonstrate this point (Preston 2010). Immigration opponents see the continued and growing number and permanence of immigrant settlement—especially among Mexican immigrants—as an assault on the American identity (Chavez 2008). The "facts" of genetics may obfuscate this point by ignoring or overshadowing the political and social processes, which generate the gendered relations and negotiations that form the basis for the resulting physical evidence of settlement and birth. However, gender remains an implicit force, shaping the meaning of the family, race, or nation by underlying the construction, collection, and evaluation of genealogies and genomic data for nation-building purposes. Thinking generally about what kinship means can help illustrate these gendered processes more clearly, which is what I turn to in the next section.

Gendered Ties and DNA

Family, race or ethnicity, and nation all have similar structural forms as types of kinship. As the anthropologist David Schneider has argued, there is nothing universal about kinship (1977; 1980). That is, there is no rule about blood, law, or affection that defines its structure or form. To this extent, we can think about kinship in a more general sense. Thus drawing from his work, I suggest that we think about the constructs of family, race or ethnicity, and nation as having two important elements: "relationship" (ties or connection) and "natural substance" (blood or genes)—both of which become codes for conduct. The "natural substance" is part of the putative claim-making, which may be touted as genetic or biological. Thus, DNA tests may provide evidentiary proof for the "natural substance." However, what relationship results from this and how it should be cataloged and formulated as code for conduct has always been up for debate. That is, the stories family members or nationalists tell about their families or nation are not made self-evident by the physical proof of the natural substance. Furthermore, as I discuss below, this substance arises from, is preserved, and is called into service through particular gendered negotiations between individuals, racial or ethnic groups, or nationalists.

DNA testing is often part of an elaborate system aimed at shaping codes of conduct, which can dictate both action and emotion. The action may include things like determining the financial support of a parent for a child or enlistment in the military during times of war. Emotion includes the affective ties that may undergird the rationale or justification for such actions—sense of responsibility, duty, or pride. Thus, what kinship tells us—how we're related and what that relationship is made of (the "natural substance")—is no small matter. They help explain, for example, what makes people love, die, or kill for nations as Benedict Anderson asked and thoughtfully answered. The nationalist appeal rests in part on the notion that the nation is "conceived as a deep, horizontal comradeship" (1991:7).

People conceive of nations as imagined communities, wherein members can conceptualize links to one another across time or generations or space that are preternatural. Thus, the ordering is not just horizontal but vertical as well. The vertical, or generational linkage is structured through the family and the gendered work that both men and women perform, which is something Anderson and other scholars of nationalism have largely ignored (Yuval-Davis 1998). Therefore, seeing the connections between family and nation may help us to answer more fully Anderson's question if we recognize the emotive ties and the notions of duty and loyalty that familial bonds can command. And as the Owusu case illustrates, these notions are shaped by gender.

We can also see the ways in which DNA testing, in the context of the family, can literally transform the family into a microcosm of the nation. This is most apparent in studies of reproductive policies and the state or in ethnic conflict and sexual violence. For example, in Ceaucescu's Romania, anti-abortion and pro-natal policies were intended to secure the continued birthing of the nation (Kligman 1998). During ethnic conflicts in Bosnia and Croatia in the 1990s or in Rwanda in 1994, raping women of the enemy ethic group helped to blur the ethno-national claims as well as familial lines as part of genocide or ethnic cleansing programs (Card 1996; Meznaric 1994). These examples highlight the importance of gender and patriarchal notions of sexuality and reproduction, which helps to obscure the lines of division between family and nation by the work that men and women's bodies perform. For example, they demonstrate how women as biological reproducers serve to mark the physical and symbolic boundaries of the nation, achieved through the symbolic and even physical use of their bodies by men or by the male-dominated state (Anthias and Yuval-Davis 1992; Bock 1991; Gal and Kligman 2000; Mostov 1995; Nagel 1998; Yuval-Davis 1998).

Efforts to regulate women's sexuality are endeavors to achieve purity *qua patriline* for a racial or ethnic group as well as for the nation. For many nationalists and racists, one equals the other to the extent that a biologically distinct and unique group of people constitutes a given nation or race. Women must be sexually pure in order to preserve the purity of the race or nation; the race or nation is pure, because the women are sexually pure. The reasoning is circular. What is significant is the use of discourse to make the symbolic connection seem natural and real. Putative claims about the "natural substance" that defines the relationship between members of a race or nation, like the family, help to make the discursive and practical link between race and nationality. Genetic testing of DNA—whether mitochondrial "maternal" DNA, or Y-chromosome (male) DNA, or other markers—becomes easily woven into the broader framing of sexuality, reproduction, and gender. Men's and women's bodies do the work of making such links between race and nation possible, thereby coupling the meanings of race and gender.

The gendered dimension of nationalist or racist projects that dictate rules for reproduction have consequences for how we interpret demographic and genetic genealogies, including the historical records of marriage and the inheritance of mitochondrial DNA. Thus, for example, antimiscegenation laws and other eugenics programs determined who could marry whom or whose reproductive capabilities would be rewarded (positive eugenic programs designed to encourage "better breeding") or violently denied (negative eugenics programs such as forced sterilization) (Kelves 1985; Stern 2005). Gendered bodies render gendered DNA. Implicitly understood in studies of family, race, or nation and genetics is the importance of gendered rules for determining kinship's dual code for conduct—relationship and natural substance.

Obfuscating Gender in Genetic Ties

As different societies grapple with the questions posed by DNA for race and for historical memory and understanding, the gendered dimensions of this collision have been pulled out of focus as geneticists and nationalists consider the meaning and utility of DNA to frame and construct our stories of national origin and national identity. For example, in Canada and in Great Britain, politicians and scientists often ignore or refute the complex gendered rules that shaped migration, intermixing, and settlement. This is evident in Amy Hinterberger's examination (in this volume) of the development of Canada's support for genomics-based biomedical research and the concomitant ways by which its multicultural policy provides both the rationale and classificatory scheme for how groups are identified and counted. Canada and its supported researchers must address tensions that exist with a multiculturalism policy that celebrates diversity and inclusion and genomics research that presumes homogeneity of its settling founders and exclusion of its native peoples. Similarly, the question of national identity and gender is evident in Nina Kohli-Laven's study of how scientists draw lines that define populations according to racial, ethnic, or ancestral logics that privilege a white, French, colonial history in Quebec, which ignores the complexities of native settlement and intermixing in the demographic reconstruction of genealogies documented by church records and DNA sampling. She shows how scientists use these forms of evidence to represent Quebec's mixed frontier society as biologically pure. In doing so, she demonstrates the affinity between scientists' rendering of population boundaries and Quebec nationalists' historiographic and political agenda. Both groups set out to narrate stories of origin and the founding of Quebec. Similarly, as Marianne Sommer explains, British scholar Bryan Sykes successfully markets genetics testing while drawing upon claims to a Celtic heritage in the British Isles that is colorfully articulated and identified as pure—a claim that denies a complex migratory history.

How can we understand such obfuscations, contradictions, and inconsistencies in the governments' and scientists' approaches to genetic genealogy in Canada and Great Britain? How do these mythic stories of origin deny marital and other intimate relations that existed in frontier society? Genetic genealogy that ignores complex gendered processes is not unlike other nation-building activities, which rely on the symbolic and physical work of men and women's bodies while denying the existence of such efforts (Yuval-Davis 1998). Genetic analysis, in this view, is not simply involved with the erasure of a mixed or multi-ethnic colonial history, but with erasing the gendered dimensions of migration and settlement in earlier times and today as well. Migration is always the expression of gendered norms, roles, and expectations about who should stay or leave, work inside or outside the family, and the valuing of productive labor over reproductive labor. These gendered arrangements determined the formation and settlement of the frontier and continue to shape immigrant communities today (Courtwright 1996; Hirata 1979; Hondagneu-Sotelo 1994).

The boundary-making and nation-making processes that lie at the heart of genetic stories of origin are the mythic narration of the "natural substance," which identifies Canada's or Britain's ethno-national history as pure. This is so despite the contradictions presented by the current identification of either country as multicultural or by diverse new immigration. Even ancient history and genetic "proof" of a more complex past are ignored. Thus, for example, Sykes can claim that the male lines in Great Britain are mainly Celtic, rendering the existence of Y-chromosomes that are Saxon, Dane/Viking, or Norman as "minorities," which makes the British Isles "stubbornly Celtic" (2006:287). This literal and figurative gendered narration of genes by Sykes is critical to his customers' link to a pure imagined community. In addition to the male lines, Sykes argues that the British female gene pool is Celtic, suggesting it has remained more or less intact. This sort of claim to an ethnic and sexual purity has long been the foundational rhetoric of nationalists (Mosse 1985; Nagel 1998).

It is notable and striking, as Priscilla Wald notes in her chapter, how women's bodies do the literal work of narrating the past and foretelling of the future. Giving literary and political dimensions to the story of genes, race, and history, Wald illustrates the expansive possibilities of genetic discourse and links these themes ultimately to the issue of colonization. Women, in her analysis, can be both the silently subjugated actors of such colonization efforts and active resistors. As Joane Nagel has argued in her study of sexuality and nationalist politics, women "occupy a distinct, symbolic role in nationalist culture, discourse and collective action, a role that reflects a masculinist definition of femininity and of women's proper place in the nation" (Nagle 1998: 252), though women often resist such definitions of themselves.

Gendered meanings are fundamental to the ways these notions of family, race or ethnicity, genetic identity, and the nation are constructed and deployed for cultural and political projects, including nation building. New scientific developments such as genetic analysis are asked to adjudicate questions about kinship ties, belonging, and boundaries—matters that have long vexed citizens, nationalists, racists, and illegitimate sons. DNA analysis is perhaps only the most recent iteration for determining eligible groups for migration and settlement or for verifying paternity. Even more significantly though, it is clear that these scientific developments—including DNA analysis and genome banks—work through gender, and thereby help to frame how kinship ties and boundaries are identified, analyzed, narrated, and remembered.

NOTES

1. Currently, the United States government does not require DNA testing for purposes of proving eligibility for immigration. However, as it has identified the growing use of fraudulent documents by would-be immigrants, the U.S. government has argued that genetic testing may be a more valid and speedy method for determining eligibility. See the Department of Homeland Security's Citizenship and Immigration Services Ombudsman's 2009 Annual Report (www.dhs.gov/xlibrary/assets/cisomb_annual_report_2009.pdf [accessed Oct. 10, 2011]) and the United States Citizenship and Immigration Services Response (www.uscis.gov/USCIS/Resources/Ombudsman%20Liason/cisomb_2009_response.pdf [accessed Oct. 11, 2011]).

WORKS CITED

Anderson, Benedict. 1991 . Imagined communities. Revised edition. London: Verso.

Anthias, Foya, and Nira Yuval-Davis. 1992. Racialized boundaries: Race, nation, gender, colour, and class and the anti-racist struggle. London: Routledge.

Bock, Gisela. 1991. Antinationalism, maternity, and paternity in national socialism. In Maternity and gender policies: Women and the rise of the European welfare states, 1880s to 1950s, edited by Gisela Bock and Pat Thane, 233–255. London: Routledge.

Card, Claudia. 1996. Rape as a weapon of war. Hypatia 11(4): 5–18.

Chavez, Leo. 2008. The Latino threat: Constructing immigrants, citizens, and the nation. Palo Alto, CA: Stanford University Press.

Courtwright, David T. 1996. Violent land: Single men and social disorder from the frontier to the inner city. Cambridge, MA: Harvard University Press.

Gal, Susan, and Gail Kligman. 2000. The politics of gender after socialism: A comparative-historical essay. Princeton, NJ: Princeton University Press.

Hirata, Lucie Cheng. 1979. Free, indentured, enslaved: Chinese prostitutes in nineteenth-century America. Signs 5:3–29.

Hondagneu-Sotelo, Pierrette. 1994. Gendered transitions: Mexican experiences of immigration. Berkeley: University of California Press.

Kevles, Daniel J. 1985. In the name of eugenics: Genetics and the uses of human heredity. Berkeley: University of California Press.

Kligman, Gail. 1998. *The politics of duplicity: Controlling reproduction in Ceausescu's Romania.* Berkeley: University of California Press.

Lee, Catherine. 2010. "Where the danger lies": Race, gender, and Chinese and Japanese exclusion in the U.S., 1870–1924. *Sociological Forum.*

Meznaric, Silva, 1994. Gender as an ethno-marker: Rape, war, and identity in the former Yugoslavia. In *Identity politics and women: Cultural reassertion and feminism in international perspective,* edited by Valentine M. Moghadam, 76–97. Boulder, CO: Westview.

Mosse, George. 1985. *Nationalism and sexuality.* New York: H. Fertig.

Mostov, Julie. 1996. "Our women/their women": Symbolic boundaries, territorial markers, and violence in the Balkans. In *Women in a violent world: Feminist analyses and resistance across "Europe,"* edited by Chris Corrin, 515–529. Edinburgh: Edinburgh University Press.

Nagel, Joane. 1998. Masculinity and nationalism: Gender and sexuality in the making of nations. *Ethnic and Racial Studies* 21:242–269.

Preston, Julia. 2010. Citizenship from birth is challenged on the right. *New York Times,* August 7.

Schneider, David M. 1977. Kinship, nationality, and religion in American culture: Toward a definition of kinship." In *Symbolic anthropology: A reader in the study of symbols and meanings,* edited by Janet L. Dolgin, David S. Kemnitzer, and David M. Schneider, 63–71. New York: Columbia University Press.

_____. 1980. *American kinship: A cultural account.* Chicago: University of Chicago Press.

Stern, Alexandra Minna. 2005. *Eugenic nation: Faults and frontiers of better breeding in modern America.* Berkeley: University of California Press

Swarns, Rachel. 2007. DNA tests offer immigrants hope or despair. *New York Times,* April 10.

Sykes, Brian. 2006. *Saxons, Vikings, and Celts: The genetic roots of Britain and Ireland.* New York: W. W. Norton.

Yuval-Davis, Nira. 1998. Gender and nation. In *women, ethnicity, and nationalism,* edited by R. Wilford and R. Miller. New York: Routledge.

PART TWO

Decoding the Genomic Age

4

A Biologist's Perspective on DNA and Race in the Genomics Era

ABRAM GABRIEL

Public awareness of DNA has reached a tipping point. In 2008, *New York Times* reporter Amy Harmon won a Pulitzer Prize for her series of articles on the implications of DNA and DNA-based technology in modern society. In this same year, revenue from publicly traded biotechnology firms was nearly $90 billion. DNA-based evidence is the gold standard in courts for proving individual identity. DNA data are used with increasing frequency to explore ancestral origins, and are particularly marketed to African Americans and others who may lack records of their specific heritage. Companies have sprung up that will analyze an individual's DNA and provide ongoing reports of possible disease susceptibilities and genetic risk factors. Every month, new gene-associations for common diseases are announced in the scientific literature, and news of these discoveries is often reported in the lay press. Both genomics (the study of the structure, evolution, and function of all of the DNA in a cell) and personalized medicine (the concept that diagnostic and therapeutic decisions can be made based on analysis of specific variations in an individual's DNA) have been endorsed and heavily promoted by the pharmaceutical industry, government agencies, and human geneticists. And to protect the public, Congress passed and President George W. Bush signed into law the Genetic Information Non-discrimination Act of 2008, making it illegal to discriminate against individuals in employment and health insurance based on information obtained from genetic testing.

It all sounds pretty exciting. As a molecular biologist, I realize that my field has entered the limelight and that knowledge about DNA is no longer the esoteric province of academic researchers. I take pride in the fact that the study of DNA and genomics has progressed so far so fast, and that the science is being recognized as a powerful tool for fundamental advances in disciplines as disparate as biomedicine and human history. But I feel trepidation, too, that the translational process is moving faster than the science itself, potentially leading to public misconceptions, oversimplifications, and unverifiable claims about the power of these discoveries, with consequent lowering of society's trust in its scientists.

In particular, genomics has reinvigorated interest in the thorny topic of the significance of DNA variation and genetic differences between and among human races. Race is a key variable in analyses of American society. Disparities in opportunity, access, income, education, and disease rates by race remain among the most pressing impediments to our becoming a more equitable nation. By examining the genomes of individuals sampled from many world populations, human geneticists have identified DNA sequence differences that can indeed predict continental ancestral origins (referred to as ancestry informative markers). Using this information, companies now offer analyses of individuals' ancestry. Some academicians and commercial interests have used the existence of ancestry informative markers to support the notion that genetic differences in disease predisposition can be linked to ancestral population groups. But it is far from obvious what DNA data reveal about race, particularly since most geneticists acknowledge that human races cannot be objectively defined (Hunt and Megyesi 2008).

The concerns of this essay are how race has become part of our current discussions of genomics and whether it belongs there. At the beginning of the twentieth century, genetics and race were conflated through the popular pseudoscientific social movement of eugenics, with its belief that complex cultural, medical, and socio-economic differences between ethnic groups could be explained by genetic differences. Although the experimentally and statistically based discipline of genetics diverged from the dubious tenets of eugenics after the 1920s, the social and political dimensions of the eugenics agenda had lasting and infamous consequences in the United States, England, and Germany. By the second half of the twentieth century, it had become generally accepted, within academic circles, that "race" cannot be defined as a biological entity, but is subjectively defined by the social and cultural milieu. But in today's scientific and popular literature, race is being equated with ancestral DNA markers and genetic causes are being ascribed to racial differences in disease predisposition. It is troubling that these links may become accepted without recognition of the limitations of the underlying science and without putting an individual's genetic makeup in the context of his or her entire life experience.

In this essay, I first discuss how the technical advances of recombinant DNA, beginning in the 1970s, and of genomics, in the last decade, have propelled the field of human genetics forward and resurrected the race connection. I then use the examples of race and genetics in ancestry testing and personalized genomics to illustrate how the public's expectations for and faith in the power of genomics may be misguided. Finally, I consider how the biotechnology industry has influenced the direction of human genetics and how the industry contributes to the public's wishful thinking and often unrealistic beliefs in the omniscience of DNA.

Human Genetics and the Recombinant DNA Revolution

The field of genetics began in the early twentieth century, when scientists redis-covered Gregor Mendel's 1865 studies of heredity and began to appreciate the consequences of Charles Darwin's theories of natural selection and evolution. Archibald Garrod reported the first inherited disorder, alkaptonuria, in 1902, and later broadened the concept of inherited biochemical abnormalities with the term "inborn errors of metabolism."(Garrod and Harris 1963) These reports pre-ceded, by more than forty years, our realization that genes (the units of inheri-tance) were physically composed of DNA. But human and medical genetics did not assume its preeminent role in biomedical research for still another forty years.

Watson and Crick's discovery of the double helical structure of DNA in 1953 inaugurated the modern era of molecular biology. The succeeding generation of researchers defined the universality of the rules and mechanisms by which genetic information is transmitted through DNA. Most of this pioneering work used bacteria and their viruses as the experimental model systems. During this period, while scientists purified enzymes and developed techniques for their own lines of research, colleagues across the hall, at scientific meetings, or reading papers in scientific journals, gleaned these technical nuggets and adapted them for their own unrelated areas of interest. By the mid 1970s biologists from many disciplines realized that this composite technical knowledge, particularly the ability to cut out a segment of DNA from one species, recombine it with a seg-ment of DNA from another species, and express it inside of a bacterium (cloning), could be harnessed to tackle genetic questions about organisms much more complex than bacteria. This collective appreciation was the start of the "recombinant DNA revolution."

Human genetics may be the area where recombinant DNA has had its greatest impact. Through the 1970s fundamental genetic discoveries made with model organisms like *E. coli* and *Drosophila* outshone the contributions of human genetics. Scientists lacked the technological and experimental tools necessary to advance human genetics. Classical genetics—the study of inheritance and muta-tions and genetic and biochemical pathways—depends on the investigator's ability to manipulate the biological system through controlled experiments, to mate individuals with various observable traits and analyze their offspring, and to use large samples to derive statistically valid frequencies on which to base theories. While geneticists could routinely manipulate model organisms, these approaches did not apply to humans. Physicians could only follow the transmis-sion of disease traits through families or observe chromosomal changes through a microscope. But observation and description did little to explain how or even which defective gene caused a disease.

The recombinant DNA revolution changed all of that. "Disease genes" are mutant versions of normal genes that cause disease because of their malfunction. Human geneticists realized that, if they could identify specific human disease genes, they could then clone them in bacteria, sequence them, and identify the causative mutations. They could generate large quantities of both normal and mutant protein products of the genes and analyze their differences. All of this might lead to treatments or even cures. Almost certainly identification of disease genes could be useful for population screening, for genetic counseling of couples, for prenatal diagnosis, and for gaining a better understanding of the pathophysiology associated with a given disease.

In 1980, Botstein, White, Skolnick, and Davis published an influential paper describing a technique to identify disease genes (Botstein et al. 1980). The technique was based on the fact that, while all humans are 99.9 percent identical at the level of DNA sequence, the 0.1 percent differences are not random, but are inherited from one's parents. These sequence differences, scattered throughout the 6 billion bases of our genomes, are called polymorphisms, with the most common type being single nucleotide polymorphisms (SNPs, pronounced "snips").

SNPs can be found within genes, where they may alter a gene's activity in obvious or subtle ways, or where they may be completely innocuous. Polymorphic versions of the same gene are referred to as alleles. Much more commonly, SNPs are found outside of genes, where they have no obvious effect on how a gene functions. Instead, like fingerprints, SNPs generally are markers of individuality. But unlike fingerprints, the pattern of polymorphisms in an individual's DNA is inherited in equal parts from his or her mother's and father's DNA, and therefore also marks lines of descent.

The chromosomes we inherit from our parents have gone through a rough shuffling process (meiotic recombination) during the production of germ cells, that is, sperm and egg. Each germ cell contains exactly one half of the parent's genome, but the composition of that half genome is different in each germ cell, due to the shuffling process. Therefore two siblings will share only 50 percent of their parents' DNA. Botstein et al. reasoned that in large extended multigenerational families that carry an inherited disease, investigators could identify the presence or absence of specific polymorphisms along each chromosome, in each family member. Polymorphisms found more commonly in individuals with the disease and less commonly in family members without the disease may be "linked" to the disease gene. Even though the linked polymorphism might be hundreds of thousands of bases away from the actual disease gene, this approach narrows the hunt for a disease gene to a particular region of a particular chromosome, which can then be explored in fine detail.

Starting in the mid 1980s, teams of human geneticists used Botstein et al.'s linkage approach to identify genes that are mutated in dozens of inherited disorders including cystic fibrosis, sickle cell anemia, neurofibromatosis, Duchene's muscular dystrophy, amyotrophic lateral sclerosis, and familial cancer predisposition syndromes. These early successes had an electrifying effect on the fields of genetics and medicine, stoking the optimism that recombinant techniques could reveal the genetic basis of any disease.

While the linkage approach has been remarkably successful in identifying mutant genes in diseases caused by the malfunction of single genes (monogenic disorders), such conditions make up only a small fraction of diseases with a genetic component. Despite valiant efforts, human geneticists have been largely unsuccessful in identifying the genetic basis for common chronic diseases using the linkage approach. Common chronic diseases, for example, depression, schizophrenia, autism, essential hypertension, type 2 diabetes, and asthma, are all multifactorial, and therefore difficult to characterize at a genetic level. Defects in several different genes may result in the same signs and symptoms. Additionally, these diseases are influenced by the environment and may be only partially manifested due to either genetic or environmental modifiers. In fact, we do not understand enough about either the genetic or the environmental components of these disorders to describe them comprehensively at the molecular level.

By the late 1980s, geneticists were looking past the linkage approach for finding disease genes and beginning to consider the potential benefits of having the entire human genome sequence at their fingertips. The Human Genome Sequencing project was carried out in part by an NIH-funded effort and in part by private companies. Chief among the rationales for this massive effort were the abilities to understand human biology, identify disease genes, and develop better predictors of disease and more individualized treatments.

At the White House ceremony in June 2000 to publicly announce the completion of the draft version of the Human Genome, President Bill Clinton, Prime Minister Tony Blair, Celera President J. Craig Venter, and National Human Genome Research Institute Director Francis Collins reiterated three points. First, that the sequence would transform medicine and mean better health and a better quality of life for mankind. Second, that the ongoing alliance of governments, universities, and biotechnology companies would be key to the future of genomics. Third, that beyond the medical dimension the sequence information illustrated "that the concept of race has no genetic or scientific basis" and that the information derived from the sequence must be used ethically and fairly. At that critical moment in the history of genetics, issues of race, commercial interests, and the future of medicine were all in the mix.

Since the 2000 announcement, the university-company-government model has dominated advances in genomics. Genome sequencing centers throughout the world, all previously involved in the Human Genome Sequencing project, have turned their sequence-reading and compiling capacity to the job of determining the genome sequence of a wide array of species. As of this writing (October 2010) complete or draft genome sequences are publicly available for more than 280 eukaryotic species, as well as more than 1,300 different bacterial species. This wealth of gene data has made comparative genomics a field unto itself.

Detailed knowledge of genome sequence has also spurred technologic advances and experimental approaches that may finally shed light on disease-causing genes in common multifactorial disorders. DNA microarrays, a relatively straightforward and reproducible technique, have become a central tool of genomic research, in part because of the massive amount of genetic information that can be collected on a single slide (Schena et al. 1995). Using DNA data derived from genome sequencing projects, academic investigators and microarray-companies have glued hundreds of thousands of unique segments of DNA (spots), representing known SNPs, to defined locations on single microscope slides. The slides are incubated with a solution containing samples of an individual's DNA, and the strength of DNA binding to each spot corresponds to the presence or absence of that SNP. Thus DNA microarrays can identify genetic variation throughout the genome of any individual.

Microarrays have been adapted to disease gene hunting through an approach termed "genome wide association studies" (Carlson et al. 2004; Iles 2008; McCarthy et al. 2008). The new method has advantages over the earlier linkage approach. Genome wide association studies do not use the rare family with generations of an inherited disorder. Instead, DNA from large numbers of people with a particular disease and their matched controls are individually analyzed for the presence or absence of specific SNPs at tens to hundreds of thousands of spots around the genome. Computer algorithms then search for SNPs that show up more frequently in the genome of people with the disease than in the controls, at a statistically significant level. As with family linkage studies, a significant difference between the SNP frequency at a particular locus in cases versus controls suggests that the surrounding genomic region is linked to a potential disease gene. If a locus looks promising, investigators can molecularly dissect it to find the potential disease gene and determine what differs between the alleles in the cases compared to those in the controls.

The power of the association method comes from being able to sample large numbers of individuals to gain statistical power and to sample so many loci along each chromosome that the potential regions of interest comprise thousands of bases, rather than the millions of bases in family linkage studies. But a disadvantage of the approach is that, with so many independent loci, false positives (that is, significant differences between cases and controls due to chance or unexpected bias) can far outnumber true positives. Choosing the populations for both the cases and controls must be done very carefully. Differences in SNP frequency might be due to differences in the two sampled populations rather than the disease being studied. These can lead investigators down blind alleys or, conversely, cause them to miss real candidates within the noise of the false positives. Further, the method is geared to finding fairly common variants. While this makes reaching statistical significance easier, such variants rarely show very large differences in disease risk when comparing cases to controls. Geneticist David Goldstein has proposed that variants associated with much greater disease risk are likely to be rare, and therefore unlikely to reach statistical significance in microarray-based association studies (Goldstein 2009). Nevertheless, many human geneticists as well as genomic companies and the National Institute for Human Genome Research are heavily invested in these types of studies. New associations between

SNPs in specific chromosomal regions and particular diseases are being reported at an annually increasing rate, though rarely are actual gene associations made.

Recently, investigators have begun to reconsider the power of genome-wide association studies. Though hundreds of statistically significant polymorphisms have already been associated with specific diseases, they can only explain a small percentage of the genetic component of these conditions (Goldstein 2009). For common diseases it is likely that many genes in many genomic and physical environments will sum up to different disease risks and different disease outcomes in individuals. In that context even a million SNPs on a very dense microarray slide will not be sufficient to categorize an individual's risks, since the slide is still only a sampling of the total 6 billion bases in each genome. If large numbers of rare variants are the true genetic bases for common diseases, extremely large numbers of cases and controls will need to be compared, to reach a level of statistical significance.

Some believe that only the complete genome sequence of each individual can provide sufficient information to identify which specific variants or combinations of variants predict individual disease risks, responses to therapies, or outcomes. While not currently feasible, this approach has inspired a new human genome technology race, epitomized by the Archon X Prize for Genomics. The $10 million prize "will be awarded to the first Team that can build a device and use it to sequence 100 human genomes within 10 days or less, with an accuracy of no more than one error in every 10,000 bases sequenced, with sequences accurately covering at least 98% of the genome, and at a recurring cost of no more than $10,000 per genome" (genomics.xprize.org). As of October 2010, eight teams, consisting of companies or company-university collaborators, have entered the competition.

How Has the Concept of Race Entered Human Genetics?

The early period of human genetics had ties to the provocative racial doctrine of eugenics. Over time, anthropologists, geneticists, and other academics came to the consensus that grouping humans into distinct races is subjective and cultural, without objective biological criteria. According to this commonly held view, although modern humans have migrated throughout the globe, they all have the same common ancestors. Between isolated populations, the frequency of different alleles of certain genes will vary, but mixing of populations has gone on throughout human history. Genetic similarities far outweigh differences and variation among humans is due to the evolutionary forces of mutation, isolation, drift, and natural selection, acting on different populations in different environments over many generations (Montagu et al. 1949).

Despite this consensus, the countervailing notion, that complex traits such as disease susceptibility or intelligence are genetically determined and apportioned by racial categories, has resurfaced with some regularity in the public arena. Along with the well publicized successes of DNA analysis and genomics has come the hope that genetics can inform this discussion. Below, I describe three situations where issues of race, variously defined in terms of geography, ancestry, or history, have been incorporated into genetic studies.

Genetic Studies of Human Population Migration

Over the past forty years, geneticists and anthropologists have used biochemical and genetic studies of individuals from many geographically or culturally isolated groups throughout the world to define the origins and historical migrations of human populations around the globe. Populations have been characterized by the frequencies of specific protein variants (Bodmer and Cavalli-Sforza 1976; Cavalli-Sforza et al. 1994), or through examination of the frequency of specific sequence differences, found either in mitochondrial DNA (inherited solely from one's mother) (Cann et al. 1987; Wallace 1994) or along the Y chromosome (inherited solely from one's father) (Armour et al. 1996; Jorde et al. 2000; Underhill et al. 2000).

These studies have converged in the Recently Out of Africa (ROA) model of human geographic history. According to the ROA model, all modern humans originated in the Rift Valley in northeastern Africa. Small groups migrated at different times during the past 100,000 years throughout Africa, as well as north to Europe and the Middle East, and east to Arabia, the Indian subcontinent, and the rest of Asia, with further migration to North and South America. Each group of émigrés carried in their genomes both a more limited set of genetic variants than was present in the larger African population and specific variants that became more frequent as the founding populations expanded throughout Europe, Asia, and the Americas.

Identification of Ancestry Informative Markers

Investigators have identified certain DNA markers whose frequencies differ significantly between populations living on different continents. For example, the FyO allele of the DARC gene is present in more than 90 percent of West Africans, but in less than 5 percent of Europeans or Asians (Hamblin and Di Rienzo 2000). A 300-base insertion (Alu sequence) at a particular locus on chromosome 7 is found in more than 50 percent of Europeans and Asians, but in less than 5 percent of Africans (Bamshad et al. 2003). Using markers such as these, researchers have sorted individuals into groups that cluster by continent of origin. Presumably these are changes in the DNA that occurred after the European and Asian migrations out of Africa.

In one influential study, Rosenberg et al. (Rosenberg et al. 2002) looked at 377 genetic loci in the DNA of 1,056 individuals, previously collected from 52 different populations. Approximately 95 percent of the genetic variation in the data set was among individuals within populations, while less than 5 percent of the variation was between populations. They interpreted this to mean that "the average proportion of genetic differences between individuals from different human populations only slightly exceeds that between unrelated individuals from a single population." Though the differences among populations were minor, Rosenberg et al. then used a clustering algorithm to divide the sample set into any number of subgroups based on their distinctive allele frequencies. When they set the number of subgroups to five, the program blindly separated the individuals into clusters that corresponded to the major geographic regions of Africa, Eurasia, East Asia, Oceania, and America. This study and others (Bamshad et al. 2003; Witherspoon et al. 2007; Xing et al. 2009) have demonstrated that, with sufficient number of markers, an individual's ancestry can be determined at the level of continental origin.

Admixture Mapping

One approach to genome-wide association studies, termed admixture mapping, explicitly uses racial differences to identify disease genes (Chakraborty and Weiss 1988; McKeigue 1998). The technique is best suited to identify gene variants for diseases whose incidence differs greatly between two populations. Investigators analyze DNA for ancestry informative SNPs in individuals with the disease and in control individuals, both groups being offspring of matings between the two populations (Seldin et al. 2004; Smith and O'Brien 2005). In general, cases and controls should share the same frequency of SNPs at ancestry informative loci, except near the disease gene locus, where cases are more likely to possess the marker associated with the high incidence population.

Admixture mapping can be carried out with any group of individuals whose recent ancestors came from two or more genetically distinct populations. African Americans have been the population most studied using this approach, because their genomes have an average admixture of approximately 20 percent European variants and approximately 80 percent African variants (Parra et al. 2001; Smith et al. 2004). Studies have also been conducted with Latin American populations, though they have a more complex mixture of European, Native American, and African ancestry, with significant differences in proportion depending on their nationality (Price et al. 2007).

To date admixture mapping of African Americans has been most definitively used to identify an allele of the *DARC* gene (nearly fixed in West African populations), that correlates with lower white blood cell counts in African Americans (see below) (Reich et al. 2009) as well as two variants of the *ApoL1* gene (present in approximately 40 percent of a Nigerian population but absent from European, Chinese, and Japanese populations) that are strongly linked to non-diabetic end-stage renal disease in African Americans (Genovese et al. 2010).

In these three examples, specific genetic variants have been used to characterize group ancestry, where group refers to continent of origin and ancestry refers to forbears that settled in different geographic locations after leaving Africa. Do these genetic markers define human races? To answer this question would require an agreement on the definition of race. But the concept of race is so dependent on its cultural context that it is difficult to conceive how to objectively define the standard human populations in genetic terms. Without this linkage, the connection between race and genetics remains murky, subjective, and potentially dangerous.

One official source of self-identified racial categories is the federal Office of Management and Budget (OMB), whose definitions are used by the U.S. Census Bureau. These categories have changed more than ten times since their inception in 1800. The year 2000 categories are based on a mixture of skin color, geographic origin, and shared language. These OMB categories are standard for the myriad studies that have documented differences in disease incidence and disease outcome among Americans by race. But does that fact also put the federal imprimatur on racial classification in biological research? As Brawley explains, "The OMB openly states that the categories are not based in scientific derivations (taxonomy or anthropology) but are sociopolitical categories. These categories are published to collect socioeconomic data. Too often, data concerning health are collected with these sociopolitical categories and scientific conclusions concerning biology are drawn from them" (Brawley and Jani 2007).

A recent report suggests that geneticists do not adequately address the racial variables in their own research. Thirty geneticists were interviewed about their use of OMB categories of race in their studies. Although the investigators acknowledged the arbitrary vagueness of the classification and its scientific inadequacy, most defended its use in their work, calling racial labels "proxy variables" (Hunt and Megyesi 2008). It's surprising that geneticists, known for their care in designing experiments, would be so willingly lax in using OMB race variables for their studies.

The value and potential consequences of using racial variables in genetic studies of disease predispositions has engendered considerable debate. Some investigators note the correspondence between clustering of individuals by ancestry informative markers and classifying them by the self-identified OMB racial categories. Given the established literature on differences in disease incidence and outcome by OMB racial categories, they conclude that this justifies the potential link between disease susceptibility and genetic background (Burchard et al. 2003). They maintain that, in cases where allelic variation between population groups does correspond to differences in disease risk, failing to acknowledge or examine these potential differences by genomic methods would be wrongheaded (Mountain and Risch 2004; Risch et al. 2002).

Other researchers worry that the presumption of genetic explanations for disease disparities will lead to a genetic determinism that minimizes more complex social considerations and environmental solutions (Duster 2005; Sankar et al. 2004). Similarly, linking race to disease could result in stigmatization of whole populations, opening a "backdoor to eugenics," according to sociologist Troy Duster (Duster 2003).

An informative case in point is the Duffy antigen, the protein found on the surface of certain cell types, including red blood cells, encoded by the DARC gene. Most West Africans carry two copies of the FyO allele of DARC in their genomes, and consequently lack the protein on their red blood cells. More than thirty years ago, Lou Miller and colleagues demonstrated that individuals lacking the Duffy antigen on their red blood cells are absolutely protected from infection by *Plasmodium vivax*, a nonlethal but often severe form of malaria (Horuk et al. 1993; Miller et al. 1976). These parasites require Duffy antigen as a receptor to enter red blood cells, where they divide and cause their greatest damage.

Recently, Reich et al. (2009) demonstrated an extremely strong association between homozygosity of the FyO allele and the previous observation that people of African ancestry tend to have lower peripheral white blood cell counts than those of European descent. This phenomenon has been termed "benign ethnic neutropenia." Comparing the DARC loci of African Americans and European Americans, they showed that the white blood cell counts of African Americans who were heterozygous for FyO at this locus (or homozygous for the European allele) were indistinguishable from European Americans. Presence of two FyO alleles, however, shifted the average white blood cell count by 1.3 standard deviations (Reich et al. 2009).

These findings regarding the FyO allele among West Africans, other Africans, African Americans, Europeans, and European Americans have important implications to the discussion of race, ancestry, and human disease. The FyO allele is nearly fixed in West Africans, but almost never observed in other populations. An allele differentiation this extreme is seen in fewer than 0.003 percent of all human genome variants (Reich et al. 2009). Thus, SNPs that carry so much information about regional ancestry are exceptionally rare. Reich's work demonstrates that the phenotype of low white blood count is predicted by the number of FyO alleles in an individual's genome, not by the individual's self-identified race. Further, it is noteworthy that, in this case of a phenotype associated with an extreme difference in allele frequency between individuals of West African descent and others, the "condition" does not in fact result in any disease. Thus, even in the presence of such a rare regional ancestry informative marker, the relationship between genetics, one's "race," and disease remains extraordinarily complex.

The Cultural and Scientific Climate in Which Race and Genetics Is Joined

In today's society, terms such as DNA, genetics, and genomics are part of the common parlance. Companies, governments, the media, and even many scientists and physicians are invested in the belief that genomic research will benefit individuals. African Americans have been particularly targeted, because of their special interest in ancestry analysis, through efforts to equate their higher incidence of many diseases in the United States with their genetic background, and by the FDA's 2005 endorsement of BiDil, the only drug approved specifically for use in a particular racial group (Ellison et al. 2008; Temple and Stockbridge 2007). But two interrelated trends in our culture make it difficult for the public to clearly judge the promises of genomics or whether the concept of race adds to our understanding of the human genome and human diversity. First, the general public has a complex relationship with biomedical science—both skeptical and rapt—which leads to less than critical evaluation of claims made by, or in the name of, scientists. Second, since the beginning of recombinant DNA technology in the mid 1970s, business interests have become increasingly involved in the fields of genetics and molecular biology.

The Ascendance of DNA in the Public Mind

Public awareness of DNA and genetics has rapidly increased over the past twenty years. Whereas DNA was once a term known only to biologists, in 2007, the *New York Times* published more than 800 articles containing the term "DNA," including 126 in the Arts Sections, 25 in the Sports Section, 4 in the Automobile Section, and even one in the Real Estate section (compared to a total of 142 references in 1987). But public familiarity with the word *DNA* does not translate into a general understanding of its biological meaning. Rather, Americans both revere and mistrust scientists, and this ambivalence leads to unrealistic beliefs about the scientific process.

On one hand, polls show that scientists and physicians are among the most respected and trusted professionals (Harris Poll #61, August 8, 2006). DNA data has proven to be the most objective source of evidence in criminal cases and in paternity determination. There is a thread of belief among many Americans that science and technology can get us out of any jam.

On the other hand, polls show that less than 50 percent of the population believes in the theory of evolution, the bedrock of all biology (Miller et al. 2006). Many people are doubtful of scientists' motives. Some of this mistrust stems from historic realities such as the eugenics movement and the participation of researchers in the Tuskegee Study of Untreated Syphilis in the Negro Male (1932–1972), or more recent revelations about conflicts of interest by several prominent academic physicians. The public may be influenced by rumored connections between vaccines and autism, nefarious origins of the AIDS epidemic, or even the frequent imagery of mad scientists, colluding with corrupt capitalists and incompetent bureaucrats, that we see in popular films, TV shows, and books, from *Jurassic Park* to the *X-Men*.

Both views express unrealistic attitudes about science and the scientific process, either overly expectant or overly skeptical. In actuality, scientific progress is incremental. Breakthroughs are unusual and sometimes only appreciated long after they were made. The timing and even the direction of advances are unpredictable. Basic research is inefficient, multifocused, only moderately directed, simultaneously cooperative and competitive, self-regulating, yet ultimately tremendously successful at advancing knowledge and society. The scientific enterprise is an example where the whole is greater than the sum of its parts.

Basic scientists, at the core of the process, are those most likely to understand the power and the limitations of their discoveries. But they are less likely to pursue the commercial applications of their work; that is not their forte. Individual scientists may be motivated by being the first to uncover new knowledge, by being passionate about a particular fundamental question, or by the hope that their work will lead to something that betters mankind. They function within a global community of investigators who exchange information and ideas. The importance of a given result is determined when other scientists reproduce it, apply it to other species or situations, and use it to extend or modify their existing concepts. Competing theories, favored by different scientists, can only be reconciled over time by seeing how well each fits the data and how predictive each is of future experimental results. Consequently, the interests and concerns of basic scientists may be quite different from those trying to popularize or apply their knowledge.

The development of innovative technology and experimental methods, interpretative models and real life applications are all components of the scientific enterprise, but they are rarely in sync with one another (McBride et al. 2008). Whereas basic scientists are more concerned with the experimental design and their models, companies are focused on the equipment and its applications. Consider recent developments in human genomics. Collaborative groups such as the HapMap Project and the Human Genome Diversity Project are mapping SNPs and sequences from large numbers of individuals in many populations, filling databases with reams of genomic information. But the techniques to make sense of the incredible diversity within the human genome are only in their early stages. Although genome-wide association studies are revealing an array of potential disease loci, very few of these associations have identified specific disease gene variants, and none have led to basic changes in our understanding of common diseases or changes in diagnosis and treatment. Human geneticists are still debating the proper methods to carry out association studies, and the field does not yet have a foundation for understanding the genetic basis of any common disease. Statistical algorithms and computational models are still being developed to interpret or even to display and fit the huge amounts of generated data (Couzin 2008; McCarthy et al. 2008).

Despite these limitations, companies are racing forward with denser microarray slides and better sequencing platforms. Other companies are marketing genomics as the key to ancestry analysis and the path to personalized medicine. Their methods, their levels of certainty, and their basic motivations are different from those of the basic researchers, yet to the public, the distinctions are fuzzy. Much of this blurring is the result of the alliance of academic research, biotechnology, and government.

The Consequences of the Commercialization of Genomics

Private investors have been stakeholders in the fields of genetics and molecular biology since the 1976 incorporation of Genentech, the first biotechnology company. Pharmaceutical companies comprise the biggest share of the biotechnology industry. The current genomics era is technology-driven and heavily dominated by a few corporate entities that produce the devices necessary for genomic research, including microarray readers, massive parallel sequencing platforms, and the consumable supplies required to run this equipment. These expensive and specialized instruments have vastly increased the amount of data obtained in a single experiment. The current mix of basic science, technology development, and biotechnology applications is a fact of life, but the composition of the partnerships has important consequences to the development of the field of genomics.

First is its impact on how science is carried out. The influence of corporate and proprietary interests narrows the wiggle room for researchers to explore, expand, and tinker. Although the pharmaceutical industry is heavily invested in "research" compared to other industries, their marketing budgets are nonetheless typically more than twice those of their research budgets (Angell 2000). Changes in corporate focus may mean that promising basic research or whole areas of investigation are dropped. Companies may decide not to invest in basic research at all, but to restrict their research budgets to applying published findings of academic researchers or obtaining intellectual property from universities through patent licensing. Short-term gains and corporate goals necessarily take precedence over the slow, haphazard, and individually inefficient but globally effective approach that was so successful in the period leading to the recombinant DNA revolution.

Second is the lure of biotechnology for academic institutions. Universities have a vested interest in exploiting the intellectual capital of their faculty and in encouraging researchers to patent their ideas. Many schools employ lawyers and businessmen to translate faculty intellectual property into licensed applications with biotechnology and pharmaceutical firms or university-financed start-up companies. Proceeds from technology transfer can be a major source of revenue for a university. In 2008, 156 U.S. institutions generated over $2.4 billion from licensing faculty inventions (www.autm.net/).

Third is the dilemma for university scientists. The incentives for academic and corporate research are at odds. Academic researchers have an imperative to publish and share their findings, while company researchers have strong motivations to be secretive about their findings and keep them out of the hands of competitors. The peer review process employed by academic scientists to judge publications and grant proposals is meant to assure that claims are evidence-based and that wishful speculation is kept to a minimum. This is the antithesis of the business model, in which limited data is used to spin the prospect of lucrative future applications and returns. For academic investigators who advise or direct companies on the side, or who have patented an idea and want a company to license it, there are real dangers of losing objectivity and risking conflict of interest.

Even the process of carrying out experiments and interpreting results can be problematic when commercial concerns are injected into the scientific process. Experiments succeed or fail for reasons that may not be clear. When interpreting data, investigators must distinguish between alternate explanations, which may only be resolved by further experiments. Experiments that work in one cell type or strain may not work in another. The careful investigator does not over-generalize from his or her results. Only by replicating the results through many experiments, using different cells and/or different conditions, can the investigator reliably generalize from observations. But the public, the shareholders, the special interest groups, and the press may not understand the limitations of the scientific process in delivering speedy or unambiguous results.

The Multiple Roles of the Federal Government

The federal government influences the directions of scientific enquiry and its connection to the private sector in many ways. The National Institutes of Health (NIH) are the leading funding source to basic scientists for genetic and genomic research. Since the government derives no direct financial benefit from discoveries or patents based on this funding, it in effect subsidizes research and development from which the private sector may eventually profit. By determining funding priorities and soliciting grants for research in particular target areas, the government broadcasts what it believes are the most pressing medical and biological priorities. In addition NIH encourages and supports academic/private collaboration and commercialization through grants for small business innovation research (SBIR) and small business technology transfer research (STTR).

As discussed previously, the federal government also influences the perception that there is a connection between race and genetics. Since 1993, government-sponsored clinical trials and studies on human subjects are required to attempt to represent women and racial minorities (based on OMB definitions), and report this information to the government. While this rule was put in place to ensure inclusion of often underrepresented groups in human research, an unintended consequence is that it appears to validate racial classifications in biological research (Epstein 2007; Lee 2009; Lee and Skrentny 2010). The same is true in the case of the drug BiDil. Based on limited studies, the FDA specifically approved the drug for use in African-Americans with congestive heart failure. The implication of this approval was that the agency accepted that self-reported racial classifications translated into biological differences in response to a pharmacologic agent.

The Problem of Using Race in Genetic Analysis of Ancestry

Many Americans can trace their pre-immigration ancestry without resorting to DNA analysis and take their geographic origins for granted. However, most African Americans have been denied knowledge of a large portion of their history and heritage, due to their ancestors' forced migration to the Western Hemisphere followed by the undocumented genetic admixture that accompanied the period of slavery. In the past decade, Harvard professor Henry Louis Gates Jr. and his PBS television show "African-American Lives" helped popularize the use of DNA testing to delve farther back into individual African Americans' genealogy. Following the success of that show, Gates founded "Africandna," a "company dedicated to offering both genetic testing and genealogical tracing services for African Americans" (www.africandna.com/). Currently, dozens of companies offer individuals DNA analysis for genealogical purposes.

The rising interest in race and DNA has occurred within the business-friendly environment of human genomics. Companies that offer DNA-based ancestry determination to individuals base their knowledge and techniques on previous basic research that identified specific variations in mitochondrial DNA or along Y-chromosomes, the two regions of the genome that correlate with matrilineal and patrilineal lines of descent, respectively. Commercial ancestry testing is an unintended spin-off from basic research, but the basic research was designed to answer questions about population migration in a probabilistic manner and not to provide concrete and detailed genealogical information to individuals. At that level, current DNA approaches are neither reliable nor truly informative.

One reason for this is the fundamental nature of inheritance of genetic markers. We each inherit half of our DNA from each parent, or stepping back a generation, we inherit, on average, a quarter of our DNA from each of our grandparents. Each of our siblings also inherits a quarter of each grandparent's DNA, but it is not necessarily the same quarter, so there will be only partial overlap between siblings. Assuming twenty-five years per generation and working back two centuries, 256 different individuals, living eight generations ago, contributed some of their DNA to each of us. Can DNA testing tell us about the geographic origins of all these 256 distant ancestors? Most companies test SNPs on either the mitochondria or Y chromosome, which at best provide information about 2 of these 256 ancestors. Other companies look at markers scattered throughout the chromosomes. But we do not know how many ancestry informative markers there are, nor do we know how many should be tested. Depending on which variants an individual has inherited from those 256 ancestors, the same DNA test could give different geographic ancestry results for siblings with the same parents.

Ancestry testing of individuals has other, more technical, problems. Population standards of allele and marker frequencies have been derived from many populations sampled at different times by different researchers using different sampling methods and different loci. Determination of ancestry beyond the level of continent of origin is a statistical exercise based on differences in frequency of variants at multiple independent loci. The presence or absence of a particular allele at any one locus is usually insufficient to determine ancestry. Variants at each locus occur at a particular mean frequency for each population, surrounded by their own confidence intervals. The job of ancestry analysis is to determine which expected pattern of variation among many tested population groups best matches the set of variants present in an individual's DNA. However, the reliability of the observed population data completely depends on the sample size and representativeness of the standard group analyzed for each population.

This is a particularly difficult problem if an individual's ancestors come from different populations. The number of useful loci capable of distinguishing between two populations depends on the degree of mating and mixing between the two populations, the time since the two populations diverged from one another, and the number of generations separating the individual from his or her ancestral population groups. The more mixing of different ancestral populations in an individual's family history, as is common for many Americans, the less similar a person's genetic pattern will be to the standard populations.

If companies stated all of these very real provisos, caveats and uncertainties, most consumers would likely be left scratching their heads and wondering what new information they had actually learned from ancestry tracing.

The Problem of Using Race in the Discovery of Disease Genes

Ancestry mapping has been referred to as "recreational genetics" (Bolnick et al. 2007), to differentiate it from genetic analysis related to the more medically important area of disease association. It is in the area of disease studies that the relationship between race and genetics becomes the most susceptible to misinterpretation and distortion. Africa contains more than 2000 different ethnolinguistic groups (Reed and Tishkoff 2006). DNA analysis of present day Africans reveals fourteen ancestral population clusters (Tishkoff et al. 2009). DNA among African populations tends to be more variable and distinct than among populations from other continents (Cardon and Abecasis 2003; Tishkoff and Kidd 2004; Tishkoff and Verrelli 2003). Work carried out by geneticist Sara Tishkoff and others makes it clear that sweeping conclusions about African Americans and disease-associated genetic variants are untenable.

These conclusions are relevant to discussions of how race, disease, and genetics are related in the United States. The notion that African Americans share some meaningful collection of specific disease alleles defies logic. Even the term African American makes no sense genetically, as it implies a unified population. The 20 percent average admixture of European alleles in African Americans, as well as the great genetic variation among different African populations, belies this biogeographic generalization. Even though the ancestors of a majority of African Americans were brought to the New World from West Africa, that region comprises many distinct populations, and a sizable proportion of slaves originated in central Africa and southeastern Africa. Since their arrival in the New World, African Americans have admixed among these different original populations, as well as with European and Native American populations.

Skin pigmentation is one of the most obvious components of self-described race used for census enumerations and medical studies in the United States. But while variation in skin pigmentation is clearly a genetically determined trait under natural selection, it is not a particularly well studied area in human genetics (Parra 2007; Rees 2003). An unknown number of genes (but probably greater than 10) are involved in determining one's skin color. One reason for the relative lack of scientific interest in the subject may be the paucity of known diseases in which skin pigmentation plays an important etiological role. Only two relatively common conditions come to mind. Skin cancers including melanoma are much more rare in African and Asian populations than in European populations, probably because of the protective effect of melanin from ultraviolet light (UV)-induced DNA damage. Conversely, nutritional Vitamin D deficiency is a more frequent problem among darker skinned individuals, since UV exposure is required to synthesize Vitamin D in the lower layers of our skin, and melanin reduces the amount of available UV.

For most diseases in the United States that differ in incidence by race, racial differences correspond to socio-economic or cultural differences. Most of the difference in incidence of asthma, hypertension, and heart disease by race can be explained by differences in income and environmental risk factors (Smith et al. 2005; Thomas et al. 2005; Thorpe et al. 2008). Each of these is a multigenic disorder. At the other end of the disease spectrum are the relatively rare inherited diseases like sickle cell anemia (incidence among African Americans approximately 1/700 live births; incidence among European Americans approximately 1/158,000 live births) (Lorey et al. 1996) or cystic fibrosis (incidence among non-whites- approximately 1/12,000 live births; incidence among whites approximately 1/3400 live births) (Kosorok et al. 1996) that are caused by mutations in single genes. These diseases appear to show the strongest links between race, disease, and genetics. They are clearly genetic disorders, caused by recessive mutations in specific genes that become a problem in one of four offspring of parents who each carry a copy of the mutant gene. Upon further scrutiny though, the apparent racial basis for these disorders turns out to be a red herring.

Sickle cell anemia is a disease that occurs when an individual inherits a specifically mutated version of the beta globin gene from each of his or her parents. (Children who inherit the mutated gene from only one parent are normal.) The mutation involves a particular base change at the position that codes for beta globin's sixth amino acid. This same mutation arose independently in different populations at least five times during human evolution, and has been designated as the Bantu, Benin, Senegal, Cameroon, and Indian haplotype (Lapoumeroulie et al. 1992).

In each place the mutation emerged, the presence of the mutant allele in a single copy likely provided a slight advantage to children from six months to two years of age in resisting the lethal effects of falciparum malaria. For human populations living in regions where malaria was endemic and a major killer of children, individuals with a single copy of the mutant gene were more likely to live to adulthood and reproduce. Over many generations, this selective advantage increased the fraction of individuals within these populations who carried the mutant allele (Allison 2004). This is a classic example of the subtle power of natural selection. Unfortunately, when a sufficient proportion of a population carries the mutant allele, the probability increases that a child will inherit a mutant allele from *both* parents and have sickle cell anemia. In pre-antibiotic times, this severe and painful form of anemia was usually fatal in childhood.

Over centuries the mutant alleles have spread, through mating, to additional populations in Africa, Europe, and the Middle East. Other population groups in

Africa, particularly where malaria was absent or only an occasional burden, have either very low or negligible frequencies of the sickle cell mutation. Coincidentally the major sources of African slaves to the Caribbean, North, and South America were from the very regions where high levels of the sickle beta globin allele were present in the population. The mutant gene was imported to the Western Hemisphere along with these individuals. An Ethiopian from East Africa or a Namibian from South Africa is no more likely to have sickle cell anemia than a person from Iceland or North Korea. From a genetic perspective, the disease is associated with individuals whose ancestors originated in specific parts of West Africa, central Africa, and central India.

We know that an individual's genetic makeup—the specific polymorphisms that make him or her unique—will influence what diseases he or she is more or less likely to develop over the course of a lifetime. We also know that in most cases genetic predisposition is heavily influenced by environmental considerations. For most common diseases in the United States, an individual's risk is linked less closely to one's genetic makeup than to factors such as age and sex, as well as environmental and behavioral characteristics like income, diet, smoking, place of residence, and maternal education. Further, genetic risk is determined not by a single variant of a single gene, but by how different variants of many different genes interact in each individual in a more or less protective manner. Given the greater genetic variation among Africans than among European or Asians, I suspect that Africans have very few significant phenotypic traits in common beyond adaptation of greater pigmentation compared to many populations that migrated out of Africa in the past hundred thousand years. Even in the extreme case of the Duffy antigen and the phenotype of vivax malaria resistance (discussed above), this is primarily associated with West African populations.

Concluding Remarks

The early history of human genetics provides a cautionary lesson in the mischaracterization of race as a biological determinant. While it is easy for us to look back in horror at this travesty, it's likely that early population geneticists with eugenic agendas, like Charles Davenport, Francis Galton, and Karl Pearson, worked in good faith within the context of their times and their social and political positions. In one of the essays accompanying Davenport's recently reissued 1911 text, *Heredity in Relation to Eugenics* (Witkowski et al. 2008), University of Washington geneticist Maynard Olson points out three red flags in Davenport's writing that should be kept in mind by today's geneticists: "[Davenport] . . . deeply commingles science and social values. . . . [His] thinking is often hopelessly muddled . . . [and he] over promises what genetics could achieve even if it were vigorously applied to societal problems" (Olson:79 in Witkowski).

As I have described in this perspective, in today's genomic environment, the dominant "social value" is capitalism. The goals and approaches of business and basic scientific research have traditionally not aligned. How will the continued commingling of science and corporate values affect the types of questions asked, the directions the science follows, the strength of data accepted, and the priorities set by funders?

"Muddled thinking" is a fact of life and an occupational hazard. For example, the impact of individual studies can be compromised when investigators lack an understanding of epidemiology and biostatistics. McCarthy et al. make a plea for improved study design and for validation and replication of genome wide association studies (McCarthy et al. 2008). We have no firm conceptual basis for characterizing the genetics of most common diseases and do not even agree on the best method for identifying the genetic components. As McCarthy et al. state, "Recent discoveries [by the genome wide association approach] are nothing more than initial forays into the *terra incognita* of our genomes."

As for "over promising" what genomics can achieve, this is reflected today in both the shaky claims of genomics companies and the ebullient optimism that colors each newly announced discovery. We have no evidence that sequencing the entire genome of every individual will result in the predictive powers that proponents of personalized medicine envisage. Nor is there evidence that healthy individuals want to know or even care about their future probabilities of contracting different diseases, particularly if the predictive powers of the tests are imperfect and nothing significant can be done prophylactically.

Science is technical and difficult to comprehend but that does not absolve scientists of the responsibility to inform the public about their work, explain their methods and their rigor, admit the limitations and areas of controversy and uncertainty, and examine its wider relevance. Conversely, the difficulty of understanding and digesting science does not absolve the general public from acknowledging its importance and its contributions. The public should not assume that the public policy aspects of scientific advances are being properly debated and regulated at the state or federal levels (for example, see a case study on the lack of regulation for a pharmacogenetic test of dubious validity in Katansis et al. (Katsanis et al. 2008), or that information received from companies will be independently verifiable or meaningful.

Personalized genomics companies would like to adapt published associations between chromosomal regions and common diseases to predict disease risk for individual consumers. But these predictions are based on case-control studies of limited populations, primarily of European ancestry. Basing prospective risk-assessments for diverse individuals on retrospective analyses of restricted populations is risky at best. Questions of how admixture in individuals might affect genetic predictions, or the way in which environmental exposures influence the genomic data, have yet to be addressed. The public should treat the stated or implied claims that companies make about current capabilities with a healthy dose of skepticism.

What would it take to derive meaningful and predictive associations between specific genomic variants and medically important diseases? Despite much wishful thinking, it is not clear that this level of personalized genomics will ever become a reality. But for microarray-based genome wide association studies to stand a chance of being validated, millions of marker loci will need to be simultaneously monitored and clustered. Databases of SNP associations will need to contain large numbers of cases and controls with various diseases, where the individuals represent the full range of human population mixing. Analysis of genomic associations will need to be done in the context of an individual's complete environmental history. Such an endeavor would be a massive undertaking and its utility in improving human health is not assured. Perhaps without the pressure and expectations of the biotechnology industry and an overeager public, scientists could proceed, at a thoughtful and careful pace, to unlock the information within individual genomes. Such an analysis would be based on an individual's idiosyncratic genetic makeup, in which case the arbitrary and nonbiological variable of "race" would be irrelevant.

ACKNOWLEDGMENTS

I am indebted to Consuelo Beck-Sague, Steve Buyske, Janet Heroux, Matthew Herper, Leonid Kruglyak, and Sarah Tishkoff, for many helpful discussions of various aspects of this paper.

WORKS CITED

Allison, A. C. 2004. Two lessons from the interface of genetics and medicine. *Genetics* 166: 1591–1599.

Angell, M. 2000. The pharmaceutical industry—To whom is it accountable? *New England Journal of Medicine* 342: 1902–1904.

Armour, J. A., T. Anttinen, C. A. May, E. E. Vega, A. Sajantila, J. R. Kidd, K. K. Kidd, J. Bertranpetit, S. Paabo, and A. J. Jeffreys. 1996. Minisatellite diversity supports a recent African origin for modern humans. *Nature Genetics* 13: 15R4–160.

Bamshad, M. J., S. Wooding, W. S. Watkins, C. T. Ostler, M. A. Batzer, and L. B. Jorde. 2003. Human population genetic structure and inference of group membership. *American Journal of Human Genetics* 72: 578–589.

Bodmer, W. F., and L. L. Cavalli-Sforza. 1976. *Genetics, evolution, and man.* San Francisco: W. H. Freeman.

Bolnick, D. A., D. Fullwiley, T. Duster, R. S. Cooper, J. H. Fujimura, J. Kahn, J. S. Kaufman, J. Marks, A. Morning, A. Nelson, et al. 2007. Genetics: The science and business of genetic ancestry testing. *Science* 318: 399–400.

Botstein, D., R. L. White, M. Skolnick, and R. W. Davis. 1980. Construction of a genetic linkage map in man using restriction fragment length polymorphisms. *American Journal of Human Genetics* 32: 314–331.

Brawley, O. W., and A. B. Jani. 2007. Race and disparities in health. *Current Problems in Cancer* 31: 114–122.

Burchard, E. G., E. Ziv, N. Coyle, S. L. Gomez, H. Tang, A. J. Karter, J. L. Mountain, E. J. Perez-Stable, D. Sheppard, and N. Risch. 2003. The importance of race and ethnic background in biomedical research and clinical practice. *New England Journal of Medicine* 348: 1170–1175.

Cann, R. L., M. Stoneking, and A. C. Wilson. 1987. Mitochondrial DNA and human evolution. *Nature* 325: 31–36.

Cardon, L. R., and G. R. Abecasis. 2003. Using haplotype blocks to map human complex trait loci. *Trends Genet* 19: 135–140.

Carlson, C. S., M. A. Eberle, L. Kruglyak, and D. A. Nickerson. 2004. Mapping complex disease loci in whole-genome association studies. *Nature* 429: 446–452.

Cavalli-Sforza, L. L., P. Menozzi, and A. Piazza. 1994. *The history and geography of human genes*. Princeton, NJ: Princeton University Press.

Chakraborty, R., and K. M. Weiss. 1988. Admixture as a tool for finding linked genes and detecting that difference from allelic association between loci. *Proceedings of the National Academy of Sciences of the United States of America* 85: 9119–9123.

Couzin, J. 2008. Genetic risk: With new disease genes, a bounty of questions. *Science* 319: 1754–1755.

Duster, T. 2003. *Backdoor to eugenics*. 2nd ed. New York and London: Routledge.

———. 2005. Medicine: Race and reification in science. *Science* 307: 1050–1051.

Ellison, G. T., J. S. Kaufman, R. F. Head, P. A. Martin, and J. D. Kahn. 2008. Flaws in the U.S. Food and Drug Administration's rationale for supporting the development and approval of Bidil as a treatment for heart failure only in black patients. *Journal of Law and Medical Ethics* 36: 449–457.

Epstein, S. 2007. *Inclusion: The politics of difference in medical research*. Chicago: University of Chicago Press.

Garrod, A. E., and H. Harris. 1963. *Inborn errors of metabolism*. London and New York: Oxford University Press.

Genovese, G., D. J. Friedman, M. D. Ross, L. Lecordier, P. Uzureau, B. I. Freedman, D. W. Bowden, C. D. Langefeld, T. K. Oleksyk, A. L. Uscinski Knob, et al. 2010. Association of trypanolytic ApoII variants with kidney disease in African Americans. *Science* 329: 841–845.

Goldstein, D. B. 2009. Common genetic variation and human traits. *New England Journal of Medicine* 360: 1696–1698.

Hamblin, M. T., and A. Di Rienzo. 2000. Detection of the signature of natural selection in humans: Evidence from the Duffy blood group locus. *American Journal of Human Genetics* 66: 1669–1679.

Horuk, R., C. E. Chitnis, W. C. Darbonne, T. J. Colby, A. Rybicki, T. J. Hadley, and L. H. Miller, 1993. A Receptor for the malarial parasite Plasmodium vivax: The erythrocyte chemokine receptor. *Science* 261: 1182–1184.

Hunt, L. M., and M. S. Megyesi. 2008. Genes, race, and research ethics: Who's minding the store? *Journal of Medical Ethics* 34: 495–500.

Iles, M. M. 2008. What can genome-wide association studies tell us about the genetics of common disease. *PLoS Genetics* 4: e33.

Jorde, L. B., W. S. Watkins, M. J. Bamshad, M. E. Dixon, C. E. Ricker, M. T. Seielstad, and M. A. Batzer. 2000. The distribution of human genetic diversity: A comparison of mitochondrial, autosomal, and Y-chromosome data. *American Journal of Human Genetics* 66: 979–988.

Katsanis, S.H., G. Javitt, and K. Hudson. (2008). Public health: A case study of personalized medicine. *Science* 320; 53–54.

Kosorok, M. R., W. H. Wei, and P. M. Farrell. (1996). The incidence of cystic fibrosis. *Statistics in Medicine* 15: 449–462.

Lapoumeroulie, C., O. Dunda, R. Ducrocq, G. Trabuchet, M. Mony-Lobe, J. M. Bodo, P. Carnevale, D. Labie, J. Elion, and R. Krishnamoorthy. 1992. A novel sickle cell mutation of yet another origin in Africa: The Cameroon type. *Human Genetics* 89: 333–337.

Lee, C.. 2009. 'Race' and 'ethnicity' in biomedical research: How do scientists construct and explain difference in health? *Social Science and Medicine* 68: 1183–1190.

Lee, C., and J. D. Skretny. 2010. Race categorization and regulation of business and science. *Law & Society Review* 3/4: 617–649.

Lorey, F. W., J. Arnopp, and G. C. Cunningham. 1996. Distribution of hemoglobinopathy variants by ethnicity in a multiethnic state. *Genetic Epidemiology* 13; 501–512.

McBride, C. M., S. H. Alford, R. J. Reid, E. B. Larson, A. D. Baxevanis, and L. C. Brody. 2008. Putting science over supposition in the arena of personalized genomics. *Nature Genetics* 40: 939–942.

McCarthy, M. I., G. R. Abecasis, L. R. Cardon, D.B. Goldstein, J. Little, J. P. Ioannidis, and J. N. Hirschhorn. 2008. Genome-wide association studies for complex traits: Consensus, uncertainty, and challenges. *Nature Reviews* 9: 356–369.

McKeigue, P. M. 1998. Mapping genes that underlie ethnic differences in disease risk: Methods for detecting linkage in admixed populations, by conditioning on parental admixture. *American Journal of Human Genetics* 63: 241–251.

Miller, J. D., E. C. Scott, and S. Okamoto. 2006. Science communication: Public acceptance of evolution. *Science* 313: 765–766.

Miller, L.H., S. J. Mason, D. F. Clyde, and M. H. McGinniss. 1976. The resistance factor to Plasmodium vivax in blacks: The Duffy-blood-group genotype, FyFy. *New England Journal of Medicine* 295: 302–304.

Montagu, A., M. Ginsberg, C. Lévi-Strauss, E. Beaglehole, J. Comas, F. Kabir, F. Frazier, and L. A. Costa Pinto. 1949. Statement on "race." In *Unesco Meeting of Experts on Race Problems.* Paris: UNESCO.

Mountain, J. L., and N. Risch. 2004. Assessing genetic contributions to phenotypic differences among "racial" and "ethnic" groups. *Nature Genetics* 36: S48–53.

Parra, E. J. 2007. Human pigmentation variation: Evolution, genetic basis, and implications for public health. *American Journal of Physical Anthropology* Suppl 45: 85–105.

Parra, E. J., R. A. Kittles, G. Argyropoulos, L. Pfaff, K. Hiester, C. Bonilla, N. Sylvester, D. Parrish-Gause, W. T. Garvey, L. Jin, et al. 2001. Ancestral proportions and admixture dynamics in geographically defined African Americans living in South Carolina. *American Journal of Physical Anthropology* 114: 18–29.

Price, A. L., N. Patterson, F. Yu, D. R. Cox, A. Waliszewska, G. J. McDonald, A. Tandon, C. Schirmer, J. Neubauer, G. Bedoya, et al. 2007. A genomewide admixture map for Latino populations. *American Journal of Human Genetics* 80: 1024–1036.

Reed, F. A., and S. A. Tishkoff. 2006. African human diversity, origins, and migrations. *Current Opinion in Genetics and Development* 16: 597–605.

Rees, J. L. 2003. Genetics of hair and skin color. *Annual Review of Genetics* 37: 67–90.

Reich, D., M. A. Nalls, W. H. Kao, E. L. Akylbekova, A. Tandon, N. Patterson, J. Mullikin, W. C. Hsueh, C. Y. Cheng, J. Coresh, et al. 2009. Reduced neutrophil count in people of African Descent is due to a regulatory variant in the Duffy antigen receptor for chemokines gene. *PLoS Genetics* 5: e1000360.

Risch, N., E. Burchard, E. Ziv, and H. Tang. 2002. Categorization of humans in biomedical research: Genes, race, and disease. *Genome Biology* 3: 1–12.

Rosenberg, N. A., J. K. Pritchard, J. L. Weber, H. M. Cann, K. K. Kidd, L. A. Zhivotovsky, and M. W. Feldman. 2002. Genetic structure of human populations. *Science* 298: 2381–2385.

Sankar, P., M. K. Cho, C. M. Condit, L. M. Hunt, B. Koenig, P. Marshall, S. S. Lee, and Spicer. 2004. Genetic research and health disparities. *JAMA* 291: 2985–2989.

Schena, M., D. Shalon, R. W. Davis, and P. O. Brown. 1995. Quantitative monitoring of gene expression patterns with a complementary DNA microarray. *Science* 270: 467–470.

Seldin, M. F., T. Morii, H. E. Collins-Schramm, B. Chima, R. Kittles, L. A. Criswell, and H. Li. 2004. Putative ancestral origins of chromosomal segments in individual African Americans: Implications for admixture mapping. *Genome Research* 14: 1076–1084.

Smith, L. A., J. L. Hatcher-Ross, R. Wertheimer, and R. S. Kahn. 2005. Rethinking race/ethnicity, income, and childhood asthma: Racial/ethnic disparities concentrated among the very poor. *Public Health Rep* 120: 109–116.

Smith, M. W., and S. J. O'Brien. 2005. Mapping by admixture linkage disequilibrium: Advances, limitations, and guidelines. *Nature Reviews* 6: 623–632.

Smith, M.W., N. Patterson, J. A. Lautenberger, A. L. Truelove, G. J. McDonald, A. Waliszewska, B. D. Kessing, M. J. Malasky, C. Scafe, E. Le, et al. 2004. A high-density admixture map for disease gene discovery in African Americans. *American Journal of Human Genetics* 74: 1001–1013.

Temple, R., and N. L. Stockbridge. 2007. BiDil for heart failure in black patients: The U.S. Food and Drug Administration perspective. *Annals of Internal Medicine* 146: 57–62.

Thomas, A. J., L. E. Eberly, G. Davey Smith, J. D. Neaton, and J. Stamler. 2005. Race/ethnicity, income, major risk factors, and cardiovascular disease mortality. *American Journal of Public Health* 95: 1417–1423.

Thorpe, R. J., Jr., D. T. Brandon, and T. A. LaVeist. 2008. Social context as an explanation for race disparities in hypertension: Findings from the exploring health disparities in integrated communities (EHDIC) Study. *Social Science and Medicine* (1982) 67: 1604–1611.

Tishkoff, S. A., and K. K. Kidd. 2004. Implications of biogeography of human populations for "race" and medicine. *Nature Genetics* 36: S21–27.

Tishkoff, S. A., F. A. Reed, F. R. Friedlaender, C. Ehret, A. Ranciaro, A. Froment, J. B. Hirbo, A. A. Awomoyi, J. M. Bodo, O. Doumbo, et al. 2009. The genetic structure and history of Africans and African Americans. *Science* 324: 1035–1044.

Tishkoff, S. A., and D. C. Verrelli. 2003. Role of evolutionary history on haplotype block structure in the human genome: Implications for disease mapping. *Current Opinion in Genetics and Development* 13: 569–575.

Underhill, P. A., P. Shen, A. A. Lin, L. Jin, G. Passarino, W. H. Yang, E. Kauffman, B. Bonne-Tamir, J. Bertranpetit, P. Francalacci, et al. 2000. Y chromosome sequence variation and the history of human populations. *Nature Genetics* 26: 358–361.

Wallace, D. C. 1994. Mitochondrial DNA sequence variation in human evolution and disease. *Proceedings of the National Academy of Sciences of the United States of America* 91: 8739–8746.

Witherspoon, D. J., S. Wooding, A. R. Rogers, E. E. Marchani, W. S. Watkins, M. A. Batzer, and L. B. Jorde. 2007. Genetic similarities within and between human populations. *Genetics* 176: 351–359.

Witkowski, J. A., J. R. Inglis, and C. B. Davenport. 2008. *Davenport's dream: 21st century reflections on heredity and eugenics.* Cold Spring Harbor, NY: Cold Spring Harbor Laboratory Press.

Xing, J., W. S. Watkins, D. J. Witherspoon, Y. Zhang, S. L. Guthery, R. Thara, B. J. Mowry, K. Bulayeva, R. B. Weiss, and L. B. Jorde. 2009. Fine-scaled human genetic structure revealed by SNP microarrays. *Genome Research* 19: 815–825.

5

The Dilemma of Classification

The Past in the Present

LUNDY BRAUN AND EVELYNN HAMMONDS

Whether the concept of race captures some degree of underlying biological or genetic homogeneity has been contested for centuries. To resolve the controversy, some biomedical researchers in recent years have called for substituting ethnicity (Institute of Medicine 1999) or micro-ethnicity (Jackson 2004) for racial categories. While efforts to develop more fine-grained methods of classification are commendable, they nonetheless remain rooted in the notion that populations, large or small, are static, or at least so slowly changing that they can be demarcated for scientific purposes. The insufficiently examined concept of "population," we suggest, underlies the notion of race deployed in various contexts, be it ancestry testing, forensic analysis, population genetics, or biomedical research.

As the geographic site of early human evolution and great human genetic diversity, Africa has assumed increasing importance for researchers interested in human origins, history, and migration, the genetic etiology of complex disease, and racial disparities in disease (Tishkoff and Williams 2002). With attention to improving past practices, African partners are eagerly sought for genetic investigations in Africa, careful thought is given to informed consent for DNA sampling, and co-authorship on publications is now the norm. But the research agenda remains that of the global north. Moreover, the Africa that informs this agenda is shaped profoundly by images of the continent constructed through travelers' experiences, media accounts generally centered on violence, famine, disease, and chaos, and the history of expert knowledge systems in the human and natural sciences. One commonality to these narratives that hovers uneasily over the science is Africa as a space for "adventure" and philanthropic zeal, peopled by geographically distinct, "remote" tribes (*The New York Times*) (Lacey, 2005)—in other words, a space of negation that is everything the West is not (Mbembe 2001).

In this paper, we focus on Africa to historicize conceptual problems that plague the notions of population and groups, whether macro or micro, and their use in genetic research. Specifically, we trace the processes by which two expert knowledge systems, linguistics and social anthropology, transformed what were (and are) fluid societies into sharply demarcated, bounded units amenable to scientific analysis. Although certainly building on earlier ideas about Africans as naturally organized into groups, we argue that the conceptualization of populations, ethnic groups, or tribes *as discrete entities* suitable for scientific definition, sampling, and classification hardened in the 1930s and 1940s. At this time social anthropologists took to the field to delineate the dynamics of African societies; the field of linguistics became professionalized; and both disciplines of study became institutionalized in Western and South African universities.

Once named and studied in depth, knowledge of African societies was further flattened as anthropologists in the United States, notably Georges Peter Murdock, constructed internationally accessible atlases and databases, thereby making natural the existence of populations as bounded entities. Murdock's grand systematizing project thus set the stage for the use of African societies in large-scale population genetic studies currently underway and also for the contemporary reinvigoration of broad claims of difference based on population identification. In acquiring the status of transnational, and thus universal, knowledge, the complexity of local knowledge systems, with their blurry boundaries and their varied contributors, was erased. Not surprisingly, the move to finer levels of group analysis has not signaled the "end of race." Indeed, many studies that deploy populations as units of analysis are easily reaggregated into what seems eerily akin to traditional racial typologies, in both the scientific and the popular imaginations.

From Race to Population: From Population to Race

To be useful in biological investigations, a population must represent "a gene pool," which is bounded, geographically, linguistically, or culturally, reproductively isolated, and relatively unchanging over a long period of time. The requirement for isolation, evident in the call by leading population geneticists in 1991 to organize a DNA survey of human diversity, known as the Human Genome Diversity Project (HGDP), has a long history, which Jenny Reardon (2005) and Amade M'Charek (2005) have so insightfully analyzed. "The populations that can tell us the most about our evolutionary past," organizers of the HGDP note, "are those that have been isolated for some time, are likely to be linguistically and culturally distinct, and are often surrounded by geographic barriers. . . . Such isolated human populations are being rapidly merged with their neighbors . . . destroying irrevocably the information needed to reconstruct our evolutionary history" (Cavalli-Sforza et al. 1991:490). This sense of urgency has been a recurring theme in the writings of Luca Luigi Cavalli-Sforza and other scientists, as well as those of linguists and social anthropologists.

Despite a long history of contest (MacEachern 2000), for organizers of the HGDP, the existence of "populations" was a given. It was simply a technical question of identifying them and assembling the requisite linguistic expertise to trace the coevolution of genes and languages and on anthropological expertise to prioritize the units for sampling and describe any cultural traits relevant to genetic research. Yet, maintaining clarity on the unit of study has been a challenge, as illustrated in "Genetic Structure of Human Populations," an article published in *Science* by Rosenberg and colleagues in 2002 using the HGDP-CEHP database.[1] On the basis of genotyping a mere 1,056 individuals from fifty-two "predefined" populations, only six of which were African, these investigators claimed that allelic frequencies clustered by continent of origin. The methods by which populations were defined did not even warrant a footnote in this article, despite the many assumptions built into *Structure*, the computer program employed to cluster DNA data from sampled populations (Bolnick 2008). What is significant for this discussion is that Rosenberg and colleagues employed the language of "population," not race, in their paper. That continental clusters, however, were thinly disguised surrogates for race was made clear when Nicholas Wade of *The New York Times* (2002) argued that the Rosenberg study proved that races did, in fact, exist. In interviews with Wade, the authors concurred, perhaps uneasily, that "these regions broadly correspond with popular notions of race." Race is thus reproduced, naturalized, and reified (Duster 2005) through complex and largely invisible mechanisms of population.

Delimiting Tribes in Africa: From Missionaries to Linguists

As historian Leroy Vail and coauthors (1989) have illustrated in their fascinating collection *The Creation of Tribalism in Southern Africa*, ethnicity is not a simple reflection of a "traditional" or tribal past, insulated from historical change. Rather, in Africa concepts of ethnicity, or "tribalism," or what Lisa Gannett (2001) refers to more broadly as "population thinking," were formed and reformed during the nineteenth and twentieth centuries in response to the internal dynamics of African societies, the rapid social, political, and economic changes triggered by colonialism and industrialization, and, of particular relevance to this discussion, intellectual work in linguistics and academic theorizing about the nature of so-called "primitive" societies. Important to note, this was not a linear process, imposed in any simple way on African peoples. Rather, what took place on the ground was more akin to what Patrick Harries (2007:3) refers to as "a swirling interaction." Nonetheless, it was the particular frame constructed by Europeans that circulated transnationally and was ultimately incorporated into international databases.

Prior to the twentieth century, in accounts that still resonate with rich, if offensive, ethnographic detail, travelers, European missionaries, and colonial administrators embraced the project of producing knowledge about Africans, publicizing their work in the metropole in museum exhibits, books, pamphlets, and the popular press and using their understandings to guide colonial policy and resolve metropolitan socio-cultural anxieties (Coombes 1995). Travelers, such as John Barrow and Mungo Park, were among the first to systematically engage in a broad project of "othering" as they described, classified, and homogenized the people they encountered (Pratt 1985). Later, working closely with African intellectuals and informants, Europeans conducted anthropological, ethnological, and linguistic studies, writing the history of tribes, constructing written African languages, and detailing the rites and customs of indigenous peoples. Indeed, even in the nineteenth century, this work was seen as urgent, as the languages and traditions of indigenous races, and their histories and relationships to one another, were thought to be disappearing rapidly.

In his magnificent history of missionaries, the development of linguistic unity, and the emergence of ethnic consciousness among Tsonga-speakers of South Africa, Harries (1989; 2007) recounts the use of names such as the Tonga to describe *heterogenous groups of migrants* speaking different language forms and holding different cultural affinities, who fled to the northern and eastern Transvaal from southern Mozambique. Migrating in successive waves in the nineteenth century to escape domination by the Zulu kingdom, civil war in Mozambique, ecological crises, and disease, the people of southern Mozambique were linked, not by language, but by their skills as traders, their diet and methods of food preparation, their social organization, and significantly their social exclusion as foreigners in the Transvaal. According to Harries, "when people from the coastal area entered the Transvaal, they brought with them a number of speech forms and *these changed and developed* as they came into contact with local languages" (2007:160; emphasis added). Signifying their foreignness, they were variously referred to as Gwambas, Koapas, Tongas, Toka, Knowbnoses, Tchekes, Bonos, and Shangaans.

By the end of the nineteenth century, codification of language was a more sophisticated and transnational enterprise. To further their evangelical work and unify their converts, Swiss missionaries worked closely with African assistants and informants to codify the diverse languages of the coastal peoples from southeast Africa (which had been influenced by Zulu, Gaza, and Swazi) into a single written language and to teach this language in mission schools. Working within a Western structure of thought, they created grammar, vocabulary, Bibles, and literature (Harries 2007). The key point for this discussion, however, is that "once grammars had been constituted, their man-made origins were forgotten and they were perceived as givens, operating according to natural laws of science" (Harries 2007:166).

Bitter debates among missionary intellectuals over the precision of classification ensued, which ignored, if not erased, the complex history of African societies. Although the missionaries failed in their efforts to impose a single written language throughout southern Mozambique and the northern Transvaal, they nonetheless categorized the various languages into distinct subgroups. Confident that speakers of these language subgroups were sufficiently cohesive, the Swiss missionary, linguist, natural scientist, and anthropologist Henri-Alexandre Junod would confer the status of "tribe" on Tsonga-speakers in 1905. Tsonga speakers experienced continued social exclusion and alienation from the land, a sharp division of labor and housing in the gold mines structured along tribal lines, a Native Affairs Department in South Africa that promoted tribalism, and a mission-educated petty bourgeoisie schooled in written Tsonga and eager to pursue their own social agendas. By the mid-twentieth century, an ethnic consciousness, which was consolidated by the Bantustan system of the apartheid government, did indeed develop among Tsonga-speakers. Yet, Tsonga is thus best understood as an identity assigned to and adopted and reshaped by a diverse group of peoples in a specific historical context.

In the 1890s in eastern Zimbabwe, the people who gathered under Chief Makoni did not understand themselves as Manyika. By 1930, a term that, in the precolonial period, referred to a narrowly circumscribed political allegiance, and which was later redefined as the Portuguese and British competed for territory, came to describe a cultural identity rooted in a primordial past of a people composed of residents and settlers in a large geographic area. This shift in identity over the course of four decades required the construction, out of an arrray of dialects, of a written Manyika language, with a standardized orthography and rule of grammar, undertaken by missionaries of the American Methodist Episcopal Church, the Anglicans, and the Trappist/Mariannhill Catholics. In so doing, "differences were exaggerated" and gradualism of "dialect zones" was erased (Ranger 1989:127).

Working in close association with'African converts, the missionaries wrote and translated religious works, folktales, and literature. Each mission worked among people who differed in their means of subsistence, interest in linguistics and literacy, and receptivity to missionary work. Despite competing interests, a Manyika identity was consolidated in the 1930s under the pressure of the migrant labor system, as residents in eastern Zimbabwe married "foreign women" and mission-influenced migrant laborers drew on this identity to survive the dislocation of migration (Ranger 1989:140).

Constructing these identities produced purity out of mixture, something of great importance to Europeans. It is certainly the case that ethnic identities have acquired profound social meaning. It does not follow, however, that these identities conform to cohesive biological or genetically circumscribed units—although it is important to note that, at the time, the arguments for cohesiveness were primarily based on cultural unity. Moreover, missionary linguists did not always produce unity. In contrast, in the case of the Zulu and Xhosa, it was rivalries between missionaries that prevented unification of the languages.

While promoting tribalism was not necessarily the intent of missionary linguistic work, missionaries were nonetheless working within a European system of knowledge that constructed reality and produced "a pattern of domination" (Harries 1987). They drew on and respected local knowledge but, authorized with scientific methodologies, technological instruments, visual diagrams, maps, and cameras, it was Europeans who were considered to be the true systematizers and producers of universal knowledge (Harries 2007:115). The leap from linguistic group to tribe, with defined and fixed characteristics and boundaries, was but a short one in ordering the universe. The pertinent point for this discussion is that the pattern of domination that produced "tribes," or populations that are the unit of study in genetic studies, erased a complex history of intermingling of heterogeneous peoples in precolonial and colonial Africa—or, in the language of population genetics, continued and constant gene flow.

Despite the persistent efforts of the missionaries, the project of standardization of African languages was not yet complete in the late nineteenth and early twentieth centuries. Fixing and maintaining the boundaries of languages required reliable institutional support, which would come as linguistics became institutionalized in South African universities in the third decade of the twentieth century, especially with the establishment of the journal *Bantu Studies,* in 1922, and the Inter-University Committee for African Studies in 1931. Of particular significance, is that professionalization of linguistics was taking place at approximately the same time and place as the ethnographic turn in social anthropology.

Social Anthropology, Ethnographic Fieldwork, and Population in Africa

The typological thinking of physical anthropology, with its emphasis on the study of racial origins, dominated scientific discourse in South Africa for the first three decades of the twentieth century, as Saul Dubow (1995) has written, whereas population-based concepts of race, based on clustering of genetic polymorphisms, characterized the post-World War II period (Reardon 2005). For this shift to take place, populations needed to be scientifically delimited.

Beginning in the 1920s and continuing into the 1960s, social anthropologists of the functionalist school, influenced both by Bronislaw Malinowski's meticulous methods of fieldwork and Alfred Reginald Radcliffe-Brown's theories of society, turned to more systematic and theoretically informed study of African societies. Now the unit of study shifted in a more focused way to *bounded* social systems— tribes, ethnic groups, or populations. Anthropologists themselves have explored the complicated history of functionalism, engaging with the many critiques of their tendency to cultural relativism, narrow focus on synchronic, ahistorical sociological problems, and complicity with colonialism (see, for example, Asad 1973; Stocking 1984; Mudimbe 1988; Gordon 1990; Kuklick 1991; Goody 1995; Kuper 1996; Hammond-Tooke 1997; Cohn 2004). Our purpose here is not to rehearse these debates or explicate the specialized details of the field of social anthropology as it changed over time. Rather, we focus our attention on the unit of study deployed by social anthropologists to illustrate how ethnographic fieldwork produced and sustained notions of populations, tribes, or ethnic groups as bounded entities, and the consequences of such conceptualizations for contemporary population genetics research. "The question of the 'unit of study,'" writes John Comaroff, "far from being a methodological nicety, is a consequential theoretical matter.

For fields of inquiry are never naturally given; they always reflect substantive assumptions about the constitution of the 'real' world" (Comaroff 1982:144).

While the intellectual core of the functionalist school is often located in Britain, it was researchers and educators in Africa, particularly southern Africa, including the liberal social anthropologists such as Godfrey and Monica Wilson, Isaac Schapera, Meyer Fortes, Max Gluckman, Winifred Hoernle, Richard and Eileen Krige, and Hilda Kuper, who, with funding from metropolitan organizations such as the International Institute of African Languages and Cultures and the Rockefeller Foundation, conducted extensive fieldwork.[2] They went on to direct institutes in Africa, such as the Rhodes-Livingstone Institute in Northern Rhodesia, and trained many of the ethnographers who would ultimately hold prestigious chairs back in the metropole (UCT Archives).

Neglecting culture, at least initially—and, of course, not totally—functionalists conceptualized human societies as decontextualized social systems, in which each element had a functional relationship to the whole. They drew on Comte, Herbert Spencer, and especially Emile Durkheim for their theories of society and on the natural sciences for rigorous methodological approaches. For the functionalists, boundedness was conferred by a social structure held together by ties of kinship and political, legal, and religious institutions created to fulfill needs, be they biological needs as in the case of Malinowski (1929; 1930) or social needs as in the case of Radcliffe-Brown (Radcliffe-Brown 1946). According to the anthropologist Jack Goody, students of Malinowski were marked by a formalism, which was realized in their use of diagrams, figures, tables, and significantly, detailed and systematic field notes, which also reflected their scientific orientation. Thus, these early ethnographies and the visual imagery they deployed served to cast societies as static and resistant to change, and the people inhabiting these social structures as without history—*even though the researchers themselves had more nuanced understandings of social dynamics.*

This is not to imply that social anthropologists were an intellectually homogeneous group, slavishly beholden to narrow theories of functionalism, insensitive to the Africans they were studying, or uniformly or absolutely ahistorical. Indeed, like missionaries and linguists, social anthropologists were a varied group from across the political spectrum, with complicated and variable relationships with indigenous people. For the most part, they spent years in the field and struggled, often with great compassion (although of a decidedly paternalistic sort) for their research subjects, to rigorously test their hypotheses and models empirically. Nonetheless, by concentrating on descent as the organizing principle of African societies and guided by the scientific method, social anthropologists' social systems were conceptualized theoretically as closed structures with static regularities and uniformities or, in the words of Radcliffe-Brown, as systems of "ordered social relations in a given collection of human beings" (Radcliffe-Brown 1946). This framework conceptually minimized movements of peoples (which for population geneticists would lead to gene flow between populations).

Change, when it occurred in "simple" societies, was conceptualized as slower than that occurring in "complex" societies and a consequence of exogenous forces (Monica and Godfrey Wilson 1945). The internal dynamics of African societies were considered less important than European contact in triggering social change. For example, in his defense of British social anthropologists, Isaac Schapera (1962) rightly claims that the relevance of history to the study of social groups depends to a certain extent on the questions being asked. Although generally skeptical of theorizing (Comaroff and Comaroff 2006), when pushed to do so, he promotes a sense of history centered on what happened after contact. "The tribes the [functionalists] studied had been so greatly influenced by contact with Europeans that to ignore the resulting changes would have led to an incomplete and distorted view of present-day social life; and study of the changes always included study of when, how, and why, they had come about" (Schapera 1962:145). The goal of the social anthropologist, Schapera goes on to write, is to "ascertain how far the traditional Native institutions persist, not only in memory or in practice; but in addition he tries to ascertain how widespread is the adoption of European elements . . . The modern anthropologist . . . tries to determine why contact with the Europeans has modified Native life along certain lines." (Schapera 1962:146) African history before colonial penetration remains an unchanging and forever inaccessible black box. The inescapable conclusion is that precontact societies were produced and therefore bounded by traditional institutions, cultures, and social structures, that persist to greater or lesser extents into the ethnographic present. Although Schapera's theorizing does not reflect his own much richer understanding of Tswana societies, this narrowing of "history" to the period after contact has epistemological consequences.

South African-born Meyer Fortes, a leading figure in British social anthropology for many decades, was quite explicit in his articulation of groups as bounded. "A group of people bound together within a single social structure have a boundary, though not necessarily one that coincides with a physical boundary or is impenetrable" (Fortes 1953:22, quoted in Cohn 2004). Structures were, according to Fortes, "resistant to change" (Fortes 1953:23). For Radcliffe-Brown, culture was not bounded but "the system of society was contained within a territorially bounded community" (Stocking 1984:172). Like organic life, social systems had a functional unity (Radcliffe-Brown 1935).

In his writing about the social anthropologists in Africa, Bernard Cohn (2004) takes a sharply critical stance, arguing that the conceptualization of African societies as organized into unchanging, bounded entities according to principles of descent was a legitimizing practice, enacted by social anthropologists, which was essential to maintenance of the social order under colonialism. "Unit, boundary, social structure, and group," Cohn writes, "are the central concepts which appear time and time again in the anthropological literature of the forties and the fifties. A unit meant something that was observable on the ground. Hamlets, villages, lineages, tribes were believed to be bounded—they were countable and mapable, had names, and above all had social structures—patterned relations between groups. Groups were made up of individuals recruited on known principles, usually genealogical connections which were thought to be 'real' i.e. met western concepts of descent traceable to common ancestors and expressed in the metaphor of 'blood'" (Cohn 2004:203).

As noted earlier, a sense of urgency characterized the fieldwork of social anthropologists of the 1930s and 1940s. They were fully aware that colonial interventions were changing indigenous societies rapidly and irrevocably. Radcliffe-Brown was so concerned by the rapid disappearance of untouched societies that he urged the Rockefeller Foundation to support a center for vanishing cultures at Yale (Stocking 1984:168). By the late 1960s, structural functionalism was in decline. But, the social anthropologists' social systems, according to "scientific" principles, survived.

George Peters Murdock: Classifying Culture

Anthropologists' and linguists' tribes could easily double as geneticists' populations. But, first they had to be incorporated into standardized datasets in the systematizing project of the American cultural anthropologist George Peters Murdock (1897–1985), a renowned comparativist from Yale. Murdock's project is of particular relevance to this discussion as his work helped to shape the conceptualization of populations that informs the HGDP.

As with earlier anthropological systematizers, Murdock had limited fieldwork experience himself. From early in his career, he focused his efforts on ordering the ethnographic knowledge of others. Interested in cultural universals and animated by the desire to place the study of society on a scientific basis, Murdock first published a summary of ethnographies in 1934 and later, in the 1930s, took on the mammoth task of creating the Cross-Cultural Survey at Yale's Institute for Human Relations, a data archive of ethnographic information, later to be the Human Relations Area Files (HRAF). It incorporated ethnographies conducted by fieldworkers operating in a variety of widely divergent and sometimes oppositional anthropological traditions, including those influenced by Franz Boas and Malinowski (who were committed to different classificatory systems). Such a systematic effort would facilitate statistical comparison of cultural traits by researchers the world over. While sometimes critical of the functionalists for their lack of attention to culture and history, Murdock nonetheless admired their ethnographic contributions for the factual social knowledge they produced (Murdock 1951). From the early years of his career, Murdock's goal was to define culture in terms of traits that could be compared globally and analyzed statistically for patterns (Murdock 1932). For this project, the work of the functionalists as well as other anthropologists would be key. Indeed, in the late 1930s, Murdock attempted to recruit Evans-Pritchard to Yale, a plan that was interrupted by the outbreak of World War II. In the same period, he brought Malinowski to Yale, where he died in 1942, shortly after his arrival (Darnell 1938).

In 1957, Murdock published the "World Ethnographic Sample," a compilation of groups worldwide with a simple coding system, in the *American Anthropologist* (Murdock 1957). In it he sought to synthesize knowledge of world cultures by detailing their distribution and carefully classifying them according to "certain standard ethnographic categories" (664). The sample was further developed in his *Outline of World Cultures*, published in 1958.

Several years later, Murdock began to compile a more comprehensive coded atlas of the world's peoples in *Ethnology*, a journal he founded in 1962, where he expanded on the number of societies available for cross-cultural analysis. The completed *Ethnographic Atlas*, which contained a summary of 239 African societies organized into 85 clusters, was published as a single volume in 1967. By codifying social, cultural, and economic characteristics, such as mode of marriage, family organization, community organization, kin groups, settlement patterns, and so on, into a simplified form suitable for entry on punch cards and later computer programs, Murdock promoted statistical comparisons of various traits of world societies and ushered in an era of new forms of ordering knowledge about Africa. At the same time, in a more hardened way than previous systematizing projects, he reduced dynamic societies to static forms and rendered invisible the more nuanced understandings of social formations held by ethnographers.

In *Africa: Its Peoples and Their Culture History* published in 1959, Murdock provides an index of African tribes based on the abundant ethnographic work accumulated on Africa in recent decades. By mapping language, culture, and tribe unproblematically onto each other, the definition of groups appears to be straightforward throughout the book. "Tribes," he writes, "are classified into groups of essentially identical language and culture, arranged numerically in alphabetical order, with reasonably complete synonymies to facilitate identification through an index of tribal names included at the end of the book" (Murdock 1959: ix). For Murdock, language was particularly informative of ancestral relationship. Recognizing that classical racial typologies were dated, he unapologetically proceeds to describe the five classically typological races—Bushmanoid, Caucasoid, Mongoloid, Negroid, and Pygmoid—that people the continent of Africa. Thus, we see here early evidence of constant, and intentional, slippage between populations and more typological notions of race that continue to plague many areas of social and natural scientific research.

Although criticized extensively by Africanists, Murdock's works influenced future genetic researchers in Africa, especially—for the purposes of our discussion— the research and syntheses of Cavalli-Sforza (MacEachern 2000). The hunter-gatherer groups described in Murdock's *Africa: Its Peoples and Their Culture History* were featured on the first page of the introduction to Cavalli-Sforza's *African Pygmies*, a detailed compilation of virtually all the studies on population structure, genetics, anthropometry, and other biological characteristics of African Pygmies. Significantly, Murdock's classification of Central African pygmies, deep in the heart of Africa, framed the conceptualization of pygmies as distinct groups and guided blood sampling. Cavalli-Sforza returns again and again to Murdock in his ambitious compendium of genetic data *The History and Geography of Human Genes* (1994) and more recently in his popular work, *Genes, Peoples, and Languages*, published in 2002.

As noted previously, some of the most prominent social anthropologists were South African, carrying out ethnographies among people referred to as Tswana, Swazi, Zulu, Xhosa, and so on. Asserting their rightful place in this transnational research agenda South African scientists are now actively using ethnographically defined populations in genetic research and creating their own databases (Soodyall 2003). Murdock's *Africa: Its Peoples and Their Culture History* appears as one of only three references in the draft document of the internationally representative sub-Saharan Working Group of the HGDP (draft document n.d.). The Xhosa as a distinct, and presumably genetically homogeneous, population appears on the Working Group's list of African populations to be studied.

While acknowledging that "neither in the present nor past is there any simple correlation between ethnicity, language, and gene pool," the sub-Saharan Working Group nonetheless decided to sample groups based on ethnicity and language, using Murdock's maps to select populations to be included on the final list. The reliance on outmoded histories to guide genetic research is all the more surprising, given the proliferation for decades of texts in history and historical anthropology that chronicle the making and re-making of ethnicity in Africa (see, for example, the special issue in the *Journal of Southern African Studies on Anthropology and History* in 1981).

While ostensibly theory-neutral, projects that order diffuse and changing societies into fixed and unchanging databases that serve as handy reference guides for researchers from other disciplines mask assumptions about those societies, erase the complexity of their dynamics and historicity, and convey a skewed sense of the world (Bowker 2000). The point here is that the very construction of databases raises important questions of knowledge and power.

Conclusion

In what is often referred to as the "Golden Age of Ethnography," university-trained social anthropologists took to the field to systematically study, organize, and order the world's diverse peoples. With its peoples "conceptualized, first and foremost, as members of groups" (Vaughn 1991: 11), Africa was the centerpiece of this enterprise. Intent on creating a scientific methodology of neutral observation, ethnographers replaced amateur travelers, traders, colonial administrators and physicians, and missionaries as authoritative producers of knowledge about the customs, beliefs, and languages of indigenous peoples. At the same time, linguists were engaged in an intensive project of construction and standardization of African languages, mapping language onto primordial "tribal" territories and cultural units.

It is important to emphasize that this was a messy and incoherent process on the ground. Mozambique was not Leopold's Congo. Nonetheless, ordering projects, be they political, anthropological, linguistic, or biological in nature, erase the complicated reality that people have always been interacting, exchanging goods, social ideas, culture, and genes (Goodman 2007). While socio-cultural exchanges took a particularly violent form in nineteenth- and twentieth-century colonial interventions in Africa, which profoundly and irreversibly shaped the constitution of groups on this continent, colonialism did not initiate the movement and mixing of peoples. Historical analysis demonstrates that populations are not now and never were isolated, bounded entities; they are in reality actively produced social formations—appearing, disappearing, and reappearing over time as part of global socio-scientific projects. Rather than a continent peopled by timeless relics of a tribal past Africa, like all continents, is built on "a mosaic of groups," which incorporates "people of different language affiliations; it involved extremely sophisticated ritual, economic, and technological accommodations to a diverse and changing natural and cultural milieu; it allowed for processes of immigration, emigration, and population interchange" (MacEachern 2000:363).

The legacy of work in the human sciences from the first half of the twentieth century, which is almost invisible and unknown to present-day researchers, profoundly shapes contemporary genetic research protocols, whether they deploy racial typologies or finer-grained micro groups. Just as nothing less than state-of-the-art statistical or basic science methodologies would be acceptable to biomedical scientists, the basic unit of analysis, this very first step in conducting population studies, must be subjected to rigorous scrutiny. This begins with the difficult process of uncovering the rich history of the making and re-making of populations and how they are defined and understood.

ACKNOWLEDGMENTS

We thank Jenny Reardon for providing us with the Sub-Saharan Working Group Draft Document, Julie Livingston for insightful comments on our presentation to the Race, DNA, and History Conference, at Rutgers University, Center for Race and Ethnicity in April 2008. This chapter is adapted from an earlier version entitled "Race, Populations, and Genomics: Africa as Laboratory," *Social Science and Medicine* 67: 1580–1588. We thank Elsiever, Ltd., for permission to publish it.

NOTES

1. This database contains cell lines from 1052 individuals in 52 populations throughout the world, from whom DNA was extracted. See supplementary material in Cann et al. (2002) for more detail.

2. This group moved continuously throughout their career between Britain and South Africa. Most participated in the famed Malinowski seminars at the London School of Economics. Only Monica Wilson remained in South Africa, holding the chair of social anthropology for over twenty years.

WORKS CITED

Asad, T., ed. 1973. *Anthropology and the colonial encounter.* New York: Humanities Press.

Bolnick, D. 2008. Individual ancestry inference and the reification of race as a biological phenomenon. In *Revisiting race in a genomic age, edited by* B. Koenig, S.S-J. Lee, S. Richardson. New Brunswick, NJ: Rutgers University Press.

Bowker, G. 2000. Biodiversity datadiversity. *Social Studies of Science* 30: 643–683

Cann, H. M., C. de Toma, L. Cazes, M.-F. Legrand, V. Morel, L. Piouffre, L., et al. 2002. A human diversity cell line panel. *Science* 296, 261–262; Supplementary material. www .sciencemag.org/cgi/content/full/296/5566/261b/DC1.

Cavalli-Sforza, L. L., ed. 1986. *African pygmies.* Orlando, FL: Academic Press.

Cavalli-Sforza, L. L. 2000. *Genes, peoples, and languages.* Berkeley: University of California Press.

Cavalli-Sforza, L. L., A. C. Wilson, C. R. Cantor, R. M. Cook-Deegan, and M. C. King. 1991. Call for a worldwide survey of human genetic diversity: A vanishing opportunity for the human genome project. *Genomics* 11: 490–491.

Cohn, B. S. 2004. African models and Indian histories. In *An anthropologist among the historians and other essays.* New Delhi: Oxford India Paperbacks.

Comaroff, J. L. 1982. Dialectical systems, history, and anthropology: Units of study and questions of theory. *Journal of Southern African Studies* 8 (2): 143–172.

Comaroff, J., and Comaroff, J. L. 2006. Portraits of the ethnographer as a young man. *Anthropology Today* 22: 9–16.

Coombes, A. 1995. *Reinventing Africa: Museums, material culture, and popular imagination in late Victorian and Edwardian England.* New Haven: Yale University Press.

Darnell, D. 1998. Camelot at Yale: The construction and dismantling of the Sapirian synthesis, 1931–1939. *American Anthropologist* 100: 361–372.

Dubow, S. 1995. *Scientific racism in modern South Africa.* Cambridge: Cambridge University Press.

Duster, T. 2005. Race and reification in science. *Science* 307: 1050–1051.

Fortes, M. 1953. The structure of unilineal descent groups. *American Anthropologist* 55: 17–41.

Gannett, L. 2001. Racism and human genome diversity research: The ethical limits of "population thinking." *Philosophy of Science* 68: S479–S492.

Goodman, A. 2007. Toward genetics in an era of anthropology. *American Ethnologist* 34 (2): 225–227.

Goody, J. 1995. *The expansive moment: Anthropology in Britain and Africa, 1918–1970.* Cambridge: Cambridge University Press.

Gordon, R. 1990. Early social anthropology in South Africa. *African Studies* 49 (1): 15–48.

Hammond-Tooke, W. D. 1997. *Imperfect interpreters: South Africa's anthropologists 1920–1990.* Johannesburg: Witwatersrand University Press.

Harries, P. 1987. The roots of ethnicity: Discourse and the politics of language construction in south-east Africa. *The Making of Class,* University of Wiswatersrand Workshop, February 9–14.

———. 1989. Exclusion, classification, and internal colonialism: The emergence of ethnicity among the Tsonga-speakers of South Africa. In L. Vail, ed., *The creation of tribalism in Southern Africa,* 82–117. London: James Currey Ltd.

Institute of Medicine (IOM). 1999. *The unequal burden of cancer: An assessment of NIH research and programs for ethnic minorities and the medically underserved,* edited by M. A. Haynes and B. D. Smedley. Washington, DC: National Academy Press.

Jackson, F. L. 2004. Human genetic variation and health: New approaches based on ethno-genetic layering. *British Medical Bulletin* 69: 215–235.

Kuklick, H. 1991. *The savage within: The social history of British anthropology 1885–1945.* Cambridge: Cambridge University Press.

Kuper, A. 1996. *Anthropology and anthropologists: The modern British school.* London: Routledge.

Lacey, M. 2005. Remote and poked: Anthropology's dream tribe. *The New York Times,* Dec. 18.

MacEachern, S. 2000. Genes, tribes, and African history. *Current Anthropology* 41: 357–384.

M'Charek, A. 2005. *The Human Genome Diversity Project: An ethnography of scientific practice.* Cambridge: Cambridge University Press.

Malinowski, B. 1929. Practical anthropology. *Africa* 2 (1): 22–38.

———. 1930. Kinship. *Man* 30: 19–29.

Mbembe, A. 2001. *On the Postcolony.* Berkeley: University of California Press.

Murdock, G. P. 1932. The science of culture. *American Anthropologist* 34 (2): 200–215.

———. 1951. British social anthropology. *American Anthropologist* 53 (4): 465–473.

———. 1957. World ethnographic sample. *American Anthropologist* 59: 664–687.

———. 1958. *Outline of world cultures.* New Haven: Human Relations Area Files Press.

———. 1959. *Africa: Its peoples and their culture history.* New York: McGraw-Hill.

———. 1967. *Ethnographic atlas.* Pittsburgh: University of Pittsburgh Press.

Pratt, M. L. 1985. Scratches on the face of the country; or, what Mr. Barrow saw in the land of the Bushmen. *Critical Inquiry* 12: 119–143.

Radcliffe-Brown, A. R. 1925. Letter to Winifred Hoernle, August 20. University of Capetown Manuscripts and Archives Collection, Isaac Schapera Papers, B.C. 1168, D.

———. 1935. On the concept of function in social science. *American Anthropologist, New Series* 37 (3), Part I, 394–402.

———. 1946. A note on functional anthropology. *Man* 46: 38–41.

Ranger, T. Missionaries, migrants, and the Manyika: The invention of ethnicity in Zimbabwe. In *The Creation of Tribalism in Southern Africa,* edited by L. Vail. 118–150. London: James Currey Ltd.

Reardon, J. 2005. *Race to the finish: Identity and governance in an age of genomics.* Princeton, NJ: Princeton University Press.

Rosenberg N. A., J. K. Pritchard J. L. Weber H. M. Cann K. K. Kidd L.A. Zhivotovsky and M. W. Feldman. 2002. Genetic structure of populations, *Science* 298: 2381–2385. Supporting online material, www.sciencemag.og/cgi/content/full/298/5602/2381/DC1.

Schapera, I. 1962. Should anthropologists be historians? *Journal of the Royal Anthropological Institute of Great Britain and Ireland* 92: 143–156.

Soodyall, H. 2003. A walk in the garden of eden: Genetic trails into our African past. Social Cohesion and Integration Research Programme, Africa Human Genome Initiative Occasional Paper Series No. 2. Cape Town: Human Sciences Research Council (HSRC).

Stocking, G. Jr. 1984. Radcliffe-Brown and British social anthropology, In *Functionalism historicized: Essays on British social anthropology,* Edited by G. Stocking, 131–191. Madison: University of Wisconsin Press.

Sub-Saharan Africa Working Group. n.d. Draft document.

Tishkoff, S. A., and S. M. Williams. 2002. Genetic analysis of African populations: Human evolution and complex disease. *Nature Reviews Genetics* 3: 611–621.

Vail, L. 1989. Introduction: Ethnicity in southern African history. *The creation of tribalism in Southern Africa,* Edited by L. Vail. 1–20. London: James Currey Ltd.

Vaughn, M. 1991. *Colonial power and African illness.* Palo Alto, CA: Stanford University Press.

Wade, N. 2002. Gene study identifies 5 main human populations, linking them to geography. *The New York Times,* Dec. 20: 37.

Wilson, G., and M. Wilson. 1945. *The analysis of social change based on observations in Central Africa.* Cambridge: Cambridge University Press.

6

The Informationalization of Race

Communication, Databases, and the
Digital Coding of the Genome

PETER A. CHOW-WHITE

In our time—at the end of the twentieth century—the crisis of race . . . is still
raging. . . . In this age of globalization, with its impressive scientific and technological innovations in information, communication, and applied biology,
a focus on the lingering effects of racism seems outdated and antiquated.
The global cultural bazaar of entertainment and enjoyment, the global shopping mall of advertising and marketing, the global workplace of blue-collar
and white-collar employment, and the global financial network of computerized transactions and megacorporate mergers appear to render any talk
about race irrelevant. (West and Gates 1997:68)

Something is happening to race. (Fausto-Sterling 2003:1)

In 2005, a series of publications signaled a new phase of the biopolitics of the
human body. In March, an evolutionary developmental biologist wrote an op-ed
piece in the *New York Times* that ran contrary to standing assumptions about race
as a social construct. He argued that new scientific evidence has been emerging
that showed genetically identifiable racial differences. The next month a story in
the same periodical described how students in an introductory sociology class
were taking a DNA test to determine their genetic ancestry by comparing their
DNA to "four parent populations, western European, west African, east Asian and
indigenous American." Finally, in October the results from the first phase of the
next human genome project, the HapMap Project, were published in the journal
Nature. In 2000, leaders of the Human Genome Project concluded that humanity
is genetically 99.9 percent the same and that race is indeed a social construct and
not a biological one. However, one of the goals of HapMap has been to map the

haplotype groups, or "neighborhoods" of genome variation, of individuals from different "population" groups: African, Asian, and European. The HapMap results showed, in figures vividly color coded in green, orange, and purple, genetic variation between these groups. Instead of following the millennium declaration that race has no biological basis, increasing numbers of scientific studies are "discovering" how race is meaningful at the genetic level.

If the late twentieth century was characterized by the deconstruction of race, then it is being reconstructed around a biomedical and informational paradigm at the beginning of the twenty-first century. This development is not simply the result of scientists acting with ideological blinders or the return of the racial science of the nineteenth century. The context for the genomic turn in racial identity lies at the convergence of race and new technologies. As race becomes twice recoded, in terms of culture or what some refer to as the new racism (Barker 1982; Collins 2004) and into the Internet and other related information and communication technologies (Hammonds 1997; Kolko et al. 2000; Nakamura 2002; 2008), discourses about race are being reimagined. Research into race and digital culture has shown how new technologies reinforce old forms of racial identity in new ways that are less obvious than previous media forms (Nakamura 2008). The conditions for identity-building have shifted, as new social, political, and economic formations emerge in and through new media- and techno-scapes, shaped most significantly by the Internet. This essay examines how the convergence of changing concepts of race with information technologies has produced a new paradigm for race. This paradigm, while it emerges in discourses of the information age that present themselves as colorblind, is, I argue, in fact productive of new regimes of racial knowledge that are oriented around the digital cultures of communication technologies, especially the Internet and databases, both in everyday practices and social institutions.[1]

An important area in which to investigate how race is being recoded via culture and technology is human genomics. This burgeoning field has been referred to as an information science because communication technologies, such as computers, the Internet, and digital databases, are essential for sequencing DNA. Without them, genome science would be virtually impossible.

It is the meeting ground for genetic, computer, and racial codes and is both challenging preconceived notions of racial meaning and reproducing racial classification. For example, where Craig Venter and Francis Collins, the leaders of the private Celera genome project and public Human Genome Project (HGP), concluded that we are all 99.9 percent the same at the genetic level, the next HGP, the International HapMap Project, is mapping differences between African, Asian, and European groups. Drawing on interviews with members of the HapMap Project[2] and textual data from biomedical and scientific journals, this study examines technological innovation and cultural and scientific discourses in genomics.[3] Utopian visions of this emerging biotechnology suggested that scientists would be able to see into the human body in new ways and begin to map and manipulate the very building blocks of life to improve health. However, genome research into group differences is also a crucial site of negotiation in the relationship between race and technology.

The Informationalization of Race

Critical scholars have divided racialization into two interdependent ontological paradigms: race as biology and race as culture. In the race as biology paradigm, racial groups are identified according to a collection of physical phenotypes, such as skin color, hair texture, shape of eyes and nose, and then tied to a hierarchical order of racial groups with whites at the top ranging to blacks at the bottom (Banton 1998; Jordan 1974; Miles 1989). The formative process of racialization has been linked to the rise of enlightenment thought (Eze 1997), spread of European colonialism (Césaire 1972; Fanon 1963, 1967; Memmi 1965), slavery (Jordan 1974), and scientific racism (Barkan 1992; Gould 1996; Mosse 1978; Stepan 1982). In the post–civil rights era, biological classification shifted to cultural codes, a development that has been referred to as the culturalization of race (Razack 1998) or the new racism (Barker 1982; Collins 2004). Group characteristics continue to be ascribed based on a symbolics of the body. Yet the real differences between groups are no longer biological but rather ethnic or cultural.

Cultural notions of race are deployed in a manner similar to those of biological ones: homogenous, dislocated from historical context, static, and containing an implicit association to group position in the social order: "a fixed property of social groups, [rather than] something intrinsically fluid, changing, unstable, and dynamic" (Gilroy 2000:266). Racial signification is rearticulated in cultural terms, where everyday talk and political statements about the cultural characteristics of a particular group often are thinly disguised racial claims. Kim argues that the move to culturally coded racial discourse has in fact stabilized white privilege in the post–civil rights era. "It is precisely because it has been revamped in nonracial language that the field of racial positions functions so effectively to reinforce White privilege today. Representing a cultural explanation for group inequalities, the field of racial positions implies that American society is substantially colorblind and that the American Dream is still viable" (Kim 1999:117). Scholars refer to the dominant racial ideology characterized by coded discourse about race as color-blind racism (Bonilla-Silva 2003) and colorblindness (Brown et al. 2003; Wellman 2003). Bonilla-Silva (2001) suggests that the civil rights movement marked a change in the racialized social system from Jim Crow racism to color-blind racism. In the former phase, blacks and other minorities were considered inferior to whites because of their biological and moral inferiority. One of the most significant changes in the post-civil right era is the nonracial and cultural terms in which racial differences are articulated in the public sphere. Bonilla-Silva (2001) describes race talk during the Jim Crow era as "direct and blunt" (68). Racial claims now tend to be made indirectly. Hockey, basketball, special interests, inner city, thug, welfare, and sickle cell disease are racially coded in a colorblind manner. Instead of the terms of inclusion and exclusion, superiority and inferiority being based in genetics, a group's success in society is reliant on their cultural competency. Many even speak of a postracial society.

In spite of the continued existence of racial inequality in terms of social, economic, and political power, what Lipsitz (1998) refers to as the possessive investment of whiteness, the turn to colorblind racism attributes differential standings of minorities to market forces, naturally occurring phenomena (segregation is natural, because people want to live with others who are like them, what Taguieff [1990] refers to as the *biologization of culture*), and cultural variations between groups (Bonilla-Silva 2003:2).

A new regime of racial signification characterized by the creation and deployment of information is emerging through the digital space of communication networks, computer codes, computational algorithms, and databases. New communication technologies increasingly make up the central media systems in which racial meanings are created, transformed, and destroyed, to borrow from Omi and Winant (1994). This networked system is not simply a delivery tool for ideas and meanings. Its very structure and scope, both hypertext and globally linked, is productive of new mechanisms of racialization. Where conventional conceptions of race have been articulated in terms of culture or phenotype, in the digital age information is the material by which racial meaning is worked on. However, *race as information* does not replace the dependency of racialization on ethnicity or skin color. Rather, as the paradigm of race as culture emerged from the paradigm of race as biology, I would argue that the paradigm of race as information has emerged from both. I call this new racial formation the *informationalization of race.*

What distinguishes race as information from other modes of racialization is the transformation of society due to globalization, the new economy, and communication technologies. Racial identity, meanings, and structures are being created through the use and shaping of new media and communication technologies. The informationalization of race acknowledges that race as a structuring device in society has not diminished in importance with the information age and has continuity with modernity. While at the same time, this research seeks to examine new mechanisms of racialization that are an effect of innovations and applications of communication technologies and the rise of information in a post-civil rights context. In one of the first books on race and new media technologies, Kolko, Nakamura, and Rodman show that, in spite of utopian visions of fluid online identities, "race matters no less in cyberspace than it does 'IRL' (in real life)" (2000:4; see also Nakamura 2002). This is significantly different from previous forms of the social construction of race as the body becomes "posthuman" (Hayles 1999). That is, the "meat" has been left behind and cultural signification has become embedded in computer programs and complex algorithms, hidden from the front end, user interfaces.

In an early example of this process, Hammonds (1997) describes a computer program that could morph people into different races and create entirely new people from an amalgam of a number of facial features of different racialized groups. Rather than deconstructing biological notions of race, she argues, they reinforce centuries-old stereotypes of racial difference and cultural anxieties of miscegenation. Ideologies of bio-race were translated into the seemingly neutral space of the digital. As a space of new media, the Internet has been used to translate racist ideology online and as a site of contestation over racialized identities. Where traditional media (film, television, etc.) have been largely one-way media that excluded or marginalized people of color, cyberspace's unique architecture enables the building of communities among minority and transnational groups across time and space.

Linda Leung (2005) explores the presence and community-building of racialized minorities in representation, production, and consumption in cyberspace. In an empirical analysis of a research project based in East London called Project @THENE, she finds that, although the World Wide Web is dominated by a white, western-centric notion of technology and media, there are significant points of participation where people from minority groups can and do challenge dominant ideologies of race and ethnicity, either directly or indirectly. Similarly, Gray (2005) shows how groups such as the Afrofuturists, a movement made up of a loose collection of artists, musicians, writers, and critics, utilize the global networked architecture of cyberspace to stitch together and create cultural production in the digital Black Atlantic (see also Nelson 2002).

The computational routines that produce racial representations are "new technologies of race," translating ideologies of bio-race into the seeming neutrality of digital space. As cultural and phenotypic signification meet computer code, the analog systems of racial signification enter the digital world, producing new modalities as well as reproducing old ones. Traditional media analyses of the mechanisms of racialization tend to focus on representation in television, film, and news. Scholars, such as Vaidhyanathan (2006), working between a number of academic fields, suggest that asking critical questions about the nature, uses, and (global) flows of information is a crucial practice in understanding emerging relationships between technologies, social norms, and democracy. The concept of the informationalization of race directs attention to the algorithms, data, and discourses produced in the hypertext communication environments of computers, databases, data mining, and the Internet.

Unlike the more visible forms of new media technologies such as the mobile phone, the laptop computer, and the iPod, or "invisible" delivery systems such as wi-fi or the Web, the database is a central innovation in the information economy (Elmer 2004; see also Cubitt 2000; Loro 1995; Manovich 1999; Poster 1991).

Similar to old media forms, like the novel, film, or television, the database is a new media technology that structures our personal and institutional experiences both symbolically and materially. Differing from these largely one-way media, databases enable a "networked multilogue" (Loro 1995:55) between producers and consumers through the process of sorting and storing data, networking information, and constructing knowledge. Data mining is a technique for searching and creating knowledge out of digital databases (KDD). Derived from the computer sciences, data mining is a step in discovering knowledge in data. Within specified parameters, computers programs search databases using mathematical algorithms to find significant patterns. Data mining techniques are made up of sophisticated algorithms, neural networks, and artificial intelligence. They can work from predetermined sets of categorical variables, or they can go beyond what a user knows in order to request and "discover" unseen patterns, facts, or relationships between the data (Danna and Gandy 2002; Zarsky 2003). As the Internet has been employed by government agencies and marketing firms to gather information on citizens and customers, the goals for data mining have increasingly moved from description to prediction (Gandy 2006). Companies across all business sectors, from grocery shopping to Amazon.com to genetic services, employ databases and data mining to find out characteristics about their clientele. In order to provide personalized services, firms collect demographic and behavioral data on individuals and groups to understand who they are, what they like, and their future buying potential.

The term "informationalization" builds on the insights of the literature on surveillance and the information society that examines the shift in societies from industrial economies to services economies due to the restructuring of capitalism, the new technological paradigm, and globalization (Webster 2002). Informationalism is a "specific form of social organization in which information generation, processing, and transmission become the fundamental resources of productivity and power" (Castells 2000:21). Traditionally, the concept of information denotes a neutral set of facts, data, or observations. When information is networked and takes on the form of an information infrastructure, such as when databases are compiled and linked or the seemingly endless pathways of the World Wide Web, it should not be treated as having a simply reflective role in the social world. Like other media forms (news, television, film) information infrastructures do not just support cultural, political, social, and scientific processes. They play a constitutive role. "It is politically and ethically crucial to recognize the vital role of infrastructures in the 'built moral environment.' Seemingly purely technical issues like how to name things and how to store data in fact constitute much of what we have come to know as natural" (Bowker and Star 1999:326). Technologies and the classification systems that use them tend to make invisible the myriad of decisions that create them. We, the users, see only the interface, the front end of a particular technology. Hidden away inside are the attitudes, values, and politics that are written into code and "the arguments, decisions, uncertainties and processual nature of decision-making" (Bowker and Star 1999:187; see also Garfinkel 2000). Put another way, the seemingly descriptive representations derived from information infrastructures in fact naturalize a whole set of practices, procedures, and ideological premises.

> Looked at historically, information seems basic to social life. . . . In modern, literate cultures, artificial signs proliferate, and are frequently associated with social order itself. Signs tell us of distant events, places, persons and processes. Information is relational, connecting by reference persons and things. . . . But whereas information might once have thrown light on reality, or even, through instructions or recipes, contributed to the transformation of reality, once technological devices become the predominant carriers of information, the distinctions blur. (Lyon 2005:225)

Information has moved from being factual, to being technical, to being a commodity and a basis for social, technical, political, and cultural organization. Castells argues that it is not only the centrality of knowledge and information that characterizes the current technological revolution, "but the application of such knowledge and information to knowledge generation and information processing/communication devices, in a cumulative feedback loop between innovation and the uses of innovation" (Castells 2000:31).

Race as information brings into the fore new forms of racialization that previous concepts, such as race as the body, race as nation, race as culture do not. When cultural codes meet computer code, programming and distributed networks have become the new sites of negotiation over norms and the terms of social inclusion and exclusion. As Galloway and Thacker suggest about the logic of the network society, "codification, not reification is the new concern" (2007:134). Where racialization has been about the reduction of cultural practices and social relations to objects, the informationalization of race looks to where bodies and practices become code. This could be in the form of state surveillance, bioprospecting, or self-expression online such as Facebook.

At all levels of society, from institutions to individual identities, information has become the material that social and political meaning is constructed in, new companies profit from, and states utilize to govern over. This is a crucial development for the study of racial formations. This research seeks to examine how innovations and applications of communication technologies and the rise of information have produced new mechanisms of racialization in a post–civil rights context. Scholars have pointed out that race has not decreased in significance, but persisted and transformed into colorblind racism. As communication technologies play an increasingly centralized role in the everyday practices and organization of a range of social institutions and industries, there are a number of sites where we can see the informationalization of race at work, such as law enforcement, biomedical research, insurance, and marketing. While each would have its own set of technologies for information storage, classification, and surveillance, they have increasingly employed a similar array of technologies to their own institutional needs and goals. Where the microscope has been a central observational tool in the biomedical sciences, actuarial tables in insurance, and fingerprinting in law enforcement, data mining techniques and the technological infrastructure that it requires are commonly used across these different sectors. Their methods of observation, classification, and knowledge production have incorporated networked, digital, and informational processes.

This research explores developments in biomedical research into DNA. In molecular biology, Mackenzie questions the usefulness and the point of tracking computational processing of sequence data, which heavily utilize new media such as the Internet and databases for storage, analysis, and distribution: "Does not bioinformatics merely support the more decisive intellectual, social, political, cultural and economics events associated with contemporary biology and genetics?" (2003:316) While scientists debate the accuracy or inaccuracy of scientific data, which is the outcome of computational and statistical routines, it is important to understand how those outcomes stitch together cultural assumptions, molecular particles, microprocesssed bits and bytes, and historical context. In what follows, I explore how genomics, the study of DNA, is an effect of the informationalization of race.

Biology as an Information Science and the Human Genome

There has been a concurrent ascendance of the information society and genetic technologies (Capra 2002; Castells 2000; Meyers and Davis 2003). Computer science and genetics have converged to the point where biologists, computer scientists, and engineers work side-by-side, borrowing from one another both methodologically and theoretically (Marturano and Chadwick 2004). Modern science relies to a very large extent on computer simulations, computational models, and analyses of large data sets where genetic data points can number in the billions, such as in the case of the Human Genome Project (Gezelter 1999).

Genetic technologies are information technologies, since they are focused on the decoding and eventually reprogramming of DNA, the information code of living matter (Moody 2004; Thacker 2004). And, more important, without "massive computing power and the simulation capacity provided by advanced software, the HGP, would not have been completed—nor would scientists be able to identify specific functions and the locations of specific genes" (Castells 2001 p 164). In addition to this, some philosophical problems arise from the view that DNA and the Human Genome are pure informational concepts. In one sense, the convergence between the biological and computing might be thought to be associated with the massive use of computer technologies in biology. Computers are convenient tools for genome and protein sequencing. However, the bioinformatics paradigm has been central to the reorganization of disciplines such as molecular biology (Holdsworth 1999). In the process, they have absorbed Shannon's technical notion of information.

Genome science has emerged as the next wave of human scientific research. There are a number of important ways that genomics differs from genetics. Genetics is the study of genes and the inherited differences and variation in DNA and its influence on phenotypes (Interview 1001; Interview 1022). The Department of Energy's Human Genome Project website defines genomics as "the study of genes and their function,"[4] as well as their interactions with environmental factors (Interview 1022). Genome Canada calls genomics "big picture science," whose central aim is to understand the "complexity of how genes interact with each other and their environment to make living organisms function."[5] Genomics is largely driven by the impetus to understand the differences in genomes, such as the variations in sequences at the same locations in a DNA strand, between different individuals and population groups, and the origins of complex diseases such as cancer. Where genetics looks at individual genes, genomics focuses on the entire collection of the six billion chemical bases, the As, Cs, Gs, and Ts, that are strung together in our 23 pairs of chromosomes. These more technical definitions based in biology miss some important technological, social, and cultural characteristics of genomics. One of the main challenges of genomics is the enormous amount of data involved in studying the 3 billion letters of code in a strand of human DNA and the sheer number of relevant variables that has necessitated an enabling link to computing. Developing from the convergence of molecular biology and computing science, genomics can also be defined as the computer-assisted comprehensive study of all genes (Interview 1001).

Like many new technologies, boosterism about its scientific potential leads into possible social benefits. Francis Collins, the former director of the National Human Genome Research Institute (NHGRI; one of the National Institutes of Health), states about the promises of genomics for society:

> Genomics has been at the forefront of giving serious attention . . . to the impact of science and technology on society. Although the major benefits to be realized from genomics are in the area of health . . . genomics can also contribute to other aspects of society. Just as the [Human Genome Project] and related developments have spawned new areas of research in basic biology and in health, they have also created opportunities for research on social issues, even to the extent of understanding more fully how we define ourselves and each other. (Collins 2003:483)

Evelyn Fox Keller (2000) has shown how the importance and prominence of gene thinking grew in scientific and popular discourse during the twentieth century. Genome thinking may be growing at an even faster rate as we have entered the "genome era" (Bonham et al. 2005:9). While genetics emerged from the insights of Mendel and the scientific practice of observation by sight, which are "analog" practices, genomics is emblematic of a cultural shift in scientific practice characterized by digital observation, data mining analysis, and computer automation. If the twentieth century was the century of the gene, then the twenty-first may well be shaping up to become the century of the genome.

Genomics Goes Global: The International
HapMap Project and Database Networks

I don't think [HapMap] could have happened without the Internet, honestly. (Interview 1016)

I think that, in fact, in many circles genomic research has been discussed as developing out of DNA technology. I think it is fair to say that the entire concept of genomics, which is really one of data rich studies in biology where you have archival quality data that is comprehensive and is shared freely, is as much about, if not more about, computers and the Internet as it is about DNA technology. (Interview 1001)

A key site to examine the intersection of science, bioinformatics, communication technologies, and racialized identity is the next HGP, the International HapMap Project. The project is a multisite, international venture between scientific teams in Canada, China, Japan, Nigeria, the United Kingdom, and the United States. The project is in the process of mapping haplotypes of human genomes. Haplotypes are identifiable block-like patterns of the DNA nucleotides, A, C, G, and T. A genome consists of individually sequenced strings of nucleotides. The aim of the HGP was to create a comprehensive map sequence of an individual's DNA. In 2001, scientists shifted the focus to haplotypes in the genome. Haplotypes are "neighborhoods" of DNA that can be identified by common genetic variants in the genome sequence, revealing an underlying structure in a genome. Identifying the locations of the variants, called single nucleotide polymorphisms (or SNPs), can facilitate and speed up subsequent research into the genetic origins of disease (International HapMap Consortium 2003). Since the project began in 2001, Phase I and Phase II of the project sampled groups from Europe, Africa, and Asia (China and Japan). Where the organizers of the HGP declared humanity's genetic similarity, HapMap searches for differences. Like the HGP before, communication technologies are at the heart of mapping, sequencing, and data gathering, storage, analysis, and distribution.

Information sharing, data transfer, and analysis operate on a global scale from the sample collection sites in Africa, Asian, and North America to the sequencing and research centers. As the project's network of labs are scattered across the globe, the only way for genome scientists to construct a haplotype map of "major geographical groups," as they are named in the project, is to disassemble DNA into digital packets, send them through the Internet, and reassemble them in a SNP database. Each team of the HapMap project sequences a portion of the genome, such as Chromosome 2 and Chromosome 4p by the McGill University/Genome Quebec group in Canada, Chromosome 7p by the group at Washington University in St. Louis and the University of San Francisco, or others, both academic labs and biotechnology companies, in China, Japan, and the United Kingdom. The data from each group is collected, curated, and stored for distribution in a database in

Bethesda, Maryland, at the National Institutes of Health and released online for public access within twenty-four hours. The scientists' most important tools for the collection, databasing, and manipulation of genome sequences are communication technologies.

With the interaction of computer science and molecular biology, genomics has moved biomedical research to computational biology (Interview 1006). Accordingly, a number of respondents agreed that, without the rich, flexible, and networked databases, as well as increasing speeds of computing, the impact of genomics would be trivial compared to what it is today. Developments in genomics are as much feats of technological management, archiving, and distribution as advances in scientific knowledge (Interview 1001). Genomics simply would not be feasible by hand, which would make it impossible to analyze a single genome or make comparisons between individuals, groups, or even species (Interview 1003; Interview 1011). HapMap participants commonly discussed two technological developments in particular, databases/data mining and the Internet. New databases have been designed to store, analyze, and distribute the data and findings. Data mining techniques and "large, easily accessible databases that would allow the extraction and comparison of data [were] absolutely essential for being able to put together any kind of sequence database" (Interview 1014). The Internet enables genome projects to move data between global locations and labs in the same building as well as providing open access for anyone interested in the data. These large-scale information infrastructures are the back end of scientific information. They are referenced, but not normally discussed, in the scientific journals and media stories about scientific discovery. Further, they have become new technologies of difference in the informationalization of race and crucial to the new information science.

According to Leroy Hood, an early developer of sequencing technology in the 1980s, the genome posed such enormous technological challenges with sequencing, mapping, computation, analysis that a new paradigm, discovery science, was needed to tackle the obstacles posed by building and analyzing a comprehensive database. Developed during the heady years of the Human Genome Project, discovery science utilizes KDD to reorganize and sequence the haplotype blocks. Much like the basic assumptions of data mining described above, discovery science takes an object of analysis, such as a strand of DNA, and defines and collects all of the elements in it, rather than sampling or sequencing only part of it, and puts all the information in a database. In contrast to the meticulous method of making theoretically sound hypothesis before collecting and analyzing data, discovery science is more of a collect first and asks questions later approach. Craig Venter and the Celera Genome Project innovated a procedure called the "shotgun method." As Internet protocols and capacity grew in the 1990s, the new communication infrastructure became a key conduit for moving data. In the HapMap Project, the Internet allowed researchers to upload data from local sites and sequencing centers to the centralized database in Bethesda.

The HapMap consortium collected samples from "populations with ancestry from parts of Africa, Asia, and Europe" (International HapMap Consortium 2003: 789). While project organizers deliberately decided to refer to the sample groups in terms of populations and not racial groups, the initial groups do match a traditional American taxonomy of race. Lee (2005) points out that choosing such geographically disparate groups accentuates any genetic distances/differences, rather than using more gradual differences between more historically proximate groups. The gradual differences, she argues, "might uproot conventional notions of racial boundaries and inspire new trajectories of research that dispense with age-old notions of racial difference" (Lee 2005: 2135). This reinforces the racial triangle of black, white, and Asian. When the National Human Genome Research Institute (NHGRI) of the National Institutes of Health (NIH) decided to build databases and a haplotype map, the scientists involved had to make a decision on which markers would be included. They decided that the groups would be labeled according to geographical, rather than racial, signifiers. I have been told that the discussions at the preliminary HapMap meetings held in the summer of 2001 were very open about the issue of racial identification. When asked about the place of race in the schedule of items being discussed and whether or not it was an important issue or a marginal one, a bioethicist in attendance commented that it was "in the fabric of the meeting." Another attendee described the discussions of race and community as at an elementary level.

> . . . it's been an educational process for some, especially the genetic scientists, but also for the people involved in all aspects. Some scientists were using . . . East Asian or even Asian as a name for the Japanese and Han-Chinese sample. We insisted that this is inappropriate, as Asia includes too many different groups; I mean thousands of different groups. China itself includes fifty groups, and you can't call people like this. Therefore we adopted the name JPT, and it was a long discussion, and I think everyone had a kind of contention on this in the end. I think the question of concern about racial discrimination and racial discrimination and classifying these HapMap samples in that way was a serious concern for everyone involved. That was the reason for the care in taking the naming of the samples. Inside Japan, I don't think the concern is of any discrimination of Japanese people in Japan; the concern for the Japanese people [is] discrimination when the population exists as a minority, for example in the Americas or Europe or Asia, [or] other Asian countries anywhere. (Interview 1011)

By making a shift from biological notions of race to geographic ones, scientists seem to be making a return to the Linnaean racial classification systems of the eighteenth century (Banton 1988). I would suggest that the impetus for this return is not entirely ideological and may be the result of the emerging ability that communication technologies enable for genome sequencing and more fine-grained analysis of genetic differences. The HapMap database is an effect of the digital age and new processes of knowledge construction in the discipline of science.

When interviewed, most HapMap members are quick to point out that they do not use race but geographical ancestry to define the population groups. Not all the members referred to the groups by geographic ancestry, however. A white statistical geneticist suggested equivalence between "the three sort of major continental groups or racial groups or whatever your preferred term is" (Interview 1002). When differences in a selected haplotype sequence (patterns of SNPs or single nucleotide polymorphisms) between these three groups are reported, this can easily suggest, especially in the context of a racialized society, the conclusion that the differences are racial, genetic, and biological. For example, Hinds et al. (2005) report on whole-genome patterns of DNA variation between these three "population groups" and examine millions of SNPs. While this number seems rather large, the total number of individuals from whom the samples were collected was seventy-one, which is a very low sample size to assess any variation between groups. Further, when scientists collect and name the samples and enter them into databases, the distinctions they make between the social and scientific meanings of race are not clear (Fullwiley 2007a; 2007b).

Lee raises a more important question, "if there is no genetic basis for race, then why do large scale mapping projects continue to use racial categories in identifying research populations?" (2005:2135; see also S. Lee, chapter 10 in this volume). The answer lies partly in the tradition of population genetics and physical anthropology that provides the scientific basis for choosing the four groups. Clearly, there was an opportunity lost in debunking the relationship between genes and race by choosing populations that are geographically distant from one another, rather than ones closer together genetically and geographically. In addition, and this is an equally important issue for identity, there are socio-political opportunities for states who participate in large-scale genome projects. China and Japan have been eager to assert themselves, not only regionally, as leading countries geopolitically in Asia, but on the world stage. Nigeria occupies a similar position in Africa. HapMap organizers chose

> groups that were either already being engaged in some genetic research or they were groups that researchers had already a relationship or a collaboration with these groups or with persons in those communities. . . . They had contacts. They re-consented most of the people who were alive or whose families were part of . . . CEPH. With the other populations, the Chinese population and the Japanese, those populations, the specific populations, the groups that were targeted, well I shouldn't say targeted, were identified and participated, were really groups where there was some contact or some existing collaboration with those groups, for some researchers who was doing some research for that group or that community or a collaborator in that community. (Interview 1022)

Choosing the research sites and initial sample populations in the case of HapMap were matters of convenience and accessibility (Duster 2005). This is a common occurrence across the natural and social sciences. As the dominant organizing principle in the information age is the network, power operates through the space of flows. In the case of HapMap, flows of scientific knowledge and social/professional networks are accessible to scholars and states who can tap into them. In the early 1990s, Gilbert warned that the proliferation of databases would create a digital divide: "The next tenfold increase in the amount of information in the databases will divide the world into haves and have-nots, unless each of us connects to that information and learns how to sift through it for the parts we need" (quoted in Lenoir 1999:18).

For example, Cambodia or Vietnam were not "chosen" or "targeted" to represent Asia, nor was Sierra Leone for Africa, because HapMap organizers did not have relationships with anyone there and state governments lacked the funds or the international political capital to participate in the new global venture. However, some members see the data coming out of HapMap as being able to overcome this kind of digital divide.

> I think it's an opportunity for the West and the industrialized economies to efficiently transfer the intellectual benefits of wealth and investment and this technology to the developing world. There's no reason that South Africa has to re-sequence the human genome to study the parts that are relevant to urban disease there, they can leverage off of what we've done internationally. So, I think that's a fantastic opportunity for international science and humanities as a whole. I think science can bridge boundaries in a way that other cultural enterprises can't do. (Interview 1016)

Conclusion

As the information age advances and analog social, cultural, and scientific practices are recoded into the digital networks of global communication, the transformation of racial identity and signifying systems pose new challenges for scholars of race and science. In the case of genomics and the HapMap Project, the informationalization of race signals a shift in the way that big science is conducted, how the materials used for analysis have become digital information, and how this process is sorting people in new, and old, ways. Many scholars and activists assumed that the decoupling of race and biology and the enclosure of racial identity in a social constructivist paradigm was a *fait accompli* at the close of the twentieth century. However, rather than destroying race as a biological category and providing conclusive proof that we are indeed all the same, as the UNESCO statements after World War II tried to establish and leaders of the Human Genome Project proclaimed fifty years later, the specter of genetic differences that distinguish human groups has not only been raised once again, but given new currency.

The context for this gene war of maneuver is not slavery and colonialization in the eighteenth century, or scientific racism in the nineteenth century, or the eugenics movement in the first half of the twentieth century; at the beginning of the twenty-first century new genomic forms of racial knowledge are emerging at the convergence of multiculturalism and the ideology of colorblindness, new database and digital communication networks, globalization, and the ascendancy of biology. Both citizens and scholars need to be a part of this struggle over the nature of defining who we are at the most basic level of human life.

The main challenges for those who are against bio-race are on two fronts, one socio-technological and one socio-scientific. First, the processes of creating, storing, and transmitting information have become resources for the production of power. The policies, politics, and procedures that make up information infrastructures are hidden in the seeming neutrality of codes and standards. We, the users, only see the interface. Information and the networks that compose a communication infrastructure are much more than the denotative transmission of facts, computer algorithms, and data. Information is not simply descriptive and reflective of the social world; the collection, storage, and analysis of information constitutes what is known and what can be imagined, both of these bases for social action.

Information in the global new economy is deeply connotative. In this respect, race as information works in a similar manner to race as culture or race as (the epidermal) body. However, due to the hypertext of the Internet and the anti-narrative logic of databases and related new media technologies, information is much more contingent and fluid. Critical scholars of race need to continue to address the role of new technologies and new media in the process of racialization and engage in larger debates about surveillance, privacy and personal information, and intellectual property.

The socio-scientific front, like the socio-techno, is well under way. The five percent of funding allocated to social science and humanities research remains in place at the NIH's National Human Genome Research Institute. Public genome projects, such as HapMap, have built into them Ethical, Legal, and Social Implications (ELSI) committees made up of interdisciplinary teams composed of scientists, NGOs, bioethicists, lawyers, sociologists, and anthropologists. The Canadian version of ELSI, called GE3LS, sets aside a similar amount of funding, while some social science researchers have managed to secure 10 percent in their collaborations with applied genomics projects. Genome British Columbia goes a step further by funding applied genomics research projects where there is an integrated social science or humanities (SSH) component. At the proposal level this has meant that the SSH researcher stands as a co-applicant. It is crucial that this type of configuration continues.

With all these provisions and points of contact between the natural and social sciences in place, we are still seeing research results from the HapMap database being reported in prominent publications, such as *Science*, with declarations such as "In Asians and whites, gene expression varies by race" (Couzin 2007:173). This startling article was followed up the next month, where a letter to the editor states, "race is truly a biological and taxonomic problem." (Billinger 2007:766) Interestingly, while many science publications, including *Nature*, have instituted editorial policies on the use of race in research, *Science* still does not. In the absence of such a policy, letters to the editor could be sent to point out the uncritical use of race and ethnicity in such articles and research reports. Similarly, at the point when scientific findings are translated to the public, usually through the news media, editors should be notified and supported when stories such as Amy Harmon's *New York Times* article "In DNA era, new worries about prejudice" (2007) are published. Similarly, we can send words of support to politicians when they make statements against racism, such as mayor of London's censure of James Watson's comments in 2007. Also, there are a number of NGOs, such as GeneWatch in the United Kingdom and the Council for Responsible Genetics and the Indigenous People's Council on Biocolonialism in the United States, who work in the public interest by monitoring scientific research, publishing working papers and newsletters, and representing various community stakeholders. While Ethical, Legal, and Social Implications (ELSI) committees attached to genome projects such as HapMap are made cognizant of issues of identity, community consent, and privacy, the role and meaning of new technologies are usually assumed to be instrumental. There is little discussion of the ethical, legal, and social implications of new communication technologies.

While the technological utopianism of the 1990s has been replaced by more tempered approaches to the benefits of Web 2.0 that alternate between empowerment and participation on the one hand and surveillance and control on the other, we have seen that the rise of the Internet has not meant the end of racial identities. As research has shown, practices of race are at the same time transcribed and transcoded into cyberspace as well as lived there and here in RL. Further, the seeming neutrality of data mining techniques and database construction is also dependent on the nature of the data and algorithms that tells programs what to do. The standards and codes that make the design infrastructure of databases and related technologies shape their function and meaning at the user interface. In the case of genome and DNA databases, race is inscribed into the front and back ends of the technology.

The need for theoretical connections between technology and race from observations of the biomedical sciences is particularly important at this time. With the turn to the 0.1 percent of the genome that differentiates one person from another there are over 3 million points of difference that are under intense scrutiny as governments and companies create public and private haplotype maps. DNA as an object of knowledge is not only of interest to molecular biologists. DNA databases are being compiled by law enforcement agencies at both the national and local levels, such as the FBI's CODIS database, and by ancestry companies and biotechnology companies working on pharmaceuticals.

The authors in this section explore DNA technologies and instantiations of the informationalization of race in a number of enterprises. Pamela Sankar discusses forensic DNA phenotyping technologies (FDP) that are being developed by law enforcement agencies to visualize DNA evidence. Where DNA evidence is used to confirm the identity of suspects, FDP, by contrast, uses genetic code to predict what the yet to be apprehended suspect looks like in terms of facial features and other observable phenotypes. In the courts, Jon Kahn argues that the validity of DNA evidence is largely taken for granted in identifying suspects and predicting race and ethnicity. His chapter highlights the lack of attention to the technical complexities of using race and ethnicity as a genetic concept by showing, in part, how the informational procedures of coding genetic regions for race have changed since the early 1990s. Lee examines how genomics databases are shaped in the field of pharmacogenomics, which is the application of human genome variation research to the development of genome-based drugs that scientists hope will increase efficacy and safety for patients and reduce adverse reactions. While this type of research has been heralded as a major step in the direction of personalized medicine, tailored to an individual's genetic code, Lee suggests that, since the expense of sequencing technology is still prohibitive for a mass market, scientists tend to focus on differences at the level of populations. This type of focus is producing a growing literature on genetic differences between groups that are coded as African, Asian, and Caucasian. The databases for theses various enterprises based on DNA information are built by both public and private organizations.

While the public projects operate under the ethos of open access in an effort to democratize the data and community consent models, private firms are under no obligation to adopt such policies. This should be cause for concern, especially as the mapping of DNA turns to the function of DNA. One of the white scientists who has been particularly outspoken about the focus on race in HapMap suggested that ongoing discussions about racialization in genomics is regressive and that people who suggest the HapMap Project and other genome mapping ventures can and will reproduce race are naysayers. However, the same scientist offered a future implication of genomics. He suggested to me, "the rubber has not really hit the road yet." For him, the ancestral information that may be contained in DNA is a superficial issue. Genome maps of human populations are not productive of or reproducing the scientific racism of the past or reifying race. Knowing where your mother came from through your mitochondria does not say much except what our geographical origins may be. This may be true if one removes social and historical context of that information. However, as I argue in this essay, such knowledge contributes to and is produced in discursive formations of the informationalization of race. The interviewee continued,

> But what is going to be problematic and we're not prepared to deal with is what if, or not what if because it will happen, what about when someone does find a gene that does affect a trait of high interest that's not medical

perhaps but sort of behavioral, and that gene variant is not equally represented across different ethnic groups, all of sudden we won't be in this confused sort of meaningless realm we've been in to some extent, we're going
to be in a new realm where there are genes that effect traits and they're
not evenly distributed across populations. Then we're going to have a real
problem. (Interview 1001)

This particular problem is (re)surfacing at a time when science, technology, and
race are interacting in new ways. The informationalization of race attempts to
understand this transformation by recognizing that technological, scientific, and
cultural change are not separate processes but are intimately bound up with one
another. In order to avoid returning to the alter of biological determinism, debates
about genomics and race need to be expanded to incorporate technology beyond
simple mentions of the presence of supercomputers in genomic research and
their usefulness for sequencing DNA faster and cheaper. Like old media forms, new
media technologies, such as databases and the Internet, are sites of negotiation
over cultural meaning, social facts, and the politics of racial representation.

APPENDIX

A number of the individuals interviewed were principal investigators of the
various research sites. A couple committee chairs also participated. Only the
participants' broad areas of expertise are included to protect their identities.

Interview 1001	Population geneticist
Interview 1003	Site project manager
Interview 1006	Microbiologist
Interview 1011	Bioethicist
Interview 1014	Human geneticist
Interview 1016	Population geneticist
Interview 1017	Bioethicist
Interview 1022	Geneticist and bioethicist

ACKNOWLEDGMENTS

Some passages of this chapter first appeared as "The informationalization of race:
Communication technologies and the Human Genome in the Digital Age" (2008)
in the International Journal of Communication.

NOTES

1. By the term *communication technologies,* I am following Castells and others to include the
   "*converging set* of technologies in micro-electronics, computing (machines and software), telecommunications/broadcasting, and opto-electronics" as well as Internet
   applications and DNA technologies (Castells 2000:29).

2. The interview protocol and procedures were conducted under IRB regulations of the University of Southern California. Identification of subjects is public knowledge and was obtained through the International HapMap Consortium publications. Subjects were recruited by letter, email, and telephone calls. Telephone and on-site interviews were conducted and recorded by the author. Even though the interviews were recorded, I also took notes to help guide questions in the interview and for reflection post-interview. When the interview was completed, I would go over the notes and make annotations for issues and items that could be addressed in subsequent interviews and/or analysis. I developed a coding schedule (which was constantly being refined in an interative fashion). Then, I used a qualitative software program, Nvivo to code the interviews. I coded three main sub-sections first and further coding was necessary until the response had been categorized sufficiently, usually no more than three levels. After identifying a broad number of sub-codes, I refined them, merging similar codes and eliminating some if there were fewer then three responses to the code. In creating a report outline, I looked at what was said and how it corresponded to the literature in the area (or not), and then tried to develop report sections that would correspond to both the literature and data.

3. This research utilizes a multi-methodological approach. I conducted the interviews for this research study in 2005, with members of the HapMap Project, which includes geneticists, lawyers, anthropologists, bioethicists, doctors, bioinformaticians, project managers, biologists, directors of NGOs, and pharmacologists. I also interviewed senior scientists from a leading biotechnology company. Archival data for textual analysis was collected from key biomedical and scientific journals such as *Science, Nature, Nature Genetics, Genomics, Genome Biology,* the *Journal of the American Medical Association,* the *New England Journal of Medicine,* and the *British Medical Journal.*

4. www.ornl.gov/sci/techresources/Human_Genome/glossary/glossary_g.shtml

5. www.genomecanada.ca/en/info/DNA/genomics.aspx

WORKS CITED

Banton, M. 1998. *Racial theories.* 2nd ed. Cambridge: Cambridge University Press.

Barkan, E. 1992. *Retreat of scientific racism: Changing concepts of race in Britain and the United States between the World Wars.* Cambridge: Cambridge University Press.

Barker, M. 1982. *The new racism: Conservatives and the ideology of the tribe.* London: Junction Books.

Bonham, V. L., E. Warshauer-Baker, and F. S. Collins. 2005. Race and ethnicity in the genome era: The complexity of the constructs. *American Psychologist* 60 (1):9–15.

Bonilla-Silva, E. 2001. *White supremacy and racism in post-civil rights era.* Boulder, CO: Lynne Rienner Publishers.

———. 2003. *Racism without racists: Color-blind racism and the persistence of racial inequality in the United States.* Boulder, CO: Rowman and Littlefield.

Bowker, G., and S. L. Star. 1999. *Sorting things out: Classification and its consequences.* Cambridge, MA: MIT Press.

Brown, M., M. Carnoy, E. Currie, T. Duster, D. Oppenheimer, M. Shultz, and D. Wellman. 2003. *Whitewashing race: The myth of a color-blind society.* Berkeley: University of California Press.

Burchard, E. González, E. Ziv, N. Coyle, S. Gomez, H. Tang, A. Karter, J. Mountain, E. Pérez-Stable, D. Sheppard, and N. Risch. 2003. The importance of race and ethnic background in biomedical research and clinical practice. *New England Journal of Medicine* 348 (12):1170–1175.

Capra, F. 2002. *The hidden connections: Integrating the biological, cognitive, and social dimensions of life into a science of sustainability.* New York: Doubleday.

Castells, M. 2000. *Rise of the network society.* 2nd ed. *The information age: Economy, society and culture.* Oxford: Blackwell Publishers.

———. 2001. Informationalism and the network society. In *The hacker ethic and the spirit of the information age,* edited by P. Himanen. London: Vintage.

Césaire, A. 1972. *Discourse on colonialism.* New York: Monthly Review Press.

Collins, F., E. Green, A. Guttmacher, and M. Guyer. 2003. A vision for the future of genomics research: A blueprint for the genomic era. *Nature* 422 (24):835–847.

Collins, P. 2004. *Black sexual politics: African Americans, gender, and the new racism.* New York: Routledge.

Cubitt, S. 2000. The distinctiveness of digital criticism. *Screen* 41 (1):86–92.

Devlin, B., and N. Risch. 1992. Ethnic differentiation at VNTR loci, with specific reference to forensic applications. *American Journal of Human Genetics* (51):534–548.

Duster, T. 2003. *Backdoor to eugenics.* New York: Routledge.

———. 2005. Race and reification in science. *Science* 307 (5712):1050–1051.

Elmer, G. 2004. *Profiling machines: Mapping the personal information economy.* Cambridge, MA: MIT Press.

Evett, I., I. Buckleton, A. Raymond, and H. Roberts. 1993. The evidential value of DNA profiles. *Journal of the Forensic Science Society* 33 (4):243–244.

Evett, I., P. Gill, J. Scranage, and B. Wier. 1996. Establishing the robustness of Short-Tandem-Repeat statistics for forensic application. *American Journal of Human Genetics* 33 (3):398–407.

Eze, E. C., ed. 1997. *Race and the Enlightenment: A reader.* Cambridge: Blackwell.

Fanon, F. 1963. *The wretched of the earth.* New York: Grove Press.

———. 1967. *Black skin, white masks.* Translated by C. L. Markmann. New York: Grove Press.

Fausto-Sterling, A. 2004. Refashioning race: DNA and the politics of health care. *Differences* 15 (3):1–37.

Fayyad, U. 1991. On the induction of decision trees for multiple concept learning (machine learning). Ph.D. dissertation, University of Michigan.

Foucault, M. 1977. *Discipline and punish: The birth of the prison.* 2nd ed. New York: Vintage Books.

———. 1978. *The history of sexuality: An introduction.* Vol. 1. New York: Vintage Books.

Fullwiley, D. 2007a. Race and genetics: Attempts to define the relationship. *Biosocieties* 2:221–237.

———. 2007b. The molecularization of race: Institutionalizing human difference in pharmacogenetics practice. *Science as Culture* 16 (1):1–30.

Galambos, L., and J. Sturchio. 1998. Pharmaceutical firms and the transition to biotechnology: A study in strategic innovation. *Business History Review* 72 (2):250–278.

Galloway, A., and Thacker, A. 2007. *The exploit: A theory of networks.* Minneapolis: University of Minnesota Press.

Gandy, O. 2002. The real digital divide. In *Handbook of new media,* edited by L. Lievrouw and S. Livingstone. Thousand Oaks, CA: Sage.

———. 2006. Data mining, surveillance, and discrimination in the post-9/11 environment. In *The new politics of surveillance and visibility,* edited by K. Haggerty and R. Ericson. Toronto: University of Toronto Press.

Garfinkel, S. 2000. *Database nation: The death of privacy in the 21st century.* Sebastopol, CA: O'Reilly.

Gezelter, D. 2005. Catalyzing open source development in science: The OpenScience Project. www.openscience.org/talks/bnl/imgo.htm [Accessed March 28].

Gilroy, P. 2000. *Against race: Imagining political culture beyond the color line.* Cambridge, MA: Belknap Press of Harvard University Press.

Gould, S. J. 1996. *The mismeasure of man.* Revised and expanded ed. New York: Norton.

Gray, H. 2005. *Cultural moves: African Americans and the politics of representation.* Berkeley: University of California Press.

Haggerty, K., and R. Ericson, eds. 2006. *The new politics of surveillance and visibility.* Toronto: University of Toronto Press.

Haiman, C., D. Stram, L. Wilkens, M. Pike, L. Kolonel, B. Henderson, and L. Le Marchand. 2006. Ethnic and racial differences in the smoking-related risk of lung cancer. *New England Journal of Medicine* 354 (4):333–342.

Hammonds, E. 1997. New technologies of race. In *Processed lives: Gender and technology in everyday life,* edited by J. Terry and M. Calvert. New York: Routledge.

Hayles, N. K. 1999. *How we became posthuman: Virtual bodies in cybernetics, literature, and informatics.* Chicago: University of Chicago Press.

Hinds, D. A., L. L. Stuve, G. B. Nilsen, E. Halperin, F. Eskin, D. G. Ballinger, et al. 2005. Whole-genome patterns of common DNA variation in three human populations. *Science* 307 (5712):1072–1079.

Holdsworth, D. 1999. The ethics of the 21st century bioinformatics: Ethical implications of the vanishing distinction between biological information and other information. In *Genetic information. acquisition, access and control,* edited by A. K. Thompson and R. Chadwick. New York: Kluwer/Plenum.

Hood, L. 2001. Under biology's hood. *Technology Review* 54 (September):52–57.

Ignacio, E. N. 2005. *Building diaspora: Filipino community formation on the Internet.* New Brunswick, NJ: Rutgers University Press.

International HapMap Consortium. 2003. The International HapMap Project. *Nature* 426 (18):789–796.

Jobling, M., and P. Gill. 2004. Encoded evidence: DNA in forensic analysis. *Nature Reviews Genetics* 5:739–752.

Jordan, W. 1974. *The white man's burden: Historical origins of racism in the United States.* New York: Oxford University Press.

Keita, S., R. Kittles, C. Royal, G. Bonney, P. Furbert-Harris, G. Dunston, and C. Rotimi. 2004. Conceptualizing human variation. *Nature Genetics* 36 (11):S17–S20.

Kim, C. 1999. The racial triangulation of Asian Americans. *Politics and Society* 27 (1):105–138.

Kolko, B., L. Nakamura, and G. Rodman, eds. 2000. *Race in cyberspace.* New York: Routledge.

Krimsky, S. 1999. The profit of scientific discovery and its normative implications. *Chicago-Kent Law Review* 75 (15):15–40.

Landow, G. 1992. *Hypertext: The convergence of contemporary cultural theory and technology.* Baltimore: John Hopkins University Press.

Lee, S. 2005. Racializing drug design: Implications for pharmacogenomics for health disparities. *American Journal of Public Health* 95 (12):2133–2138.

Leung, L. 2005. *Virtual ethnicity: Race, resistance, and the World Wide Web.* Burlington, VT: Ashgate.

Lipsitz, G. 1998. *The possessive investment in whiteness: How white people profit from identity politics.* Philadelphia: Temple University Press.

Loro, L. 1995. Everyone's talkin' in the "multilogue." *Advertising Age* 66 (35):28.

Lowe, A., A. Urquhart, L. Foreman, and I. Evett. 2001. Inferring ethnic origin by means of an STR profile. *Forensic Science International* (119):17–22.

Lyon, D. 2002. Everyday surveillance: Personal data and social classifications. *Information, Communication and Society* 5 (2):242–257.

———. 2003. *Surveillance as social sorting: Privacy, risk and digital discrimination.* London: Routledge.

102 PETER A. CHOW-WHITE

——. 2005. The sociology of information. In *The Sage handbook of sociology*, edited by C. Calhoun, C. Rojec, and B. Turner. London: Sage.

Mackenzie, A. 2003. Bringing sequences to life: How bioinformatics corporealizes sequence data. *New Genetics and Society* 22 (3):315–332.

Manovich, L. 1999. Database as symbolic form. *Convergence: The Journal of Research into New Media Technologies* 5 (2):80–99.

Marturano, A., and Chadwick, R. 2004. How the role of computing is driving new genetics' public policy. *Ethics and Information Technology* 6:43–53.

Memmi, A. 1965. *The colonizer and the colonized*. New York: Orion Press.

Meyers, C., and Davis, S. 2003. *It's alive: The coming convergence of information, biology, and business*. New York: Crown Business.

Miles, R. 1989. *Racism*. London: Routledge.

Moody, G. 2004. *Digital code of life: How bioinformatics is revolutionizing, science, medicine, and business*. Hoboken, NJ: John Wiley and Sons.

Mosse, G. 1978. *Toward the Final Solution: A history of European racism*. New York: H. Firtig.

Nakamura, L. 2002. *Cybertypes: Race, ethnicity, and identity on the Internet*. New York: Routledge.

——. 2008. *Digitizing race: Visual cultures of the Internet*. Minnesota: University of Minnesota Press.

Nelkin, D., and L. Tancredi. 1989. *Dangerous diagnotics: The social power of biological information*. New York: Basic Books.

Nelson, A. 2002. Introduction: Future texts. *Social Text* 20 (2):1–15.

Omi, M., and Winant, H. 1994. *Racial formation in the United States: From the 1960s to the 1990s*. 2nd ed. New York: Routledge.

Poster, M. 1991. *The mode of information: Poststructuralism and social context*. Chicago: University of Chicago Press.

Rantanen, T. 2005. The message is the medium: An interview with Manuel Castells. *Global Media and Communication* 1 (2):135–147.

Rasmussen, T. 2000. *Social theory and communication technology*. Aldershot: Ashgate Publishing.

Razack, S. 1998. *Looking white people in the eye: Gender, race, and culture in courtrooms and classrooms*. Toronto: University of Toronto Press.

Risch, N. 2006. Dissecting racial and ethnic differences. *New England Journal of Medicine* 354 (4):408–411.

Rosenberg, N., M. Murata, Y. Ikeda, O. Opare-Sem, A. Zivelin, E. Geffen, and U. Seligsohn. 2002. The frequent 5,10-methylenetetrahydrofolate reductase C677T polymorphism is associated with a common haplotype in whites, Japanese, and Africans. *American Journal of Human Genetics* 70 (3):758–762.

Rosenberg, N., J. Pritchard, J. Weber, H. Cann, K. Kidd, L. Zhivotovsky, and M. Feldman. 2002. Genetic structure of human populations. *Science* (298):2381–2385.

Rotman, D. 2005. Race and medicine. *Technology Review* 107 (4).

Royal, C. and G. Dunston. 2004. Changing the paradigm from "race" to human genome variation. *Nature Genetics* 36 (11):S5–S7.

Said, E. 1978. *Orientalism*. New York: Vintage.

Schiller, D. 1999. *Digital capitalism: Networking the global market system*. Cambridge, MA: MIT Press.

Stepan, N. 1982. *The idea of race in science: Great Britain, 1800–1960*. London: Macmillan.

Taguieff, P. A. 1990. The new cultural racism in France. *Telos* 83 (spring):109–122.

Thacker, E. 2004. *Biomedia*. Minneapolis: University of Minnesota Press.

Tishkoff, S., and K. Kidd. 2004. Implications of biogeography of human populations for "race" and medicine. *Nature Genetics* 36 (11):S21–S27.

UNESCO. 1953. *The race concept: Results of an inquiry.* Paris: UNESCO.

———. 1969. *Four statements on the race question.* Paris: UNESCO.

Wade, Nicholas. 2007. Studies find more genes underlying diabetes. *New York Times*, April 26, Online.

Waldrop, M. Mitchell. 2001. Data mining. *Technology Review* (January/February). Online.

Webster, F. 2002. *Theories of the information society.* London: Routledge.

Wellcome Trust Case Control Consortium. 2007. Genome-wide association study of 14,000 cases of seven common diseases and 3,000 shared controls. *Nature* 447 (7145): 661–678.

Wellman, B. 2004. The three ages of Internet studies: ten, five, and zero years ago. *New Media and Society* 6 (1):123–129.

Wellman, D. 2003. Color blindness as color consciousness. Paper read at Color-Blind Racism Conference, October 3, at Stanford University, Palo Alto, California.

West, C., and H. Gates. 1997. *The future of the race.* New York: Vintage.

Zarsky, T. 2003. "Mine your own business!": Making the case for the implications of the data mining of personal information in the forum of public opinion. *Yale Journal of Law and Technology* 5:1–57.

7

Forensic DNA Phenotyping

Continuity and Change in the History of Race, Genetics, and Policing

PAMELA SANKAR

At the 2004 Forensic Bioinformatics conference in Ohio, a speaker announced that a new software program, DNAwitness, had triggered the start of the revolution in forensics.[1] Ushering in the new era would be the program's capability to decipher "an individual's race" "from crime scene DNA." Based on analysis of "the heritable component of race," referred to as biogeographical ancestry, the program would produce a "precise estimation" of the percentages of different types of ancestry present in the DNA sample, including Indo European, Sub-Saharan African, East Asian, or Native American and, using these estimates, produce a description of a person's appearance that police could use to narrow down a pool of suspects.

While DNAwitness and its parent company DNAPrint have not had the success they hoped for, the genetic technology on which the program relies, referred to broadly as forensic DNA phenotyping (FDP), has continued to develop in Europe as well as in the United States.[2]

In addition to analysis of genetic ancestry, DNAPrint and other companies are working to identify genotypes associated with gait, voice, and predisposition to behavioral traits such as smoking or to medical conditions such as diabetes. FDP technology, should it come into general use, would fundamentally transform the existing function of DNA in law enforcement, limited now to confirming a suspect's identity. FDP efforts to find genetic markers that are associated with physical appearance seek to get past this limit and bring the power of DNA to the antecedent task of predicting who the suspect will be. Law enforcement refers to the capacity to produce information rather than only confirm it as using DNA for "intelligence purposes."[3]

Unlike DNA-typing, there are no accepted standards for procedures or calculations to anchor the results produced by FDP analysis. The few published examples of FDP-based descriptions, such as "largely West African"[4] or "a light

104

skinned black,"[5] are notably vague and presumably would require police to rely on implicit stereotypes in order to apply them. Still FDP has succeeded in effectively redirecting investigations by shifting police attention from suspects in one racial grouping to those in another.[6] It is important to examine these outcomes and consider what they mean relative to the broader claims of FDP.

FDP's premise that phenotype is predictable from genotype draws attention to the disjuncture between the relative specificity and measurability of genotype and the more continuous nature of phenotypes, which makes them difficult to categorize and describe. The challenges encountered in moving from genotype to phenotype, absent only in a handful of single gene disorders, are not new. But because FDP operates in law enforcement, these challenges raise issues that go beyond the problems raised in medical genetics. In light of persistent, well-documented racial biases in arrest, conviction, and incarceration rates in the United States, the technology's focus on predicting a suspect's race is particularly worrisome.[7]

Potential social and ethical drawbacks of FDP have not been widely discussed by the technology's proponents, but some have spoken to these issues. One presentation, for example, cited possible demands to use the technology inappropriately, such as for pre-implantation diagnosis,[8] while another conceded that racial stereotyping concerns might be plausible.[9] Left unaddressed however is the issue of what it means practically for police to be able to claim to be able to predict a suspect's appearance based on a "heritable component of race."[10]

In this essay I examine and refute claims that FDP can reliably predict race and, on this basis, appearance. The failure lies less in the basic thrust of the claim, however, than many might suppose. In other words there are demonstrable relationships between certain genetic markers and a person's self-identified race and, under specific research conditions (such as using a limited number of self-identified races from which subjects can choose), self-identified race roughly corresponds to observer-assigned race. The problem lies instead with the practical details entailed in the series of claims or steps that FDP requires, starting with the predictability of phenotype from genotype and continuing on to the idea that phenotype can be objectively described and understood in such a way that police can use it to routinely and reliably distinguish who might and who might not be a suspect in a particular crime.

Arguably the most troubling step in the series is the final one: presuming that police can effectively interpret and judiciously apply a description such as "light skinned-black man."[11] This is not because police are somehow less skilled or less trustworthy as a group. It is rather that the nature of their training and demands of their job work against effective use of such information. Furthermore there are substantial problems with the steps prior to police actually applying FDP descriptions, including the nature of genetic markers that FDP uses and its reliance on individual inferences from population-level data, that argue strongly against allowing the technology to get that far.

FDP Accounts

There are few publicly available detailed accounts of police reliance on FDP. Indeed it is even difficult to get a realistic estimate of how often police have used it. In 2007, DNAPrint claimed that it had provided FDP analysis in over 200 cases since 2003, but the basis for the claim is unstated.[12] Nonetheless, by reviewing two cases that have been reported in depth by the media, we can get some sense of the circumstances in which FDP has been used and its results.

The first is DNAPrint's first case reported in the United States, which also appears to be one of the few that has resulted directly in arrest and conviction. The second is an ongoing case in southeastern England of a serial rapist, dubbed the Night Stalker.

The U.S. case concerns a serial murderer-rapist in southern Louisiana, believed active for more than a decade. Despite repeated audacious daylight attacks, the suspect left few eyewitness accounts. Based on what evidence they could gather, police believed they were seeking a white man in a white van. As the murders continued, police grew frustrated with their lack of success in zeroing in on a suspect and began to contact various outside agencies for help. Eventually they got in touch with DNAPrint and arranged for an FDP analysis of DNA retrieved from one of the murders.[13]

To guard against potential bias, the Louisiana state police crime lab sent to DNAPrint DNA from twenty people whose race they had independently determined, along with DNA from the crime scene. Less than two weeks later DNAPrint returned racial descriptions for all twenty-one samples. Those based on the known samples were judged accurate. The description returned for the perpetrator surprised investigators.

FDP analysis suggested that the sample belonged to someone whose ancestry was 85 percent sub-Saharan African and 15 percent Native American and who most likely was a "lighter skinned black man."[14] This finding forced the police to reconsider evidence they had previously dismissed as unrelated to the case and pointed the investigation in a new direction that led to the capture of Derrick Todd Lee, an African American. In 2004, Lee was convicted of two murders and DNA evidence linked him to at least five more. He was sentenced to death and awaits execution.

The British Night Stalker case is similar to the Lee case in that the suspect has succeeded in making repeated attacks while evading capture and escaping observation by potential eyewitnesses. The brutal sexual and physical assaults, largely against older women, have spanned nearly twenty years. Similarly frustrated with their lack of progress, British police decided to try DNAPrint's services. They too submitted multiple samples as a guard against potential bias influencing the analysis of the perpetrator's sample. The finding they were given suggested that the likely suspect had "strands" of DNA that were Native American, European, and sub-Saharan African.[15]

A detective chief inspector from the investigation concluded that this meant the offender probably came from the Caribbean, most likely an island that was a former British colony. He went on to say that further tests could be done to "break down the rapist's biological code so precisely that he could be linked to a particular Caribbean island."[16] Efforts to more precisely identify the perpetrator's ancestral home led police officials to seek DNA samples from several hundred of their own officers of Caribbean descent, a request that many refused and that led to considerable controversy among members of London's Metropolitan Black Police Association.[17] Additional analysis conducted by a government scientist reported that the perpetrator was from the Windward Islands, specifically Trinidad.[18] Eventually a team of police officials actually traveled to Trinidad and gathered DNA samples from willing inhabitants. Upon hearing how the British police had interpreted his company's report, the technical director of DNAPrint took issue with their claims, stating, "That's not what our test indicated." As he elaborated, "although broad ethnic ancestry can be determined from DNA, geneticists cannot say with any certainty that an individual comes from a specific country."[19] The suspect remains at large and attacks attributed to him continue to be reported.

Ancestry Informative Markers

Both of these FDP cases and the handful of others publicly reported[20] rely on analysis of ancestry informative markers (AIMs), which are a particular category of genes distinguished by having "several polymorphisms that exhibit substantially different frequencies between races."[21] The existence and basis of such genes, or alleles, was demonstrated in admixture mapping research well before their use in these cases, but it is testament to the evolving interest in race and genetics that they are now called "ancestry informative."[22] The reasoning behind using AIMs to produce race-based identifications is a bit circular, but important to understand. AIMs can be used to distinguish races because AIMs vary by race. The circularity goes to the heart of complaints about FDP, but does not in itself entirely invalidate claims about using FDP to identify a person's race. It does, however, suggest that these claims do not pass muster for use in law enforcement.

The basis for treating a particular set of alleles as "ancestry informative" lies in the link between human genetic variation and population migration. Changes in the human genome that result from mutations, natural selection, or genetic drift are shared and spread through reproduction, which requires contact. As populations fanned out from Africa 40,000 years ago to inhabit the globe, those who traveled the greatest distances from one another had less contact and were less likely to share genetic changes passed down through reproduction. Those who lived closer to one another were more likely to have contact and to share changes.[23] As a result, certain genes or alleles are more common among people whose ancestors come from the same geographic region. Such alleles are rarely wholly absent in other groups, and rarely universal within groups where they do appear. It is, rather, that *statistically* they appear more often in some groups than in others.

For some researchers these findings justify claiming that race has a genetic basis.[24] Some, among them FDP proponents, go a step further and claim that some of the alleles found to vary in this way are expressed phenotypically in a person's physical appearance in a way that predictably conforms to socially constructed categories of race. While there are certain practical and logical bases to these assumptions, there are also several mistakes that are particularly pertinent to understanding what is at stake if FDP were introduced into routine policing in the United States.

First, not all alleles that might appear to be AIMs actually are. Alleles that vary across geographic regions might also have developed in relation to similar environmental exposures as some alleles related to malaria resistance appear to have. As a result, a shared allele might reflect similar environmental exposures on the part of ancestors, but not shared ancestry.[25] Second, the presence or absence of a particular allele in a person's DNA in itself does not necessarily indicate something about the person's ancestry. This is because findings that show geographic or continental variation in alleles are probabilistic. They exist at a certain frequency within a population. While research has repeatedly demonstrated that certain alleles are more common in certain populations, it provides no basis on which to predict whether any particular individual in that population will or will not have a certain allele. Further, research has shown that the predictability of the link between a particular allele and self-assigned race is even more likely to be wrong among individuals from admixed populations, meaning that their family history draws from two or more ancestral populations.[26] Third, even people who do share AIMs that are known to influence physical appearance do not necessarily look the same. Gene expression depends on complex interactions with the environment, broadly construed, and the potential for similar phenotypic expression made possible by shared alleles is not always realized. And just as significant, to the extent that it is realized, insufficient research exists to provide a basis for accurate prediction of physical appearance based on genotype. For these reasons, although there is a relationship between AIMs and popular categories of race, it is neither predictable nor robust. Further, none of this speaks to the challenge of translating racial designations (whatever their basis) into verbal descriptions of personal appearance that could be useful in police work. There are no standards for classifying or recognizing a person as light-skinned or as having dark eyes.

This review of AIMs helps to clarify certain things about the Louisiana and British FDP cases. First it explains why FDP might work. In the Louisiana case, FDP analysts indicated that the suspect was a "light-skinned black man." This statement surprised investigators who had been led by witnesses to look for a white man in a white van. Investigators redirected their inquiry, reconsidered information they had collected but thought irrelevant, and realized that an African-American man associated with another case fit the profile for this case. Police arrested this man and found that his DNA matched crime scene samples. However, FDP's success in Louisiana doesn't mean that it will work elsewhere, nor does it even help to predict how often or in what cases it might prove useful. The results might just as easily have led officials to ignore the real suspect if they judged him too light or too dark to qualify as a "light-skinned black man." Misapplied, the results might also have led to the arrests of innocent men.

Proponents argue that concerns about misidentification based on FDP are unimportant, because the technology is used only to identify, not to prosecute, a suspect.[27] If the arrestee's DNA turns out not to match the crime scene DNA, the police simply release the person. While logically true, this is scarcely reassuring to people under arrest, especially members of racial or ethnic minorities who, according to a U.S.-based study, are "approximately five times more likely than white suspects, per capita, to die at the hands of a police officer."[28]

Little information about mistaken arrests in Britain's Night Stalker case is available, so it is difficult to judge the potential for damage there. However there is information about how FDP information has shaped the investigation in other ways.

The Night Stalker Case

A comprehensive review of the Night Stalker case conducted by the British government in 2006 states that the police used the FDP analysis to "re-prioritise the inquiry," to "avoid questioning those uninvolved," and instead to "approach relevant individuals."[29] While this use mirrors the stated purpose of FDP, exactly how the "re-prioritizing" unfolded bears scrutiny. It was not, as one might suppose, based on FDP proponents' claims about the predictability of physical characteristics putatively associated with FDP-identified ancestry. It seems, rather, that FDP analysis provided police in the Night Stalker case with a stereotype onto which they could project social information. For example, police statements located the perpetrator's ancestors historically, stating that they "originate[d] from slave-trade Africa,"[30] and politically, as having at some point resided in Trinidad. Another police statement claimed that both of the perpetrator's parents must have "originated from the Caribbean area."[31] Police also used the FDP analysis to make assumptions about the perpetrator's current life and to justify concentrating their inquiries in London neighborhoods that the police recognized as having a high number of Caribbean-identified residents.[32] In light of the complex and lengthy relationship between Great Britain and the Caribbean, dating to the early 1600s, the move from a handful of AIMs to a particular twenty-first-century London neighborhood is a leap. The assumption that there will be some visible or publicly knowable contemporary manifestation of this person's putative heritage is difficult to justify. Yet despite their apparent failure to produce a suspect, it would seem that police have continued to rely on such assumptions.

Incidents attributed to the Night Stalker in June and October 2008 suggest that he remains as active as ever.[33] The June incident led to the release of the first police artist's sketch of the perpetrator, itself a major breakthrough in the case, accompanied by the statement, "The victim saw the suspect in dark conditions but states he is a light skinned black man, with markings on the side of his face. These could be a number of things such as freckles, scarring or spots."[34] The sketch (fig. 1) occasioned some comment about the likely racial identity of the person depicted, with one citizen querying, "Why does the photofit not look like a black man when the offender is? surely [sic] this is misleading."[35]

Whether this image, downloaded from the web, accurately reproduces the original police sketch is unclear, both to me and to at least some of the people commenting on it in related blogs. Assuming for the moment that it is accurate, one question of concern to the elderly women and the population of southeastern England at large is whether the sketch resembles the perpetrator sufficiently to facilitate his capture. A rather different question of interest here, is what relationship the sketch bears to mental images of the suspect the police have relied on for the last four years? The person depicted in the sketch could well trace his ancestry to the Caribbean but, if so, he apparently would not match the stereotype at least some people have of what a person with Caribbean descent looks like.[36] Of course, this begs the questions, what is a person of Caribbean descent supposed to look like? Or, using DNAPrint's language, what is a person with "strands" of DNA described as Native American, European and sub-Saharan African supposed to look like? [37] And more to the point, what does the Night Stalker, with his unique personal history, look like?

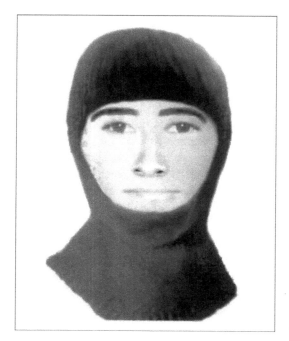

FIGURE 1 Police artist sketch of British serial rapist, dubbed the Night Stalker. The sketch was accompanied by the statement that the subject was probably a "light-skinned black man," a description that some observers thought was at odds with the image.

London Metropolitan Police, UK/PA Wire (Press Association via AP Images).

Perhaps the Night Stalker's capture will settle some of these questions. But it is not clear if it will matter then, as the point of FDP is to help predict a suspect's identity, not to confirm it after he is caught. It is possible, of course, that the police know more than they let on and that the public presentation of the inquiry is strategically misleading. Regardless, the point stands. The exact relationship between AIMs and ancestry for a specific person cannot be stated any more than can the relationship between AIMs and that person's appearance. And even if such a prediction could be made more precise, the interpretation of the description still eludes standardization. Would most people have recognized the person in the sketch as a "light-skinned black man," or as someone with a Caribbean background, or whose parents are from Trinidad? Specifically, would the police or potential witnesses have recognized him as such?

It is not that there is no relation between AIMs and popular race categories, which is why the simple criticism that race is a social not a genetic construct does not suffice against FDP. It is rather that the relationship is based on the frequency and probability of certain historic events in a population. Evidence of these events is predictable at the population level, but not for any one person. And while this point relates most directly to assertions made about the basic premise that AIMs link predictably to ancestry, it also provides a needed caution for all of the steps implied by FDP use in law enforcement, including that ancestry links to appearance and that appearance described by one person is understood by another as pertaining to the same person. And this caution is that, while any of these predictions or inferences might sometimes work, as they did in the Todd case, they often will not. And at this stage there is no way of knowing which prediction is which. The magnitude of uncertainty underlying FDP predictions suggests that it is unsuitable for its proposed use in law enforcement.

NOTES

1. T. Kessis, "Racial Identification and Future Application of SNPs," Forensic Bioinformatics, 3rd Annual Conference: DNA from Crime Scene to Court Room: An Expert Forum, August 21, 2004 (University of Dayton School of Law, Dayton, OH, 2004).

2. U.S. Department of Energy, Midwest Forensics Resource Center, [Accessed November 7, 2008].

3. B.-J. Koops, M. Prinsen, and M. Schellekens, "Wanted: A Tall Blond Dutchman. Does the Netherlands Set the Stage in Regulating Forensic DNA Phenotyping?" *Tilburg Foreign Law Review* 13, no. 3 (2006):206–227.

4. M. Shriver, T. Frudakis, and B. Budowle, "Getting the Science and the Ethics Right in Forensic Genetics," *Nat. Genet* 37 (2005):449–450.

5. T. Frudakis, *Molecular Photofitting: Predicting Ancestry and Phenotype Using DNA*. (Burlington, MA: Academic Press, 2007).

6. Ibid.

7. J. Correll, B. Park, C. M. Judd, B. Wittenbrink, M. S. Sadler, and T. Keesee, "Across the Thin Blue Line: Police Officers and Racial Bias in the Decision to Shoot," *Journal of Personality and Social Psychology* 92, no. 6 (2007): 1006–1023; Department of Justice, *Policing and*

   Homicide, 1976–1998: Justifiable Homicide by Police, Police Officers Murdered by Felons (NCJ 180987) (Washington, DC: Bureau of Justice Statistics, 2001).

8. P. M. Schneider, "DNA-Based Prediction of Physical Traits—A New Dimension for Forensic Genetics, or a First Step Towards Violation of Privacy Leading to Genetic Discrimination?" 22nd Congress of the International Association for Forensic Genetics (Copenhagen, Denmark, August 23, 2007).

9. T. Frudakis, *Molecular Photofitting: Predicting Ancestry and Phenotype Using DNA* (Burlington, MA: Academic Press, 2007).

10. Kessis, "Racial Identification and Future Application of SNPs."

11. S. D. Mustafa, T. Clayton, and S. Israel, *I've Been Watching You: The South Louisiana Serial Killer* (Bloomington, IN: AuthorHouse, 2006).

12. M. Newsome, "A New DNA Test Can ID a Suspect's Race, But Police Won't Touch It," *Wired Magazine* (December 20, 2007), www.wired.com/politics/law/magazine/16–01/ps_dna.

13. Mustafa, Clayton, and Israel, *I've Been Watching You.*

14. Frudakis, *Molecular Photofitting.*

15. P. Jacobson, "Investigation: Stalker in the Suburbs," *The Times* (January 30, 2005).

16. Ibid.

17. D. Bascombe, "Swab Squad," *The Voice* (March 29. 2005), www.voice-online.co.uk/content.php?show=6373.

18. "Burglary Linked to Sex Attacker," *BBC News* (November 16, 2007), news.bbc.co.uk/1/hi/england/london/7097797.stm.

19. K. Staley, *The Police National DNA Database: Balancing Crime Detection, Human Rights, and Privacy* (GeneWatch UK, 2005).

20. Frudakis, *Molecular Photofitting.*

21. *Nature Reviews Genetics*: Glossary Terms [Accessed January 22, 2008].

22. M. D. Shriver, E. J. Parra, S. Dios et al. "Skin Pigmentation, Biogeographical Ancestry, and Admixture Mapping," *Human Genetics* 112, no. 4 (2003):387–399.

23. M. Bamshad, S. Wooding, B. Salisbury, and J. Stephens, "Deconstructing the Relationship between Genetics and Race," *Nature Reviews Genetics* 5 (2004):598–609.

24. N. Risch, E. Burchard, E. Ziv, and H. Tang, "Categorization of Humans in Biomedical Research: Genes, Race and Disease," *Genome Biology* 3, no. 7 (2002):1–12; N. Rosenberg, J. Pritchard, J. Weber et al., "Genetic Structure of Human Populations," *Science* 298 (2002):2381–2385.

25. D. Bolnick, D. Fullwiley, J. Marks et al., "The Legitimacy of Genetic Ancestry Tests: Response," *Science* 319 (2008):1039–1040.

26. C. L. Pfaff, J. Barnholtz-Sloan, J. K. Wagner, and J. C. Long, "Information on Ancestry from Genetic Markers," *Genetic Epidemiology* 26, no. 4 (2004):305–315.

27. Frudakis, *Molecular Photofitting*; Schneider, "DNA-Based Prediction of Physical Traits."

28. Department of Justice, *Policing and Homicide.*

29. D. Johnston, *The Use of DNA in Operation Minstead* (Metropolitan Police Authority; September 7, 2006).

30. J. Bennetto, "DNA Breakthrough in Hunt for Britain's Worst Sex Offender," *The Independent* (April 28, 2004), www.independent.co.uk/news/uk/crime/dna-breakthrough-in-hunt-for-britains-worst-sex-offender-561513.html.

31. Jacobson, "Investigation: Stalker in the Suburbs."

32. "South London 'Nightstalker' E-Fit released," *London Daily News* (June 9, 2008), www.thelondondailynews.com/south-london-nightstalker-efit-released-p-766.html.

33. U. Khan, "94-Year-Old Woman is Latest Victim of "Night Stalker" Serial Rapist," *Telegraph* (October 24, 2008), www.telegraph.co.uk/news/newstopics/politics/lawandorder/ 3250295/ 94-year-old-woman-is-latest-victim-of-Night-Stalker-serial-rapist.html [Accessed November 19, 2008].

34. "New 'Night Stalker' Image Released," *METRO.co.uk.* (June 9, 2008), www.metro.co.uk/ news/article.html?in_article_id=168047&in_page_id=34 [Accessed November 19, 2008].

35. "BROMLEY: Night Stalker Could Have Struck Again," *This Is Local London* (August 6, 2008), www.thisislocallondon.co.uk/news/topstories/2418513.BROMLEY__Night_Stalker_ could_have_struck_again/.

36. Ibid.

37. Jacobson, "Investigation: Stalker in the Suburbs."

8

Forensic DNA and the Inertial Power of Race in American Legal Practice

JONATHAN KAHN

I. Introduction: Race, Genes, and Justice

The time has come to ask how and when, if ever, is it appropriate to use race in the presentation of forensic DNA evidence in a court of law.[1] Recently much attention has been devoted to some of the ethical, legal, and social issues presented by the emerging use of DNA typing to produce phenotypic "profiles" of crime suspects based on DNA samples found at the scene of a crime. Of particular concern is the growing tendency to use so-called "ancestry informative markers" (AIMs) to predict a suspect's race or ethnicity. While important and well deserving of such concern, these discussions largely overlook the conceptually distinct and far more prevalent, indeed standard, use of race in the development and presentation of forensic DNA evidence in criminal trials.

In contrast to DNA profiling, which is used to try to identify a suspect, DNA evidence is presented at a trial to try to convict a suspect who has already been apprehended. DNA presented as forensic evidence in a trial tries to establish a "match" between DNA found at a crime scene and DNA obtained from an apprehended suspect. This match is based on finding an identity across thirteen genetic loci, which, in contrast to AIMs, were explicitly chosen for their purported lack of any connection to phenotypic traits. In this context, race is used to help calculate odds regarding the probability that the same DNA profile might match a random individual in the population other than the suspect. One might say that, in such calculations, race is used to generate odds, whereas in DNA profiling odds are used to generate race.

Forensic experts have framed DNA evidence in terms of race almost since its inception in the late 1980s. The original justifications for using race involved efforts to refine the accuracy of the evidence. Early applications of forensic DNA generally typed individuals at only four distinct loci and then used statistical methods to generate probabilities that a match between two samples actually implicated the defendant. In order to refine the odds, forensic experts generated tables calculating the frequencies of each allele in diverse "ethnic" or "racial" population groups. The idea here was that groups sharing distinct ancestries would have distinct frequencies of these highly variable alleles. Using these racially identified population databases would, it was believed, provide more accurate odds that the DNA found at the crime scene did, in fact, come from the defendant. Many assumptions about the utility and appropriate use of race were questioned early on, but the use of race in forensic DNA analysis soon became normative. Hence race was injected into the science and law of forensic DNA from its outset.

Subsequent technological developments greatly enhancing the discriminating power of DNA analysis have largely rendered such concerns moot. As a practical matter, race now adds no relevant refinement to the odds that a match implicates a defendant. Yet the practice of using race persists. It has become commonplace, even standard, in the generation and presentation of DNA evidence to juries.

The recent and representative California case of *People v. Wilson*,[2] clearly illustrates the point. In that case, the prosecution presented the following race-specific probabilities that the DNA at the crime scene would have come from someone other than the defendant: Caucasian—1 in 96 billion; Hispanic—1 in 180 billion; and African Americans—1 in 340 billion. One might well ask, if there are only six and half to seven billion people in the whole world, what can possibly be gained from presenting odds of a random match that differentiate among "Caucasians," "Hispanics," and "African Americans," when those odds range from 1 in 96 billion to 1 in 340 billion? Given such a range, it is clear that the prosecution could have produced probabilities with astronomically high denominators without any reference to race. Any loss of precision occasioned by the use of probabilities for a non-racialized general population would have been forensically inconsequential. The question then becomes, why has the use of race persisted long past the time when technological advancement obviated the (questionable) need to use it?

Part II of this essay will provide some background to the history and technical aspects of both forensic DNA analysis and the debates regarding the relation between race and genetics. It will begin by introducing some of the basic technical details of early forensic DNA practices and procedures. It will also examine early debates over the appropriate use of racial categories in generating statistical match probabilities. In the early years of forensic DNA analysis, the late 1980s and early 1990s, these debates did not involve questions of *whether* to use race, but rather *how much* race to use. The concern of some early forensic DNA analysts was that using too broad a population group would generate random match probabilities—or RMPs—that were unfairly low. Advocates of using broad racial categories argued that they provided a pragmatic and useful means to generate more accurate statistics than using an undifferentiated general population database, while still providing RMPs that were fair to a defendant. Critics of this approach argued that since there is more genetic variation within racial groups than between them, databases should be characterized by smaller subgroups within the larger racial designation, in order to provide even better information about RMPs. This part of the article will also consider how these arguments relate to broader issues concerning the nature of race in relation to genetics. It moves from these early debates to current scientific opinion regarding the propriety (or lack thereof) of using racial categories in relation to genetic research and practice. This section then concludes by moving back to the mid-1990s to examine how the debates over using race to calculate RMPs were ultimately resolved in favor of using broad racial categories, which then became the norm for forensic DNA practice in the United States.

Part III will examine the current standards and protocols for conducting forensic DNA analysis and consider how, where, and when forensic experts inject race into their practices. This section begins with an examination of DNA databases, focusing on the FBI's Combined DNA Index System (CODIS), which began as a pilot project in 1990 and has since evolved into a major database, with over 5 million DNA profiles from convicted offenders nationwide. It reviews technological developments that have greatly increased the power and efficiency of forensic DNA analysis, and considers the selection of thirteen genetic loci that have become the standard for generating DNA matches and calculating random match probabilities.

Part IV contrasts the elaboration and standardization of such technical protocols for DNA analysis with the protocols, (or lack thereof) for producing and using racial and ethnic categories in forensic DNA analysis. Here I argue that the use of racial categories is woefully under-conceptualized and wholly inadequate—especially when contrasted with the great care taken to elaborate the technical protocols of DNA analysis itself. I argue that similar care of the data should be given to methods for using racial categories in a genetic context. I put forward the use of general, non-racial reference population databases as the obvious solution to this problem. This section moves on to examine what I call the "inertial power of race" to remain in a system of practice and analysis long after the initial reasons for using it have faded. It considers, as well, some of the dangers, beyond the courtroom, of allowing race to persist in a context that inappropriately reifies it as genetic.

The essay concludes with a brief review of the basic arguments for why there is no longer a place for race in the generation or presentation of forensic DNA evidence in criminal trial proceedings.

II. Race and the Early Development of Forensic DNA

Origins of Forensic DNA Testing

DNA is made up sequences of four nucleotides: adenine, cytosine, guanine, and thymine—commonly represented as A, C, G, and T. Each nucleotide base is paired through a process known as hybridization: A is always paired with T; C is always paired with G. There are approximately three billion of these "base pairs" in the human genome (Butler 2005:2–3, 18–20n18). There are two major steps in using DNA for purposes of forensic identification. First, a sample left at the crime scene by the perpetrator is compared to a sample from a suspect. Second, if there is a "match" then statistics must be used to calculate to frequency of that DNA "profile" in an appropriate reference population (Kaye 1993:101. 104). This latter step is required because, although every person's DNA is unique, it is impractical to compare the full three billion nucleotide base pairs between two samples for forensic purposes. Therefore, two samples will be compared only at a limited set (usually between four and thirteen) of "loci," or specific parts of the genome. For this practice to be effective, it is necessary to find loci that are highly variable between individuals and test only for them. Humans, however, are essentially identical in about 99.5 percent of their DNA.[3] Finding the specific points of variation among individuals, therefore, can be difficult.

In 1985, English geneticist Alec Jeffreys first described a method for developing a DNA "profile" of a person in a manner that might be used for purposes of forensic identification (Butler 2005:2–3; see also National Commission on the Future of DNA Evidence 2002:14–15). Jeffreys's innovation consisted of observing that, in particular regions of the human genome, short segments of DNA—the ACGT nucleotide sequence—are repeated between 20 to 100 times (Butler 2005:2–3n18; Lewonti and Hartl 1991:1745). These repeat regions became known as "variable number of tandem repeats" or VNTRs. Different VNTR "alleles"—or variations—are composed of different numbers of repeats. In order to examine and visualize the VNTRs, Jeffreys employed a technique known as restriction fragment length polymorphism (RFLP), which uses a restriction enzyme to cut the regions of DNA surrounding the VNTR (Butler 2005:2–3n8). By looking at VNTRs from several distinct loci on the genome, it is possible to calculate the probability that a particular genetic profile comprised of distinct sets of VNTRs will appear in one or more individuals in a particular population. A standard way to estimate the frequency of a particular profile is to count occurrences in a random sample of an appropriate reference population and then use classical statistical formulas to place upper and lower confidence limits on the evidence (National Research Council 1992:10). The resulting conclusion of identity or nonidentity between two samples is therefore necessarily probabilistic (Lewontin and Hartl 1991: 1745–1746n; Cho and Sankar 2004:S8, S9). In conducting the comparison, investigators came to adopt the "product rule"[4] for determining the "random match probability" (RMP)—the probability of finding the same DNA profile identified in the crime scene sample in a randomly selected, unrelated individual (Butler 2005:481n18; Lewontin and Hartl 1991:1745n21).[5] Any given VNTR may be calculated to occur at a certain frequency in a random population. By the early 1990s the standard was to test for VNTRs at four independent loci on the genome. The product rule allows for multiplying each independent genotype frequency together to produce an overall probability of a match at all four loci (Lewontin and Hartle 1991:1746n).

Jeffreys's innovation was first used in a forensic setting in England in 1986 (Butler 2005:3n18). Forensic DNA testing was first used in the United States in 1987 (Maclin 2006:163). Soon thereafter some commercial laboratories made use of this "fingerprinting" procedure, and in 1988 the U.S. Federal Bureau of Investigation implemented forensic DNA techniques (National Commission on the Future of DNA Evidence 2002:14–15n18). Critical to the acceptance of forensic DNA in courts was the development of standards of technical proficiency and accuracy in generating RMPs. The product rule was one such standard, requiring that each chosen loci be understood as being inherited independently of the others. Also important were basic crime scene management techniques for the identification and handling of DNA samples.[6]

Early Questions and Challenges

Questions about the reliability of DNA evidence surfaced as early as 1989, in cases such a *People v. Castro*[7] in New York and the Minnesota case of *Schwartz v. State*.[8] Partially in response to these cases, several federal agencies called upon the National Research Council (NRC), an arm of the National Academies of Science (NAS), to study and recommend guidelines for the production and use of DNA evidence (Jasanoff 2004:339–340n30). The NRC created a Committee on DNA Technology in Forensic Science, which issued a report in 1992. It is in the context of the production of this report that race first enters the story front and center.

The committee covered an array of issues relating to the forensic use of DNA technologies. Among its most controversial findings were those relating to reference populations and the appropriate methodology for calculating RMPs. In order to calculate the odds of any particular VNTR allele appearing at a given locus on the genome, one must have an appropriate reference population. The product rule depends on the assumption of statistical independence of the alleles tested—that is that they do not tend to occur in groups (National Research Council 1992:12).

Generally speaking, the more "related" a person is to a particular population group, the higher odds are of finding shared alleles—or, alternatively stated, the less independence there is among alleles. Siblings would likely share more DNA than cousins; cousins more than others in the same isolated village; members of the same isolated village more than others in the same region; and so forth. Higher odds favor a suspect or defendant because they indicate a greater likelihood that some other person may have left the DNA sample found at a particular crime scene. The choice of reference population, therefore, can play a critical role in shaping the weight and authority of DNA evidence. The choice, however, is not always straightforward. Indeed, some of the earliest and most contentious controversies involving the use of DNA technology in forensic science involved choosing the appropriate population against which a suspect's DNA should be compared and defining just how the suspect may be "related" to this population (see, generally, Butler 2005:455–519). Concepts of race played a central role in these debates and continue to frame the way forensic scientists, law enforcement, and the bar produce and interpret DNA evidence to this day.

The basic issue is whether or to what extent racial or ethnic categories should be used to characterize reference populations against which particular DNA samples could be compared in order to generate RMPs. The use of such categories may be particularly problematic in the arena of forensic DNA analysis because racial groups, especially those delineated in the U.S. Census, are fundamentally *social* not *biological* categories.[9] Indeed, at least since the 1970s scientists have understood that race will statistically explain only a small portion of genetic variations (Lewontin 1972:381). As an editorial in *Nature Genetics* put it, "scientists have long been saying that at the genetic level there is more variation between two individuals in the same population than between populations and that there is no biological basis for 'race'" (Editorial 2001:239). Nonetheless, to the extent that certain population geneticists understand particular racial groups as sharing a common genetic ancestry—usually by using race as a crude surrogate for geographic or continental ancestry—members of those groups can be viewed as more "related" to each other (like an extended family) than to individuals from other groups. This problematic understanding of relatedness can then affect the calculation of RMPs. Generally speaking, the more fine-grained the characterization of a particular reference population, the higher the odds of a random match—again, higher odds favoring the suspect/defendant. In the early years of forensic DNA analysis, there were concerns that using a general, undifferentiated population database would produce inappropriately low RMPs. The decision to use race in constructing and categorizing reference populations was introduced into forensic DNA analysis in belief that it would improve the precision of the calculations that generate RMPs (Cho and Sankar 2004:S9).

In early 1991 two pairs of eminent population geneticists squared off against each other in the pages of *Science*, a highly influential scientific journal, to debate the problem of using racial categories in forensic DNA analysis. On one side were Professors Richard Lewontin of Harvard University and Daniel Hartl of the University of Washington (described by an editorial accompanying the article as "two of the leading lights of population genetics" [Roberts 1991:1721]). On the other side were Ranajit Chakraborty of the University of Texas and Kenneth Kidd of Yale University. Their dispute did not revolve around the question of *whether* to use race but rather *how much* race to use in constructing reference population databases from which to calculate match probabilities.

Lewontin and Hartl questioned the then current practice of calculating allele frequencies in the racial categories used in the Census such as "Caucasian," "Black," or "Hispanic" to provide the basis for calculating RMPs (Lewontin and Hartl 1991:1747n). They argued that such groupings were too broad, and that substantial "genetic substructuring" occurred *within* the broad racial groupings that should be taken into account in calculating match probabilities. Using the broad racial groupings could produce RMPs with substantially lower odds than those that might be produced using more fine-grained ethnically identified sub-populations (ibid.). These concerns grew logically out of Lewontin's earlier path-breaking work showing how genetic variation *within* socially identified racial groupings was actually greater than variation observed *between* such groups (Lewontin 1972:381). This work laid the foundations for understanding that race was incoherent as a genetic concept, or at best, an overly-crude surrogate for genetic variation that improperly tended to reify race as genetic.[10] Thus Lewontin and Hartl observed,

> Among genes that are polymorphic in European national or ethnic groups, the magnitude of the differences in allele frequency among subpopulations differs from one gene to the next. . . . For example, there are striking geographical clines of allele frequency across Europe for the ABO blood groups: the frequency of the B allele is 5 to 10% in Britain and Ireland, increases across Eastern Europe, and reaches 25 to 30% in the Soviet Union; the frequency of the O allele is 70 to 80% in Sardinians, Irish, and Scottish populations, but lower in Eastern European populations. These clines reflect the migrations and political history of Europe over the last few thousand years. (Lewontin and Hartl 1991:1748n)

Problems were even greater for the "heterogeneous assemblage" known as "Hispanic," which was perhaps "the worst case for calculating reliable probabilities" (ibid.:1749). Consequently, they concluded that using reference databases organized by the broad racial groupings "Caucasian," "Black," and "Hispanic" was "unjustified" (ibid.:1747).

Chakraborty and Kidd argued that Lewontin and Hartl exaggerated both the extent of ethnic substructuring in America and its significance for calculating match probabilities (Chakraborty and Kidd 1991:1735). While conceding that some substructuring existed, they argued that its effects upon frequency estimates generated by using the broader racial databases was "trivial." Chakraborty and Kidd did not deny that using finer-grained ethnic reference populations might produce more precise allele frequency estimates. Rather, their point was that such an approach was unnecessary—and unnecessarily burdensome. Current technology and understandings of population genetics, they asserted, justified the use of broad racial and ethnic categories, which were, additionally, far more practical and currently available (ibid.). Race was at the center of this early debate. But, again, for these eminent scientists, it was not a question of *whether* to use race but *how*, or more specifically *how much* (that is, how fine-grained) race to use.

This debate took place while the NRC committee was conducting its study of DNA technology in forensic science. Its report, issued in 1992, discussed both sides of the issue without specifically taking sides. It did, however, choose "to assume for the sake of discussion that population substructure may exist and to provide a method for estimating population frequencies in a manner that may account for it" (National Research Council 2002:13). The report recognized that "population genetic studies show some substructure within racial groups for genetic variants. . . . Thus, North American Caucasians, blacks, Hispanics, Asians, and Native Americans are not homogeneous groups" (ibid.:80). In effect, this approach reflected the concerns expressed by Lewontin and Hartl, recognizing that social categories of race did not map neatly onto discrete genetically definable population groups. The NRC's 1992 report created problems for prosecutors because, by taking cognizance of the difference of scientific opinion regarding the appropriate calculation of allele frequencies and RMPs, it seemed to assert that forensic DNA technologies lacked the sort of scientific consensus needed to support the introduction of such expert evidence (Kaye 1993:102–103n). Thus, for example, in the 1992 case of *People v. Barney,* the California Court of Appeal cited the NRC Report in concluding disagreement and uncertainty in the scientific community regarding the selection of appropriate reference populations precluded the admission of DNA evidence based on the product rule.[11]

By April 1993, the director of the FBI asked the National Academies of Science to conduct a rapid follow-up study to resolve these uncertainties. The NRC then appointed a second committee (NRC II) late in 1994, with a specific mandate to update and clarify discussions of population genetics and statistics as they applied to DNA evidence (Kaye 1993:397). Meanwhile, the debate continued in the scientific community. The position advocated by Chakraborty and Kidd received a major boost in 1994 when Eric Lander of MIT, previously a vigorous critic of the lack of adequate standards in DNA typing, paired with Bruce Budowle, one of the principal architects of the FBI's DNA typing program, to write an article in the journal *Nature,* declaring "DNA fingerprinting dispute laid to rest" (Lander and Budowle 1994:735). The article argued that applying the product rule to the frequency estimates for four independent VNTRs generated odds of such magnitude that any technical statistical differences observed between the use of the broad racial databases (as advocated by Chakraborty and Kidd) versus more fine grained ethnic subgroup databases (as advocated by Lewontin and Hartl) were "of no practical consequence to the courts" (ibid.). As Lander and Budowle observed,

> In the vast majority of cases, jury needs to know only that a particular DNA pattern is very rare to weigh it in the context of a case: *the distinction between frequencies of 10^4, 10^6 and 10^8 is irrelevant in the case of suspects identified by other means.* . . . The most extreme positions range over a mere two orders of magnitude: whether the population frequency of a typical four-locus genotype should be stated, for example, at 10^5 or 10^7. *The distinction is irrelevant for courtroom use.* (ibid.:738; emphasis added)

Lander and Budowle were not arguing that racial subgroups themselves were not needed or desirable in calculating RMPs. The "distinction" they saw as "irrelevant" was the one between ethnic subgroups, such as "Irish," and larger racial groups, such as "Caucasian." Thus, they were legitimating the then-current standard FBI practice of using broad racial groups, such as "Black" and "Caucasian," as reference databases for generating allele frequencies for calculating RMPs. Significantly, Lander and Budowle did not argue for doing away with racial databases altogether in favor of using an undifferentiated general population database. Given the current state of forensic technology, which generated RMPs from examining VNTRs at four loci, they deemed race relevant. They simply did not want too much of it—that is, they did not want law enforcement forced to undertake the burdensome task of developing elaborate databases that reflected the wide array of genetic population substructuring that actually occurs across the globe. Given the odds generated by testing at four VNTR loci, they deemed the broad racial categories of the Census more than adequate.

Lander and Budowle made a critical distinction between statistical and legal relevance. Though hardly the first to do so (see, e.g., Trautman 1952:385), the distinction played a central role in allowing Lander and Budowle to quiet both the scientific debates and the legal uncertainties swirling around this new and powerful forensic technology.[12] Another critic of the NRC I report, David Kaye, made a similar distinction in a 1993 article in the *Harvard Journal of Law & Technology*. Kaye, who would sit on the NRC II Committee, wrote that in calculating RMPs, "the real issue . . . is not 'statistical significance' but rather practical or substantive significance" (Kaye 1993:101, 127–128). The difference was critical for Kaye and others because it provided the basis validating then-current law enforcement practices of using broad racial reference population databases. By distinguishing between statistical and logical or practical significance, Kaye and others did not refute Lewontin and Hartl so much as bracket off their concerns as irrelevant to the applications of forensic DNA technology in courts. Of most immediate significance in terms of the unfolding story of the use of race in forensic DNA technology, is the fact that this distinction played a central role in the NRC's second report, *The Evaluation of Forensic DNA Evidence* (NRCII), issued in 1996.

NRC II: Questions of Race Laid to Rest?

The NRC II report focused primarily on updating and clarifying issues related to population genetics and statistics as they applied to DNA evidence. It argued directly for "using separate databases for different racial groups" even while it acknowledged Lewontin's underlying argument that "the variability among individuals within a population is greater than that between populations." (National Research Council 1996:22). Recognizing the uncertainties inherent in calculating RMPs, the report noted that "the accuracy of the estimate will depend on the genetic model, the actual allele frequencies, and the size of the database" (ibid.:33). It was confident, however, that "when several loci are used, the probability of a coincidental match is very small" (ibid.:34). Nonetheless, the report recommended incorporating a ten-fold margin of error in RMP calculation, stating, "if the calculated probability of a random match between the suspect and evidence DNA is 1/100 million, we can say with confidence that the correct value is very likely between 1/10 million and 1/billion" (ibid.:34).

At first glance, such a range may strike the reader as rather large, but the report legitimizes it by returning to the distinction between statistical and legal relevance. "The proper concern," it asserted, "is not whether the probability is large or small, but how accurate it is. Probabilities are not untrustworthy simply because they are small. In most cases, given comparable non-DNA evidence, a judge or jury would probably reach the same conclusion if the probability of a random match were one in 100,000 or one in 100 million" (ibid.:56). In other words, the large range presented earlier in the report was of little practical or legal significance, so long as it was *good enough* to guide a judge or jury in their deliberations. It was good enough for two reasons: first, because it was *accurate*—accuracy here was crucially distinguished from *precision* which the large range of probabilities certainly lacks; second, because the lower end of the range still presented odds so vanishingly small as to render it indistinguishable from the upper end of the range *as a practical matter*—that is, the difference was deemed to be insufficient to have any practical effect on the conclusion a judge or jury would reach in using the evidence.

And yet, even accepting this huge range of variance, the report persists in using races as organizing categories in calculating RMPs. Thus, even while acknowledging that "some assert the word race is meaningless" in a genetic context, the report adopted the categories "white (Caucasian), black (African American), Hispanic, East Asian (Oriental), and American Indian (Native American)" as designated "racial groups" as a matter of "convenience, uniformity, and clarity" (ibid.:57). It justified this choice by asserting that, "there are reproducible differences among the races in the frequencies of DNA profiles used in forensic settings, and these must be taken into account if errors are to be minimized" (ibid.:57). It is instructive to note here just where it is that "difference" makes a difference in the calculation of RMPs. Difference is deemed insignificant when it manifests as a thousand-fold range for an "accurate" calculation using the product rule to compare a single sample against a single reference population database— that is the "difference" between 1 in 100,000 and 1 in 100 million makes no practical difference for use of the data in a court of law. To be fair, as noted above, the NRC II report recommended calculating RMPs with a margin of error limited to ten fold in either direction (ibid.:34)—but this still translates into a variation of one-hundred-fold between the lowest and highest estimate. But when race is at issue in the NRC II report, the "difference" of frequencies among racial reference populations becomes critical and "must be taken into account if errors are to be minimized" (ibid.:57).

Looking forward to the case of *Wilson v. California*, we see there the following range of variance among racial databases: one of 96 billion Caucasians, one of 180 billion Hispanics, and one of 340 billion African Americans.[13] The range of variation here is less than fourfold, yet the court in Wilson, just like the NRC II report, deemed this variation relevant, even while accepting that, internal to each estimate, the RMPs may vary as much as a hundredfold from lowest to highest.

Race enters into people's consciousness in complex and often unanticipated ways. The NRC II report clearly focused on issues of race in response to the questions raised by the debate between Lewontin/Hartl and Chakraborty/Kidd. That debate involved the relation between social groups of race and genetic variation. Both sides recognized that racial categories were crude surrogates for capturing genetic variation across groups, but Chakraborty and Kidd were, in effect, arguing that race was nonetheless not "too crude"—that is it was good enough for practical use in law enforcement because of the ability to generate astronomically low RMPs, even allowing for a substantial range of variation. As a practical matter, the debate cast into doubt the admissibility of DNA forensic evidence in courts, hence the FBI's urging that the issue be revisited by a second NRC Committee. The NRC II Report, therefore, aimed to quiet the dispute, rendering it irrelevant to the practical application of forensic DNA technologies in law enforcement. Yet, it is unclear why the NRC II report characterized difference between racial reference populations as meaningful "error" while it deemed the hundred-(or even thousand-) fold range of variance within a single reference population to be of no practical significance. This seems largely to be an artifact of the report's focus on addressing the issues raised by Lewontin and Hartl in manner that would allow forensic DNA testing to proceed unimpeded by concerns of the accuracy of using racial reference populations to calculate RMPs. The report needed to show that RMPs generated by using racial categories were good enough for practical use in courts of law. The utility and/or validity of using a general population database without reference to either race or ethnic subgroups was never really at issue.

In the end, the report issued the following formal recommendation for estimating RMPs: "In general, the calculation of a profile frequency should be made with the product rule. If the race of the person who left the evidence-sample DNA is known, the database for the person's race should be used; if the race is not known, calculations for all the racial groups to which possible suspects belong should be made" (National Research Council 1996:5). The NRC II report thus legitimized the then-standard practice of using race to generate RMPs. In rejecting Lewontin and Hartl's concerns about broad racial databases, it seems also implicitly to have rejected—or at least failed fully to appreciate—Lewontin's cognate concerns about the incoherence of race as a genetic category and the dangers of reifying race as genetic.

III. Current Standard Practices Regarding Race and
Forensic DNA Analysis

The Impact of NRC II

The NRC II report became tremendously influential in shaping forensic DNA techniques and their acceptance in courts of law. It established new norms for calculating RMPs generally and for using race-specific databases in particular.

Following the NRC II recommendation, it has since become standard practice to present race-specific RMPs (see, e.g., Butler 2005:474–517n). Thus, for example, in the 1999 case of *People v. Soto*,[14] the California Supreme Court noted that the dispute regarding population substructuring that had been at the heart of the 1992 case of *People v. Barney* had "been eclipsed by subsequent important scientific developments, most notably the publication of a completely new report by the NRC" (Butler 2005:515–516).[15] The court concluded that use of the product rule as applied to broad racial databases "has gained general acceptance in the relevant scientific community." Similarly, in *People v. Wilson* the criminologist from the California Department of Justice who presented the forensic DNA evidence to the court testified that the "to help juries understand the significance of a DNA match, the Department followed the statistical approach recommended by [the NRC II report] . . . for presenting the frequency with which genetic profiles occur."[16]

In cases such as *Soto* and *Wilson* we see that the use of racial databases characterized by the broad terms of the U.S. Census categories had emerged as normative referents for the calculation of RMPs. Thus, for example, in justifying its calculation of RMPs in *Wilson*, the State of California argued that the lower court "correctly approve[d] the California Department of Justice's *generally accepted* method for generating match probability statistics using reference data from major racial and ethnic groups. *Typically*, a range of statistics if provided using three major U.S. population databases: African-American, Caucasian, and Hispanic. This method . . . is supported by NRC II."[17] By the time of *Wilson*, incorporating race into forensic DNA analysis had thus emerged as standard, normative practice in the aftermath of the NRC II report. As representative of current practice, *People v. Wilson* shows how fully integrated race has become in the conceptualization and practice of forensic DNA analysis. The use of race is understood as requiring no justification other than that is had become "generally accepted" and is "typical."

CODIS and the Move from VNTRs to STRs

The NRC II report itself was based largely on an assessment of the then-current practice of testing samples at four VNTR loci. Ironically, by 1997, barely a year after the report had been issued, a new technology had emerged to replace the four loci VNTR analysis using restriction fragment polymorphism (RFLP) methods of analysis. In 1985 Kary Mullis and members of the Human Genetics group at the Cetus Corporation discovered a technique known as polymerase chain reaction (PCR), which enabled scientists to make millions of copies of a specific sequence of DNA in a matter of hours (Butler 2005:63n). The ability to amplify segments of DNA is critical to forensic analysis. PCR is sensitive, rapid, and not limited by the quantity of DNA, as are RFLP methods. PCR enabled a shift in focus from VNTRs to sections of DNA known as "short tandem repeats" (STRs). VNTRs are typically 10–100 bases in length. STRs (also known as microsatellites) are regions of DNA only 2–6 base pairs in length (Butler 2005:85n). STRs highly variable between individuals and are easily amplified by PCR, thus making them very effective for purposes of human identification.

Beginning in 1996, the FBI commenced an effort to develop a set of core STR loci to be used as standard referents for the calculations of RMPs in forensic DNA analysis (Butler 2005:94n). In November 1997, the FBI settled on thirteen core STR loci, which were chosen to be the basis of the CODIS (Combined DNA Index System) national DNA Database, which was launched in 1998 (ibid.:13, 85n). New technologies allowing for "multiplex" testing of multiple loci at once were soon capable of regularly generating RMPs rarer than one in a trillion (Butler 2005:95n; Budowle et al. 2000). The Minnesota State Department of Public Safety has noted that "STRs are very discriminating for single-source samples. Typically, a complete DNA profile might be found in less than one in one hundred billion people. A typical DNA report would read 'This profile would not be expected to occur more than once among unrelated individuals in the world population.'" By 2000, the FBI laboratory and many others stopped using RFLP analysis altogether in favor of PCR analysis of the thirteen CODIS STRs (Butler 2005:13n). Because of their use in the FBI database, the thirteen CODIS STRs have become a national (indeed international) standard and have come to "dominate the genetic information that has been collected to date on human beings" (Butler 2006:253).

CODIS was initially authorized by the DNA Identification Act of 1994 and became operational in 1998.[18] As described by the FBI,

> CODIS is implemented as a distributed database with three hierarchical levels (or tiers)—local, state, and national. NDIS is the highest level in the CODIS hierarchy, and enables the laboratories participating in the CODIS Program to exchange and compare DNA profiles on a national level. All DNA profiles originate at the local level (LDIS), then flow to the state (SDIS) and national levels. SDIS allows laboratories within states to exchange DNA profiles. The tiered approach allows state and local agencies to operate their databases according to their specific legislative or legal requirements. (Federal Bureau of Investigation, CODIS: Mission statement; see also Maclin 2006: 165, 166)

As of October 2007, there were over 5 million DNA profiles in CODIS (Federal Bureau of Investigation, NDIS statistics). The profiles themselves are not classified by race. Rather they are primarily used, much like a database of fingerprints, to aid in the investigation of crimes by providing matches or "hits" to DNA evidence left at crime scenes (Butler 2005:439n).[19] In the context of establishing an initial match using the CODIS database, race is therefore irrelevant.

Nonetheless, race has come to pervade the characterization of forensic DNA data generated using the standard thirteen CODIS loci. This is because establishing a match is only the first step in applying forensic DNA technology. Once a match is found, whether using the CODIS database or not, law enforcement must still take the further step of calculating an RMP for any given DNA profile. It is at this stage that race enters CODIS—and in a more powerful way than ever before. In addition to the basic CODIS database, the FBI has generated a population file to estimate allele frequencies according to specifically identified racial or ethnic groups (Butler 2005:439n). This population file is based on a 2001 study led by the FBI's Bruce Budowle, which typed allele frequencies for the thirteen CODIS loci from forty-one population data sets. Budowle classified the results in terms of five "major population groups": "African American, U.S. Caucasian, Hispanics, Far East Asians, and Native Americans" (Budowle et al. 2001:453). These allele frequencies have since become the standard reference database for calculating racially identified RMPs (Butler 2005:439n). Thus, in *People v. Wilson*, criminologist Nicola Shea referenced the Budowle study, when noting that the California Department of Justice "used databases that the Federal Bureau of Investigation published in the Journal of Forensic Sciences reflecting profile frequencies in the Caucasian, Hispanic, and African-American populations."[20]

IV. Race, Technology, and "Care of the Data"

Race versus Technology

The care (or lack thereof) taken in presenting and interpreting racial data in professional discussions of forensic DNA stands in marked contrast to the meticulous care taken concerning the more technical aspects of DNA extraction, amplification and analysis.[21] The discussions of each in a 2005 article by Peter Vallone, Amy Decker, and John Butler, of the National Institute of Standards and Technology's (NIST) Human Identity Project team, are fairly typical.[22] This particular article involved the characterization of allelic frequencies for seventy SNPs (single nucleotide polymorphisms) in DNA samples taken from three racially marked groups: U.S. Caucasian, African American, and Hispanic. The article presents its techniques for racially identifying the DNA samples as follows: "Anonymous liquid blood samples with self-identified ethnicities were purchased from Interstate Blood Bank, Inc. (Memphis, TN) and Millennium Biotech, Inc. (Ft. Lauderdale, FL). Vallone, Decker, and Butler 2005:279). In short, "self-identification" provides the sum total of all care and technique devoted by Vallone and his colleagues to characterizing genetic samples by race. Contrast this with their discussion of the more apparently technical aspects of how they manipulated the samples once in the lab (this is quoted at length to heighten the contrast):

2. DNA extraction
Blood samples were extracted using a modified salting out procedure.

3. Quantification
Extracted DNA was quantified using UV spectrophotometry followed by a PicoGreen assay to adjust concentrations to approximately 1 ng/ml.

4. SNP markers

The 70 autosomal SNP markers are listed in Table 1 (see also http://www .cstl.nist.gov/biotech/strbase/SNP.htm). The PCR primer sequences were obtained from Orchid Cellmark (personal communication, Jeanine Baisch, Orchid Cellmark Dallas). The exact chromosomal locations were ascertained using BLAT (http://genome.ucsc.edu/cgi-bin/hgBlat) and dbSNP (http://www .ncbi.nlm.nih.gov/SNP/) and are based on the July 2003 assembly of the human genome. All of the SNPs are C/T transitions.

5. PCR amplification

For each sample, the 70 SNP markers were typed in 11 unique 6-plexes and a single 4-plex PCR. The final concentrations of the 6 (or 4) PCR primer pairs were present at 0.5 mM for all multiplex PCRs. Amplifications were performed in reaction volumes of 10 ml using a master mix containing 1X GeneAmp1 PCR Gold buffer (Applied Biosystems, Foster City, CA), 4.5 mmol/ 1 MgC12, 250 mmol/ldeoxynucleotide triphosphates (dNTPs; Promega Corporation, Madison, WI), 0.16 mg/ml bovine serum albumin (BSA) fraction V (Sigma, St. Louis, MO), and 0.5 unit of AmpliTaq Gold1 DNA polymerase (Applied Biosystems).

The thermal cycling program was carried out on a GeneAmp 9700 (Applied Biosystems) using the following conditions in 9600-emulation mode (i.e., ramp speeds of 1 8C/s):
  95 8C for 10 min
  Three cycles of {95 8C for 30 s, 50 8C for 55 s, 72 8C for 30 s}
  18 cycles of {95 8C for 30 s, 50 8C for 30 s +0.2 8C per cycle,
  72 8C for 30 s}
  11 cycles of {95 8C for 30 s, 55 8C for 30 s, 72 8C for 30 s}
  72 8C for 7 min
  25 8C until removed from thermocycler
Following PCR amplification, unincorporated primers and dNTPs were removed by adding 4 ml of a Exo-SAP enzyme cocktail consisting of 1.4 ml Exonuclease I (10 U/ml) and 2.6 ml (1 U/ml) of shrimp alkaline phosphatase (SAP; USB Corp., Cleveland, OH) to each 10 ml PCR reaction. Reactions were mixed briefly and incubated at 37 8C for 90 min and then 80 8C for 20 min to inactivate the enzymes.

6. Allele specific primer extension (ASPE)

ASPE reactions were also carried out in eleven 6-plexesand a single 4-plex. Multiplex primer extension reactions were conducted in a total volume of 10 ml using 2.5 ml of ABI Prism1 SNaPshotTM multiplex kit mix (Applied Biosystems), 0.5 ml of 10X AmpliTaq Gold1 PCR buffer, 3 ml of PCR template, 3 ml of water, and 1 ml of a stock solution of extension primers, which contained empirically balanced primers (approximately 1 mM each). Extension reactions were incubated as follows: 25 cycles of 96 8C for 10 s, 50 8C

for 5 s, and 60 8C for 30 s. Excess fluorescentlylabeled ddNTPs were inacti-
vated by addition of 1 ml of SAP (1 U/ml). Reactions were mixed briefly and
incubated at 37 8C for 40 min then 90 8C for 5 min.

7. Electrophoresis and typing

A 1.0 ml aliquot of each SAP-treated primer extension product was diluted in
14 ml Hi-DiTM formamide and 0.4 ml GS120-LIZ internal size standard
(Applied Biosystems) and analyzed on the 16-capillary ABI Prism1 3100
Genetic Analyzer (Applied Biosystems) using filter set E5 without prior denat-
uration of samples. Samples were injected electrokinetically for 13 s at 1 kV.
Separations were performed in approximately 30 min on a 36 cm array using
POPTM-6 (Applied Biosystems). Automated allele calls were made in Geno-
typer1 3.7 using an in-house macro based on fragment size and dye color.

8. Analysis of data

The data were analyzed with PowerMarker v3.07. Allele frequencies,
expected heterozygosity values and p-values (based on an exact test with
1000 reshufflings) for each marker are provided in Tables 2–4 for the three
U.S. sample groups. (Vallone, Decker, and Butler 2005:279–280)

The point here is not to assess (or even understand) the intricacies of the technical analysis performed by Vallone et al. on their DNA samples. Rather it is to contrast the extreme care and detail devoted to elaborating the techniques performed
in the lab with the casual and perfunctory discussion of how the samples came to
be racially marked in the first place. As scientists, Vallone and his team understandably go into greatest detail with respect to techniques and practices in which
they are professionally trained and proficient. This reflects their reasonable
understanding that the extraction, amplification, and analysis of DNA take great
care and expertise. The contrasting lack of care taken in characterizing the racial
identity of the genetic samples indicates an implicit assumption that such characterizations are obvious, uncomplicated, and take no special expertise. This contrast may be understood more broadly as reflecting a conceptual separation of the
world of the "social" from that of the "natural," where the former is understood to
contain transparent categories accessible to all, while the latter requires specialized knowledge and expertise for proper analysis and interpretation. In other
words, race is seen as easy and obvious; DNA is seen as difficult and complex.[23]

Social versus Genetic "Race"

Ironically, this separation of the social from the natural is enabled by the work of
geneticists such as Lewontin, who, together with a wide array of social scientists,
have worked diligently since World War II to reconfigure race from a biological
into a social construct (Lewontin 1972:381–384).[24] It is precisely because race is currently widely understood as a social phenomenon that forensic scientists are able
to effectively marginalize it from their analysis of the biological construct of DNA.

As a result, their care of the data extends only to the analysis of DNA samples, while wholly overlooking the complexities of using racial categories in relation to genetics.

In effect, forensic scientists have simply adopted the broad categories of race and ethnicity used in the U.S. Census in order to organize their genetic data. The Census, in turn, is based on the Office of Management and Budget's Directive 15 on "Standards for Maintaining Collecting, and Presenting Federal Data on Race and Ethnicity," which provides the following categories as a minimum standard for maintaining, collecting, and presenting data on race and ethnicity for all Federal reporting purposes: American Indian or Alaska Native; Asian; Black or African American; Hispanic or Latino; Native Hawaiian or Other Pacific Islander; and White (Office of Management and Budget 1997:100; see also U.S. Census Bureau 2002).

These federally mandated standards emerged as a consequence of major governmental programs and legal initiatives instituted since the 1960s. The OMB categories provide the basis both for census information and also for access to a variety of governmental goods and services that are contingent upon membership in a particular racial or ethnic group (Nobles 2000:75–79). For example, federal users of racial data provided by the census include: the Department of Education, Department of Justice, Department of Labor, Equal Employment Opportunity Commission, Federal Reserve, Department of Health and Human Services, Housing and Urban Development, Department of Agriculture, and the Veterans Administration (U.S. Census Bureau 2002). Alice Robbin notes, "groups must be counted in order to make credible claims for political representation, demonstrate discriminatory practices against them, seek and obtain legal remedies, receive governmental assistance for a host of social programs, and evaluate current, as well as develop new, public policy" (Robbin 2000b:431, 435). Additionally, they provide the framework for evaluating school desegregation, electoral districting, and other civil rights initiatives (Omi 1997:7–24; Robbin 2000a:129, 148–150).

Given the social and political uses which such standards were designed to serve, it should come as no surprise that Directive 15 explicitly acknowledges that the categories it provides are social in character, not biological or genetic (Office of Management and Budget 1997:2). Using these same categories in the context of genetic research, however, presents issues of a different order. As Lee et al. note, "Research utilizing race serves to 'naturalize' the boundaries dividing human populations, making it appear that the differences found reflect laws of nature. In fact, the use of race and ethnicity in biomedical research is problematic because it is caught in a tautology, both informed by, and reproducing, 'racialized truths'" (Lee et al. 2001:33, 55). This dynamic reinforces what sociologist Michael Omi has characterized as an "interesting dilemma" facing scientists in the United States: "On the one hand," Omi asserts, "scientists routinely use racial categories in their research. . . . On the other hand, many scientists feel that racial classifications are meaningless and unscientific" (Omi 1997:7).

A recent article by anthropologist Duana Fullwiley, provides an illuminating example of this dynamic in the context of biomedical genetic research. In an ethnographic study of laboratory practices dealing with the racial characterization of genetic databases, Fullwiley explores a curious situation where scientists conducting a "Study of Pharmacogenetics in Ethnically Diverse Groups" (SOPHIE) found significant discrepancies among three genetic data sets typed according to racial identification of the samples Fullwiley 2007: 14–15). One of the SOPHIE projects involved comparing DNA from donors at the Parkinson's Institute in Sunnyvale, California, to DNA samples from SOPHIE's own data set and samples from the Human Variation Panels maintained by the Coriell Institute for Medical Research on behalf of the National Institute of General Medical Sciences (NIGMS). As Fullwiley relates,

> The researchers in question hoped to compare the Sunnyvale Parkinson donors' DNA against 'a healthy control' in order to isolate a variant associated with the disease. Taking the values that the lab had for these variants in the 'Caucasian' Coriell panel, the student heading the study soon discovered that the Coriell panel (Caucasian and, according to what the team deduced from Coriell's location, 'most likely from New Jersey') differed from the Sunnyvale samples regarding the frequency of one key transporter variant. . . . The student and the lab were surprised to find that SOPHIE 'Caucasians' and Coriell 'Caucasians,' who were both healthy, differed more than the Coriell versus the Sunnyvale Parkinson's disease population for the variant in question. The student then added that this difference was furthermore 'statistically significant.' (ibid.:14)

That is, two data sets marked "Caucasian" by different labs had different frequencies of a particular allele related to Parkinson's disease. Note that variation in allele frequency across race is also the underlying rationale for using racially marked data sets (or "reference populations") for generating RMPs in forensic contexts. Fullwiley goes on to provide the response of one of the project directors (a professor at the University of California, San Francisco's Department of Biopharmaceutical Sciences) to this discrepancy:

> I did try and find out the ethnic stratification of the Caucasian DNA that we collected here in SOPHIE as well as in Coriell, but that's not easy to get. They're just 'European-Americans.' So whether in fact the ones from Coriell came from Ireland or Finland, and ours are all from Italy and Spain, I don't know. . . . One of the main differences between Coriell and SOPHIE is the way that they were collected [self-report versus family history of identifying as that group for three generations]. I would say we should take a close look at this because people may not want to be using Coriell if it is contaminated. (ibid.:15)

Most striking here is that the Coriell Repository is used worldwide as a basic resource for genetic research. Both it and the Department of Biopharmaceutical

Sciences at the University of California, San Francisco can be presumed to be at the forefront of responsible practices in the analysis of DNA samples. Yet even here, at the pinnacle of biomedical research, there appear to be significant discrepancies in the allele frequencies for two data sets both marked "Caucasian." The explanation may be the way race assigned to the samples, or the way they were handled—or it may simply be that correlating genetic variation with broad census-based racial categories such as Caucasian is inherently problematic. If some of the most advanced laboratories in the world can produce discordant results concerning race-specific allele frequencies, what does this say about the samples used for the influential Budowle article—where no protocols for the collection of samples or assignment of race were specified?

The Obvious Solution: A Non-Racial, General Population Database

Race was originally introduced into the calculation of RMPs in the early years of forensic DNA analysis in hopes of providing more refined statistical calculations. The rationale was grounded in the reasonable observation that there is a modicum of genetic variation across certain human populations. Capturing this variation might provide more accurate RMPs. Greater accuracy was important in the early years of forensic DNA analysis when generating RMPs using only four VNTR loci. With such limited data, the variation of RMPs generated using different reference populations could be of forensic significance.

Today the situation has changed significantly. With the advent of multiplex assays testing for the thirteen standard CODIS loci, forensic scientists are now capable of regularly generating RMPs with denominators far in excess of the entire world's population. As another article with Bruce Budowle as lead author put it as early as 2000, "By typing these [thirteen] STR loci, the random match probability for a multiple locus profile will be exceedingly small. The average random match probability for unrelated individuals for the 13 STR loci is less than one in a trillion, even in populations with reduced genetic variability" (Budowle 2000). The article goes on to note that, "in many forensic cases processed routinely today, a sufficient number of highly polymorphic markers are used so that the reciprocals of random match probabilities exceed the world population many fold" (ibid.). Under such circumstances the concerns originally expressed by Lewontin and Hartl, that using broader racial categories will not produce accurate enough RMPs, fade into irrelevance (Lewontin and Hartl 1991). When one is dealing with odds in the hundreds of billions or trillions, the more fine-grained characterizations of genetic variation among ethnic subgroups called for in their original 1991 article in *Science* simply are not necessary as a practical matter.

The issue then shifts from *how much* race to use, to *whether* to use race at all. As is made evident by the range of odds generated in cases such as *People v. Wilson* (1 of 96 billion Caucasians, 1 of 180 billion Hispanics, and 1 of 340 billion African-Americans),[25] the use of a nonracially marked general reference population would still generate RMPs whose reciprocals would still exceed the world population many-fold. Under such circumstances, any differences between RMPs generated by using race-specific reference populations vs. a general population are without forensic significance. Thus, it is no longer necessary even to use the broad racial reference populations advocated by Chakraborty and Kidd back in 1991.

The possibility of abandoning racial reference populations in favor of a general population database was broached in a 2000 report by the National Institute of Justice's National Commission on the Future of DNA Evidence. In the context of discussing the rise of testing for STRs in contrast with the older method of VNTR analysis, the report noted that, "It is already apparent that most of the STR variability is within groups. Although groups differ, the mean differences between groups are less than the individual differences within groups; profiles that are rare in one group tend to be rare in others. *With enough loci it may be possible to have a single database for all the major groups in the United States*" (National Institute of Justice 2000:27; emphasis added). Given the ability to generate RMPs in the trillions, it seems obvious that we currently have enough loci to have a single non-racial reference population database. The question remains, why do we continue to use race?

The Inertial Power of Race

There is no easy answer to this question. I would like to suggest that there is an inertial power to race in American society that propels its continued use long after any original rationale for its introduction may have faded. In particular, I would like to consider three possible dynamics contributing to the persistent use of race in the presentation of forensic DNA evidence, even after current technology has obviated the need for race-specific databases: (1) the persistent conceptualization of race as genetic; (2) the confusion of statistical with forensic significance; and (3) the deep seated American identification of violent crime and race.

First, with respect to genetics, in spite of decades of efforts on the part of social and natural scientists to sever the ties between race and biology, large segments of American society continue to conceptualize race primarily in genetic terms (Lee 2006:443, 447–448). The rise of modern genomics was supposed to resolve the dispute. Upon the completion of the first draft of the human genome in 2000, President Clinton declared, "After all, I believe one of the great truths to emerge from this triumphant expedition inside the human genome is that in genetic terms all human beings, regardless of race, are more than 99.9 percent the same" (qtd. in *New York Times* 2000). At the same press conference, Craig Venter, president and CEO of Celera Genomics, reinforced Clinton's message, asserting that "the concept of race has no genetic or scientific basis" (ibid.). Yet, ironically, since this historic press conference, genetic conceptualizations of race seem to have reemerged with a vengeance. As anthropologist Sandra Lee has noted,

the current trajectory of genomic research is increasingly focused on the 0.01 per cent genetic difference that is believed to separate one individual from another. The search for functional genetic variability is increasingly taken up in populations that are identified by conventional notions of 'race.' This trajectory is the result of a confluence of factors, including a growing infrastructure of research materials that are racially categorized through the creation of biobanks. Such sorting practices reflect the ongoing conflict over the meaning of 'race' in science and medicine. In the emerging era of the new genetics, in which super-computer technology has given way to an explosion of human genetic data, biobanks that utilize taxonomies of race in the classification, storage, and distribution of DNA samples become 'racializing technologies' that promote notions of racial biology in research protocols designed to discover group difference. (Lee 2006)

Sociologist Troy Duster has further argued that "new claims that DNA analysis of crime scene data will assist criminal investigations" and have led to a "molecular reinscription of race in the biological sciences" (Duster 2006:427). The same technology underlying the creation of racialized forensic DNA databases is also being used for drug development and to market new genetic ancestry tracing services (see, e.g., Kahn 2005:105–106; Kahn 2007:353; Bolnick et al. 2007:399). There have thus emerged both structural and commercial incentives to continue to use race in relation to genetics. This dynamic under girds the inertial power of race in forensic DNA analysis by providing a broader context in which race is understood somehow to be naturally or logically connected to genetics. This dynamic is further reinforced by the tendency of forensic DNA experts, to take race as an obvious, unproblematic category that does not require the same care and analysis as genetic data.

Second, the technical ability to generate statistically significant variation in RMPs across racial databases has led to the unquestioned assumption that such variation is also legally significant. Using the thirteen CODIS loci, forensic experts around the world have characterized allele frequencies for numerous ethnically and racially marked populations (National Institute of Standards and Technology 2007). Modest frequency variation at each individual locus, when multiplied across loci by the product rule, can lead to apparently significant variations in RMPs across races. Thus, in cases such as *People v. Wilson*, the variation in RMPs across race-specific databases may appear, at first blush, to be important. In that case, RMPs varied from 1 in 96 billion Caucasians, to 1 in 180 billion Hispanics, and 1 in 340 billion African Americans.[26] According to the databases, Wilson's genetic profile was more the three times as likely to occur in a Caucasian as an African American—an apparently significant difference. But in the forensic context, this statistically significant difference has no real practical importance. When the world's population is under 7 billion, the difference between an RMP of 1 in 96 billion and an RMP of 1 in 340 billion provides no meaningful distinction for a finder of fact. Both are astronomically low probabilities. Nonetheless, the experts' ability to generate statistically significant differences across races seems to have propelled the continued use of racial databases; even when these differences are of no practical legal significance.

Ironically, the reverse logic is used by law enforcement to support the rising use of race to generate suspect profiles from DNA evidence left at the scene of a crime. This sort of genetic racial profiling uses allele frequencies to generate an estimate of the likely racial or ethnic background of an as yet unidentified perpetrator. In this context, Troy Duster notes that law enforcement officials themselves have made a distinction between theoretical and practical significance of racial difference in genetics. Thus, as Duster notes,

> When representative spokespersons from the biological sciences say that 'there is no such thing as race,' they mean, correctly, that there are no discrete racial categories that come to a discrete beginning and end, that there is nothing mutually exclusive about our current (or past) categories of 'race,' and that there is more genetic variation within categories of 'race' than between them. All this is true. However, when Scotland Yard or the Birmingham police force or the New York Police Department wants to narrow the list of suspects in a crime, they are not primarily concerned with tight taxonomic systems of classification with no overlapping categories. That is the stuff of theoretical physics and philosophical logic, not the practical stuff of crime-solving or the practical application of molecular genetics for health delivery via genetic screening, and all the messy overlapping categories that will inevitably be involved with such enterprises. That is, some African Americans have cystic fibrosis even though the likelihood of that is far greater among Americans of North European descent and, in a parallel if not symmetrical way, some American Whites have sickle cell anaemia even though the likelihood of that is far greater among Americans of West African descent. But in the world of cost-effective decision-making, genetic screening for these disorders is routinely based on commonsense versions of the phenotype. The same is true with regard to the quite practical matter of naming suspects. (Duster 2006:435–436)

Here the scientific understanding that race is not genetic is trumped in practice by the purported ability of some genetic tests to estimate the likelihood that a suspect belongs to one or another socially identifiable race. Law enforcement is using race because it is perceived as of practical significance—even if not scientific. Yet, in the courtroom context the reverse is the case—race is used because it is perceived as scientific—even if not of practical significance.

Race persists largely because it has become normative, an unquestioned, standardized practice that persists long after the rationale for it has faded. In *Wilson*, the State argued for the legitimacy of using race-specific RMPs, primarily on the grounds that such was the "standard practice"[132] and the "generally

accepted method for generating match probability statistics"[133] and that "typically" the state and federal labs used "three major U.S. population databases:
African-American, Caucasian, and Hispanic."[27] General acceptance, typicality, and
standardization—these all powerfully drive the inertial power of race.

Third, there is the unfortunate but well documented tendency in the United
States to identify race and violent crime. In their book *Whitewashing Race*, Michael
Brown et al. discuss a cultural shift that began in the 1960s, when the image of "the
brave little girl walking up to the schoolhouse door in the face of jeering white
crowds was replaced by fearsome young black men coming down the street ready
to take your wallet or your life" (Brown et al. 2003:132). In the context of the rising
racialization of crime in the United States, Rothenberg and Wang observe that
"[f]rom 1990 to 2004, blacks were five times more likely than whites to be incarcerated, and in 2000, blacks and Latinos comprised 63 percent of incarcerated
adults, even though together they represented only 25 percent of the total population" (Rothenberg and Wang 2006:343, 352). Similarly, while examining the
impact of DNA technology on the criminal justice system, Simon Cole concludes
that, "At the endpoint of this system is a carceral system that embodies gross race
and class disparities, even if differential rates of offending are taken into account:
two thirds of people in prison are racial and ethnic minorities, one in eight black
males in their twenties are in prison or jail, three-quarters of persons in prison for
drugs are people of color" (Cole 2007:95, 98). Considering the dynamics that have
produced such inequalities, Brown et al. review an array of historical, legal, and
sociological data on race and crime in the United States. Discussing a classic
observational study of police responses to juveniles in a midwestern city in the
1960s, they note that police justified their different treatment of black youths on
"epidemiological lines," concentrating on "those youths whom they believed were
more likely to commit delinquent acts." They argue, however, that "the results of
this 'actuarial' reasoning . . . is to exacerbate the very differences that are invoked
to justify the racially targeted practices in the first place. This in turn helps to
cement the public's image, and the police's image, of the gun-toting gangster or
drug dealer as black or Latino. And this confirms the validity of the police focus on
youth in the same kind of vicious circle . . . described a generation ago" (Brown
et al. 2003: 149–150, 151). The same sort of actuarial reasoning is at work in
Duster's identification of the use of genetics in the "practical matter of naming
suspects" (Duster 2006:435–436). The association of crime and race produces
more racialized crime. As Dorothy Roberts has noted, the resulting mass incarceration is "iatrogenic"—by damaging social networks, distorting social norms, and
destroying social citizenship, the disproportionate incarceration of minorities has
produced a vicious cycle of crime and repression that further reinforces the identification of race and crime in the public mind (Roberts 2004:1271, 1297; see also
Brewer and Heitzeg 2008:625).

Taken together, the persistent conceptualization of race as genetic, the confusion of statistical with forensic significance, and the deep-seated American

identification of violent crime and race may be understood to frame and facilitate the inertial power of race to perpetuate itself as a salient category of forensic DNA analysis long after its practical legal utility has passed.

V. Conclusion

Race has been present in forensic DNA evidence since its inception. Over the past twenty years, the use of race-specific RMPs has become a normative, routine, and largely unquestioned practice. Whatever justifications may have originally been proffered for this practice have long since been superseded by basic technological developments that allow for the calculation of extremely powerful RMPs without reference to race. In relation to the presentation of forensic DNA evidence to juries, race is simply a concept whose time has passed. Its use persists largely due to inertia and a consistent lack of care given to compiling and interpreting racialized data. The current standard practice of using race-specific RMPs thus needlessly injects race into a context that already connects genetics and violent crime. This is a volatile mix that presents a significant (and unjustifiable) danger of unfairly prejudicing jury deliberations in particular as well as distorting broader social perceptions of relations among race, genes, and violence.

NOTES

1. I do not attempt to provide a set definition of "race" in this article. Rather I focus primarily on how actors in specific legal and scientific contexts have used the term. In the interests of economy and manageable syntax, in the remainder of this article I will often refer only to "race" when speaking generally of racial and ethnic categories. I am assuming both to be socially constructed categories that nonetheless have come to have biological implications as they play out in real world biomedical and forensic contexts. I will use the terms "race" and/or "ethnic" when referring to specifically marked groups. Thus, for example, the U.S. Census codes "White" or "Asian" as racial categories and "Hispanic" or "Latino" as ethnic categories. In the context of forensic practice, Hispanic is also sometimes referred to as a racial group. Ethnic groups are often also discussed as sub-groups within races. For example, Italian or Irish might be understood as ethnic sub groups within the racial category of Caucasian.

2. 38 Cal.4th 1237 (2006).

3. Older analyses typically put the figure at 99.9 percent, but a more recent study indicates that 99.5 percent may be a more accurate finding. See Weiss 2007:A1.

4. Richard Lempert (1993:1n3) defines the product rule as follows:

    According to the product rule, the probability of two independent events equals the probability of the first event times the probability of the second; with n independent events the separate probabilities of each of the n events are multiplied together to give the probability of their joint occurrence. Thus if the probability that a person had allele A = 1/10 and the probability that he had allele B = 1/10 and the probability that he had allele C = 1/10, and if the probability that the person had one of these alleles was not affected by whether or not he had either or both of the others, the probability that the person would have alleles A, B, and C would be 1/10 × 1/10 × 1/10, or 1/1000.

5. That the individual be "unrelated" is significant, because related individuals will have a higher likelihood of sharing a greater percentage of DNA, hence altering the probabilities of a random match.

6. This latter area of concern was brought front and center in 1995 in the highly publicized murder trial of O. J. Simpson, where defense lawyers undermined apparently airtight evidence connecting Simpson to the crime by calling into question the methods (or lack thereof) employed by the Los Angeles Police Department in collecting and handling of relevant DNA samples. See, e.g., Lazer 2004:4; and Jasanoff 2004:340–345.

7. 545 N.Y.S.2d 985 (Sup. Ct. 1989).

8. 447 N.W.2d 422 (1989).

9. For example, federally mandated racial and ethnic categories are not biomedical in origin. Rather, they derive from the Office of Management and Budget's 1997 "Revisions to the Standards for the Classification of Federal Data on Race and Ethnicity." These standards set forth five minimum categories for data on race: American Indian or Alaska Native, Asian, Black or African American, Native Hawaiian or Other Pacific Islander, and White. There are two categories for data on ethnicity: "Hispanic or Latino," and "Not Hispanic or Latino." These categories provide the basis for the classification of all federal data on race and ethnicity, most notably, the census. The OMB Standards, however, contain an important caveat: "The racial and ethnic categories set forth in the standards should not be interpreted as being primarily biological or genetic in reference." These categories were developed to serve social, cultural, and political purposes.

10. For a brief discussion of the conception of reification of race, see Duster 2005:1050–1051.

11. *People v. Barney*, 8 Cal.App.4th 798, 819; 10 Cal.Rptr.2d 731, 743 (Ct. App.1992). David Kaye (1993:103n20) notes that this case was followed in *People v. Wallace, 17 Cal. Rptr. 2d 721 (Ct. App. 1993)*; *Commonwealth v. Lanigan*, 596 N.E.2d 311 (Mass. 1992) (finding that product rule calculation method not prescribed by NRC panel for calculating frequency of DNA pattern is not generally accepted among population geneticists); *State v. Vandebogart, 616 A.2d 483 (N.H. 1929)* (same); *State v. Cauthron*, 846 P.2d 502 (Wash. 1993) (finding error in allowing expert to testify that defendant was the source of the incriminating DNA and yet excluding testimony of frequency of the DNA pattern given that the NRC panel had proposed a generally accepted method of calculation); cf. *State v. Bible*, 858 P.2d 1152 (Ariz. 1993) (holding method as applied to 1988 database not generally accepted); *Springfield v. State*, 860 P.2d 435 (Wyo. 1993) holding frequency re-calculated with "the most conservative" NRC method admissible under relevance standard); *People v. Atoigue*, DCA No. CR 91–95A (Guam Dist. Ct. App. Div. 1992) (method not generally accepted among population geneticists).

12. This distinction continues to play a role throughout the continuing development and application of DNA technology up to the present day cases such as *People v. Wilson* 38 Cal. 4th 1237, 1239–40 (2006).

13. *People v. Wilson*, 38 Cal.4th 1237, 1241, 45 Cal.Rptr.3d 73, 76 (2006).

14. 21 Cal.4th 512, 981 P.2d 958, 88 Cal. Rptr. 2d 34 (1999).

15. Further on in the case, the court notes that significant developments since *Barney* included an FBI world survey of genetic variation in 1993, the publication of the article in *Science* by Lander and Budowle, and "of greatest significance," the National Research Council report of 2006 (Butler 2005:539).

16. *People v. Wilson.* Answer Brief on the Merits. No. S130157, November 18, 2005. 2005 WL 3956844.

17. Ibid.; emphasis added.

18. DNA Identification Act of 1994, codified at 42 U.S.C. §14132. Pub. L. 103–322.

19. The database is also used to aid investigations in identifying human remains.

20. *People v. Wilson,* 38 Cal.4th at 1241.

21. For an elaboration of the concept of "care of the data," see Fortun and Fortun 2005:44, 49–50.

22. Vallone, Decker, and Butler 2005: 279. Other similar treatments of both race and technique in forensic DNA analysis can be found in Butler et al. 2003:1; Budowle et al. 2001:453; Budowle and Moretti 1999. The Human Identity Project at the NIST is funded by the National Institute of Justice to improve forensic DNA testing methods (National Institute of Standards and Technology, "DNA measurements").

23. This lack of comparable care is not restricted to the arena of forensics. For example, a recent survey of biomedical studies using race as a variable found that 72 percent of 268 reports analyzed did not explain their methods of assigning race or ethnicity as independent variables (Shanawani et al. 2006:724).

24. For an excellent overview of the history of scientific and cultural understandings of race, see generally Marks 1995. For some influential statements on race by professional social science organizations, see, e.g., American Anthropological Association 1997, 1998; American Sociological Association 2003.

25. *People v. Wilson,* 38 Cal.4th 1237, 1241, 45 Cal.Rptr.3d 73, 76 (2006).

26. *People v. Wilson,* 38 Cal.4th 1237, 1241, 45 Cal.Rptr.3d 73, 76 (2006).

27. *People v. Wilson,* 38 Cal.4th at 1243; Answer Brief on the Merits. No. S130157. November 18, 2005. 2005 WL 3956844; Answer Brief on the Merits. No. S130157. November 18, 2005. 2005 WL 3956844.

WORKS CITED

American Anthropological Association (AAA). 1998. Statement on race. www.aaanet.org/stmts/racepp.htm [Accessed Nov. 8, 2005].

———. 1997. Response to OMB Directive 15: Race and ethnic standards for federal statistics and administrative reporting. (Sept.). www.aaanet.org/gvt/ombdraft.htm [Accessed Jan. 7, 2006].

American Sociological Association (ASA). 2003. The importance of collection data and doing social scientific research on race. asanet.org/galleries/default-file/asa_race_statement.pdf [Accessed Nov. 8, 2005].

Bolnick, Deborah, et al. 2007. The science and business of genetic ancestry tracing. *Science* 318 (Oct.):399–400.

Brewer, Rose, and Nancy Heitzeg. 2008. The racialization of crime and punishment. *American Behavioral Scientist* 51:625–644.

Brown, Michael, Martin Carnoy, Elliott Currie, Troy Duster, David Oppenheimer, Marjorie Schultz, and David Wellman. 2003. *Whitewashing race: The myth of a color-blind society.* Berkeley: University of California Press.

Budowle, Bruce, Ranajit Chakraborty, George Carmody, and Keith Monson. 2000. Source attribution of a forensic DNA profile. *Forensic Science Communications* 2 (July). www.fbi.gov/hq/lab/fsc/backissu/july2000/source.htm#Introduction [Accessed May 27, 2007].

Budowle, Bruce, and Tamyra Moretti. 1999. Genotype profiles for six population groups at the 13 CODIS short tandem repeat core loci and other PCRB-based loci. *Forensic Science Communications* 1 (July). www.fbi.gov/hq/lab/fsc/backissu/july1999/budowle.htm [Accessed July 27, 2007].

Budowle, Bruce, Brendan Shea, Stephen Niezgoda, and Ranajit Chakraborty. 2001. CODIS STR loci data from 41 sample populations. *Journal of Forensic Science* 46:453–489.

Butler, John. 2006. Genetics and genomics of core short tandem repeat loci used in human identity testing. *Journal of Forensic Sciences* 51:253–265.

———. 2005. *Forensic DNA typing*. 2d ed. New York: Elsevier.

Butler, John M., Richard Schoske, Peter M. Vallone, Janette W. Redman, and Margaret C. Kline. 2003. Allele frequencies for 15 autosomal STR loci on U.S. Caucasian, African American, and Hispanic populations. *Journal of Forensic Sciences* 48 (May):1–4.

Chakraborty, Ranajit, and Kenneth Kidd. 1991. The utility of DNA typing in forensic work. *Science* 254 (December):1735–1739.

Cho, Mildred, and Pamela Sankar. 2004. Forensic genetics and ethical, legal, and social implications beyond the clinic. *Nature Genetics* 36:S8–S12.

Cole, Simon. 2007. How much justice can technology afford? The impact of DNA technology on equal criminal justice. *Science and Public Policy* 34 (Mar.):95–107.

Duster, Troy. 2006. The molecular reinscription of race: Unanticipated issues in biotechnology and forensic science. *Patterns of Prejudice* 40:427–441.

———. 2005. Race and reification in science. *Science* 307 (Feb.):1050–1051.

Editorial. 2001. Genes, drugs, and race. *Nature Genetics* 29:239–240.

Federal Bureau of Investigation. CODIS: Mission statement and background, www.fbi.gov/hq/lab/codis/program.htm [Accessed Sept. 27, 2007].

———. CODIS National DNA Index System, *www.fbi.gov/hq/lab/codis/national.htm* [Accessed Jan. 30, 2008].

———. NDIS statistics, www.fbi.gov/hq/lab/codis/clickmap.htm [Accessed Jan. 30, 2008].

Fortun, Kim, and Mike Fortun. 2005. Scientific imaginaries and ethical plateaus in contemporary toxicology. *American Anthropologist* 107 (Mar.):43–54.

Fullwiley, Duana. 2007. The molecularization of race: Institutionalizing human difference in pharmacogenetics practice. *Science as Culture* 16 (Mar.):1–30.

Jasanoff, Sheila. DNA's identity crisis. In *DNA and the criminal justice system,* edited by David Lazer. Cambridge, MA: MIT Press.

Kahn, Jonathan. 2005. From disparity to difference: How race-specific medicines may undermine policies to address inequalities in health care. *Southern California Interdisciplinary Law Journal* (fall):105–129.

———. Race-ing patents/patenting race: An emerging political geography of intellectual property in biotechnology. *Iowa Law Review* 92 (Feb.):353–394.

Kaye, David. 1993. DNA evidence: Probability, population genetics, and the courts. *Harvard Journal of Law & Technology* 7 (fall):101–172.

Lander, Eric, and Bruce Budowle. 1994. DNA fingerprinting dispute laid to rest. *Nature* 371:735–738.

Lazer, David. 2004. Introduction. In *DNA and the criminal justice system,* edited by David Lazer. Cambridge, MA: MIT Press.

Lee, Sandra. 2006. Biobanks of a 'racial kind': Mining for difference in the new genetics. *Patterns of Prejudice* 40 (Sept.):443–460.

Lee, Sandra, Joanna Mountain, and Barbara Koenig. 2001. The meanings of 'race' in the new genomics: Implications for health disparities research. *Yale Journal of Health Policy Law & Ethics* 1:33–76.

Lempert, Richard. 1993. The suspect population and DNA identification. *Jurimetrics* 34 (fall):1–8.

Lewontin, Richard C. 1972. The apportionment of human diversity. *Evolutionary Biology* 6 (fall):381–386.

Lewontin, Richard C., and Daniel Hartl. 1991. Population genetics in forensic DNA typing. *Science* 254 (Dec.):1745–1750.

Maclin, Tracey. 2006. Is obtaining an arrestee's DNA a valid special needs search under the Fourth Amendment? *Journal of Law, Medicine & Ethics* 34 (summer):165–187.

Marks, Jonathan. 1995. *Human biodiversity: Genes, race, and history.* Edison, NJ: Aldine Transaction.

Minnesota Department of Public Safety. *Guide to DNA analysis.* www.bca.state.mn.us/Lab/Documents/DNAbroco3.pdf [Accessed November 16, 2007].

National Institute of Justice, National Commission on the Future of DNA Evidence. 2002. *The future of forensic DNA testing.* Washington, DC: National Institutes of Justice.

———. 2000. *The future of forensic DNA testing: Predictions on the Research and Development Working Group.* www.ncjrs.gov/pdffiles1/nij/183697.pdf.

National Institute of Standards and Technology. DNA measurements. www.cstl.nist.gov/div831/DNATechologies/Human_Identity.htm [Accessed Feb. 4, 2008].

———. Population survey. www.cstl.nist.gov/div831/strbase/population/PopSurvey.htm [Accessed Sept. 28, 2007].

National Research Council. 1992. *DNA technology in forensic science.* Washington, DC: National Research Council.

National Research Council, Committee on DNA Forensic Science. 1996. *The evaluation of forensic DNA evidence.* Washington, DC: National Research Council.

New York Times. 2000. Reading the book of life: White House remarks on decoding of genome. *New York Times* (27 June), query.nytimes.com/gst/fullpage.html?res=9502E1D81230 F934A15755C0A9669C8B63 [Accessed Jan. 9, 2007].

Nobles, Melissa. 2000. *Shades of citizenship: Race and the census in modern politics.* Palo Alto, CA: Stanford University Press.

Office of Management and Budget (OMB). 1997. Revisions to the standards for the classification of federal data on race and ethnicity. www.whitehouse.gov/omb/fedreg/ombdir15.html [Accessed Dec. 5, 2005].

Omi, Michael. 1997. Racial identity and the state: The dilemmas of classification. *Law & Inequality* 15:7–24.

Robbin, Alice. 2000a. Classifying racial and ethnic group data in the United States: The politics of negotiation and accommodation. *Journal of Government Information* 27:129–156.

———. 2000b. The politics of representation in the US national statistical system: Origins of minority population interest group participation. *Journal of Government Information* 27:431–453.

Roberts, Dorothy. 2004. The social and moral cost of mass incarceration in African American communities. *Stanford Law Review* 56 (Apr.):1271–1305.

Roberts, L. 1991. Fight erupts over DNA fingerprinting. *Science* 254 (Dec.):1721–1723.

Rothenberg, Karen, and Alice Wang. 2006. The scarlet gene: Behavioral genetics, criminal law, and racial and ethnic stigma. *Law & Contemporary Problems* 69 (winter/spring): 343–365.

Shanawani, H., L. Dame, and D. A. Schwartz. 2006. Non-reporting and inconsistent reporting of race and ethnicity in articles that claim associations among genotype, outcome, and race or ethnicity. *Journal of Medical Ethics* 32 (Dec.):724–728.

Trautman, Herman. 1952. Logical or legal relevancy—A conflict in theory. *Vanderbilt Law Review* 5 (spring):385–413.

U.S. Census Bureau. 2002. Racial and ethnic classifications used in Census 2000 and beyond. www.census.gov/population/www/socdemo/race/racefactcb/html [Accessed Apr. 16, 2002].

Vallone, Peter M., Amy E. Decker, and John M. Butler. 2005. Allele frequencies for 70 auto-somal SNP loci with U.S. Caucasian, African-American, and Hispanic samples. *Forensic Science International* 149 (May):279–286.

Weiss, Rick. 2007. Mom's genes or Dad's? Map can tell. *Washington Post* (Sept. 4): A1, www.washingtonpost.com/wp-dyn/content/article/2007/09/03/AR2007090301106.html [Accessed Sept. 5, 2007].

9

~~~~~~

Making History via DNA, Making DNA from History

Deconstructing the Race-Disease Connection in Admixture Mapping

RAMYA RAJAGOPALAN AND JOAN H. FUJIMURA

Admixture mapping is an approach in population genetics that has gained some recent notoriety because of the use of some of its tools in the growing industry of direct-to-consumer genealogy and ancestry testing, as well as in biomedical research. In particular, some social scientists have criticized the increasing focus on race in medical and genetics research, arguing that such projects essentialize race as biological, attributing health differences to innate differences among race groups. In this chapter, we explore the ways admixture mapping technologies (mis)use race and race groups and how they connect race groups to stories of continental origins. Focusing on the race-disease connections that are made through admixture mapping practices, this chapter examines and critiques the conceptual frameworks of admixture mapping (also known as mapping by linkage disequilibrium, or MALD), especially as used in biomedical studies of genetics and disease.

Our interest in admixture mapping stems from our ongoing project that examines the use of notions of population—including race and ancestry—in contemporary biomedical research. In the twenty-first century, the search for biological contributions to complex diseases has increasingly meant a turn within science to genetic readings of disease etiology. In the process, geneticists have cast bits of DNA in the genome as medically relevant, and these bits gain new weight and importance as they circulate inside and outside laboratories. Genomes, as biological information, are increasingly the focus of explanations for the disease conditions of bodies, and genomes as inherited substances are held accountable for the passing on of disease or (increasingly) disease risk across generations, from "ancestors" to "descendants."

Geneticists employ concepts of genetic history, ancestry, and theories of human genetic variation in various ways to search for disease susceptibility markers in human populations. In the last four years, for example, genome-wide association studies (GWAS) researchers have used the concept of "ancestry" to try to distinguish disease-related genetic differences from non-disease-related differences between groups, and they have developed methods to account for these different differences, using comparisons of genetic markers.

Although no method is devoid of cultural politics, some GWAS technologies designed to account for ancestry at least attempt to avoid the use of race categories (Fujimura et al. 2010; Fujimura and Rajagopalan, 2011). In contrast, admixture mapping tools and methods employ group categories generally considered by many in the United States to be socio-cultural race categories—categories whose biological and health relevance is and has been hotly contested. Our study identifies multiple problems and circular assumptions about the relationships linking race, population, and ancestry at each step in the theory and method of admixture mapping. What follows is an analysis and critique of how researchers in admixture mapping studies, attempting to identify disease-associated regions of the genome, deploy particular socio-cultural genealogical stories within the "ancestral origins" labels they attach to "chunks of DNA."[1] We demonstrate how discourses of race and continental ancestry are deeply entangled in the construction of genetic technologies in this research.

Genetics, Relatedness, and Race

The concept of "relatedness" has been an important heuristic tool in geneticists' search for disease genes, driven by the idea that DNA is inherited, passed on from one generation to the next. For over a hundred years, family linkage studies have followed groups of closely related individuals to track the inheritance of DNA that seems to be associated with particular phenotypic characteristics or disease symptoms.[2] These studies have often been limited to diseases that were later shown to be strongly heritable, and thought to be caused by defects in one gene. Such single-gene hereditary diseases include, for example, Tay-Sachs disease, sickle-cell disease, and cystic fibrosis. The past decade has significantly changed this scene through the invention of methods and instruments of genetics that now allow researchers to begin to conduct studies of diseases on a genome-wide scale.

Coalescing around the major genomics projects at the turn of the century, these new technologies and genetic tools (such as faster and cheaper genotyping technologies, the Human Haplotype Map, and databases with human genome sequence and annotations) have facilitated the move from the study of single-gene diseases to the much more complicated analysis of diseases assumed to have multifactorial etiologies; that is, diseases that may be affected by many genetic factors as well as environmental factors. These genetic tools have been used in the search for genes related to common complex diseases like heart disease, cancer, and Type II diabetes. Significantly, common complex diseases tend to occur in all human groups, not just in particular families who share similar genetic profiles.

What distinguishes these new approaches in genetics is that they have not required that the sampled participants be selected on the basis of their familial relations, and an important question is, why not? Part of the reason is because some of these studies make conclusions about similarities and differences in DNA based on assumptions of relatedness within and between groups, rather than families.

Admixture mapping is a research approach that in some sense occupies a middle ground between family linkage studies that use classical genetics methods and tools to look at a few loci in the genome, and resource-intensive approaches that look more comprehensively across the genome and across many unrelated individuals (Cooper et al. 2008). It is important to note that, while admixture mapping incorporates analysis of genetic markers spread throughout the genome, it examines far fewer points in each genome than, for example, GWAS studies.[3] It looks at individuals who are not necessarily familially related, but who self-report as belonging to the same race category.

This is related to two other points critical to our analysis. First, admixture mapping methods assume a particular form of relatedness and unrelatedness among and between the individuals they study. That is, they use socio-culturally defined categories of race to infer a higher level of relatedness among people in one race category and a lower level of relatedness between people in different categories. Unlike family linkage studies, admixture mapping researchers do not require that their samples come from related individuals. Nevertheless, they do still assume that distant relationships among people who identify in the same race category will make their search for medically relevant genomic loci more efficient. In this effort, they have delineated a set of assumptions and practices that weave notions of continental ancestry and race with socio-cultural ideas about geohistorical origins.

Second, admixture scientists inextricably link particular groups of purportedly related humans to particular diseases. This by itself does not set it apart from other kinds of genetic studies. But in admixture mapping the link between disease and group is a product of the scientists' assumptions about relatedness within race groups.[4] We explore and deconstruct these assumptions below.

Deconstructing "Admixture" in Admixture Mapping

In an admixture mapping study, particular groups become linked to particular complex diseases, both before the study begins, through the practices and processes of the study, and through the study outcomes. Researchers have designed admixture mapping studies around group-disease correlations, which have often been generated by epidemiological studies that suggest that particular groups have an elevated risk or incidence of a particular disease. For example, epidemiological data has been mobilized in admixture mapping to argue that African Americans have an elevated risk of prostate cancer over white Americans (Freedman et al. 2006), and Hispanic Americans have an elevated risk of asthma over non-Hispanic Americans (Burchard et al. 2003). Genetic researchers have argued that socioeconomic or environmental factors can explain some, but not all, of the elevated risk of such diseases, and much of the work of contemporary medical genetics is devoted to finding genetic contributors to these and other common complex diseases.

Epidemiological data are often collected and analyzed according to U.S. census categories of race and ethnicity, for a variety of historical and institutional reasons. Admixture mapping researchers use these categories as they try to construct appropriate study groups. They base their study on two premises. The first is that if a potential study group—defined by race—appears to have an elevated incidence of a disease compared to another race group, then genetics may be part of the explanation. This is where the categorization of samples by race or ethnicity in epidemiological studies has implications for the study of genetics and disease. Second, they only study groups that they describe as genetically "admixed," with a mix of DNA inherited from two "ancestral" groups. We will next interrogate the ideas of genetic admixture that admixture mapping researchers work with.

Admixture mapping geneticists have cast "admixture" and "admixed populations" in particular ways. (Here, it is necessary to emphasize that admixture as a term has a long history of its own, and this essay will focus only on uses of the concept in the context of American biomedical genetics.) Although encounters among many peoples throughout human history have resulted in mixtures of genetic material, researchers do not consider all groups as suitable subjects for the admixture mapping approach. They only work with study subjects that they feel comfortable describing as members of populations descended from encounters between two previously "geographically isolated" groups.

Further, admixture mapping geneticists distinguish "recent" admixture from other kinds of admixture, and study only "recently admixed" groups. This choice is based on the theory of DNA exchange occurring every generation between the two copies of each chromosome in a human genome, one copy of which is inherited from the maternal ancestors and the other of which is inherited from paternal ancestors. The theory holds that over a large number of generations, the DNA exchange process makes it increasingly difficult to trace any particular piece of DNA, let alone whole chromosomes, to either the maternal or paternal side. For the purposes of distinguishing the lineages that contribute to present-day genomes, admixture mapping geneticists have decided that they have to examine admixtures that occurred in the last twenty generations. They thus specify "recently admixed" groups as those whom they believe are descendants of two "ancestral" and "isolated" populations that "mixed" within the last twenty generations.

In short, scientists' constructions of the populations they deem to be well-suited to these studies illustrate how their views of history, and the timescale of that history, enter into and shape scientific practice. In the latter part of the twentieth century, professional historians argued that histories may differ, depending on the available evidence and the storyteller. Biological scientists are no different from the rest of us in their reliance on these stories of the past. Thus, for example, admixture mapping scientists employ particular preestablished definitions of groups and categories to produce genetic understandings of these groups. They gain these ideas of groups and categories from stories in other disciplines. For example, they use sociocultural discourses on geography, history, and migration of human groups written by archaeology, physical anthropology, linguistic anthropology, and social anthropology. Genetics then is not a stand-alone discipline, basing its research only on its statistical techniques. Biological scientists' knowledge and their research outcomes are also steeped in fields of research that study pieces of bones, pottery, and language phonemes. And just as there are debates in anthropology about how to make meaning of these materials, so too must we address these issues with respect to the field of population genetics.

How do these stories become embedded in the materials of population genetics? The idea motivating admixture mapping is that, if the admixture is "recent," then some large chunks of the genome can be inherited virtually unchanged, because of the small number of generations since admixture. The contentious issue arises when scientists trace these chunks back through time to one of two "continental lines of descent." Typically, they label these DNA chunks with identifiers that describe continental origins, such that some chunks become labeled, for example, "African," and others "European." In this way, stories of human migration patterns become etched into descriptions of DNA, even though these stories often simplify very complicated exchanges and "mixing" of DNA throughout history.

Equally thorny is the description of the "ancestral populations," which are thought to have mixed, giving rise to the admixed population. Researchers define ancestral populations as having been largely geographically, and thus reproductively and genetically, isolated from each other prior to the historical events that facilitated large-scale "mixing" of these groups. For example, admixture mapping researchers believe that people who self-identify as African Americans possess both African and European ancestry, as a result of colonial encounters in which Europeans brought people of African ancestry to the Americas and subsequent mixing between these groups during the period of slavery in the United States. We note that this research does not consider any other kinds of "mixing" that could have happened prior to this large-scale transfer of peoples, including mixing within Africa, where population geneticists hypothesize that "ancestral" peoples had much greater genetic variation compared to groups on any other continent.

Further, admixture mapping researchers assume two ancestral contributions, for the sake of simplicity. Thus, they consider African Americans to have combinations of segments of "African" inherited genes and "European" inherited genes. When studying groups that researchers assume to have multiple ancestries (for example Hispanic groups, whom they describe as descended from white Europeans, native/indigenous groups in America, and Africans), these scientists typically examine only two of these ancestries at a time.

Our respondents (including population geneticists and genetic epidemiologists) felt they could define admixture and admixed populations because they felt comfortable distinguishing ancestral populations from each other. Of course, they also *defined* in advance the requirements of an ancestral population, for the purpose of their studies. Thus, while one of our respondents noted that "the available admixed populations are fairly limited," our analysis is that this limitation is the outcome of admixture geneticists' decisions about what constitutes a "population" and what constitutes the boundaries of a population, in space and in time. That is, these scientists *co-constitute* populations and the rules for what constitutes a population.

As noted above, admixture scientists base their definitions of ancestral populations on population genetics and anthropological stories of historical and geographical isolation and subsequent mixing of groups. One set of stories revolved around geographic boundaries such as those that separated continents (and presumably populations). Another set of stories is based in theories of migration patterns, histories of colonization or invasion events, and histories of slave trades in the last five hundred years of human history. These definitions of ancestral populations group peoples along continental divisions. This casts inhabitants of a continent as a relatively homogenous ancestral population. The problem is the implication that at some time in the past, "isolated pure types" existed. But other histories, overlooked in admixture mapping, suggest that peoples have been mixing for centuries prior to the colonial expansion of peoples from Europe, which calls into question the possibility of ever distinguishing a continent-specific ancestral contribution. The typological categories that admixture mapping scientists have devised for organizing their ideas of ancestral populations are similar to continental race categories, such as those first proposed by Blumenbach (1795).

In a similar way, stories and theories built in other disciplines are used to mobilize contemporary groups as study populations for the admixture mapping approach. These "admixed" populations are produced and operationalized intentionally by researchers, in such a way that they emerge as seemingly suited to the goal of linking disease to a particular continental ancestry. Researchers define suitable admixed groups as a "mix" of two ancestries, but also as retaining discernible and separable traces of each of the ancestries. In the U.S. biomedical context, the construction of admixed populations as recently descended from the mixing of two previously isolated continental populations has resulted in a focus on groups thought to trace their history to "mixing" during colonial encounters. The groups that have been described as admixed for the purposes of this research overlap considerably with race groups such as Latino/Hispanic groups, African Americans, and to a lesser extent, Native or indigenous groups. This ignores the fact that people who self-identify in these groups do so based on their lived experiences, which includes present-day experiences as well as their own sense of their histories, which may or may not include colonial encounters either in the present-day U.S. or elsewhere.[5]

Why is this use of race categories problematic? Many have criticized the view that race categories are a useful shortcut for characterizing genetic or biological similarity in biomedical studies of disease. Critics of race-based research have argued that the search for biological and/or genetic contributions to racially stratified health outcomes may distract clinicians and public health officials from more proximate social causes and more effective social interventions to redress these inequities (Cooper et al. 2003; Ossorio and Duster 2005). Other critics have warned that, while race may be expedient as a proxy for anything from diet to ancestry, contemporary biomedical uses are often incorrect, misleading, or able to cause more harm than good (Sankar and Cho 2002). Their primary concern was that the conflation of race categories (especially in the United States) with biomedical research categories has the potential to reinstitute and reify these race categories as biological (Duster 2003; Kahn 2006; Marks 1995; Wailoo and Pemberton 2006). Others have suggested that, while race as a sociopolitical construct is appropriate for monitoring health disparities, race and race categories are not appropriate analytical constructs for genetic studies of complex diseases (Feldman 2006; Fujimura and Rajagopalan 2011; Shields et al. 2005). For these reasons, the link that admixture mapping makes between social histories and the genetics of disease not only may potentially re-stabilize race categories, but may be misleading for understanding human disease.

As we will show next, these qualitative assumptions of admixture become embedded in and quantified in the tools and algorithms of admixture mapping that are used to link continental ancestry and disease during the analysis of genotypes in disease-affected patients.

How Race Is Read into DNA: The Making of Ancestry-Informative Markers (AIMs)

We have described how admixture mapping researchers study populations that they define as having two ancestral lineages. In order to differentiate two ancestral contributions to the DNA of study subjects, admixture mapping scientists have devised a method for generating genetic markers they label as "ancestry-informative." The production of these "ancestry-informative markers" or AIMs, is a clear example of how admixture mapping begins with socio-cultural categories and groups and produces genetic understandings of these groups.

The AIMs are a subset of genomic markers known as SNPs, or single nucleotide polymorphisms. They are sites in the genome that vary between different people. Geneticists estimate that there are about 10 million SNPs in a human genome, and of these, researchers have deemed a few thousand informative for ancestry, which they call "AIMs." Some population geneticists and some genetic epidemiologists consider subsets of these AIMs to be "informative" for different ancestries, for example, European ancestry, African ancestry, or Native American ancestry.

Researchers have designated AIMs as "special genetic markers" that are able to distinguish between groups, as one respondent described: "An ancestry informative marker has more information about ancestry on average than a random marker on the genome. And you can say how much more information it has about ancestry. We can quantify that."

How do researchers make AIMs? Admixture mapping researchers begin with an "admixed population"—with all the qualifications we discussed above—in which to study disease, and postulating the two ancestral populations that gave rise to it. Then they construct a particular set of AIMs to use in studying that admixed population. They call this set an "admixture map" for that population. For example, to study disease in African Americans, a collaboration of scientists at over twenty institutions created a map they believed to be specific for African American groups. This map has since been used in many recent studies (Smith et al. 2004). An admixture map, then, is a set of AIMs that are specifically built and put together for the purposes of studying disease in a predefined admixed population. We argue that this is a circular process and demonstrate this circularity next by showing in detail how an admixture map is constructed.

As described above, AIMs are a subset of SNPs, so-called polymorphic sites in the DNA at which more than one of the DNA "bases" (abbreviated as "A," "T," "G," and "C") appears when human genomes are compared. For example, at a non-SNP position in the genome, all people will have the same letter, but at a SNP position, some people will have one base, others will have another base. These different base possibilities are known as "variants."For the purposes of building an admixture map, researchers focus their efforts on determining the *frequencies* of SNP variants. For example, at a SNP position at which some people have "A" and others have "C," the frequency of the "A" variant is the percentage of people in a group who have "A" at that position. Many SNPs in human genomes have been estimated to occur with similar variant frequencies in different groups. This means that, at many SNP markers, variant frequencies are believed to *not* differ across groups. In contrast, however, admixture mapmakers claim that AIMs have comparatively "large" variant frequency differences between groups. They argue that at an AIM, one of the two possible variants is much more common (or much less common) in certain populations compared to other populations. It is these sorts of statistical assessments that admixture mapping researchers use to label markers as diagnostic or "informative" of a particular continental ancestry at particular points in the genome.

Admixture mapping researchers believe that such "large" frequency differences can be used statistically to differentiate "ancestral populations." But the meaning of "large" matters here, since admixture scientists distinguish AIMs from other SNPs based on their frequency differences. For example, in constructing the previously mentioned admixture map used to study African American groups, researchers were searching for AIMs to differentiate between groups they called West Africans and European Americans. They constructed AIMs with variants that, on average, differed in frequency by about 56 percent between their two groups of samples.

Thus in admixture mapping, the construction of groups and the construction of markers for distinguishing those groups are tightly connected. We have already discussed some concerns about the practices of delineating admixed and ancestral groups in admixture mapping. How do researchers' assumptions about these groups get built into the technologies of the admixture map and reinforce ideas of difference between groups?

For one, the process of admixture mapmaking illuminates the contingent ways in which researchers conceive of "ancestral" groups, as well as "ancestral" and contemporary DNA. In practice, ancestral DNA samples do not exist or are inaccessible. So, admixture mapping researchers use *contemporary samples* to estimate the frequencies of SNP variants, and select those SNPs with "large" frequency differences as AIMs for their admixture maps. We note that SNP frequencies are always estimates, calculated either by genotyping purported representatives of a group, or computationally estimated. For example, in selecting AIMs for the previously mentioned admixture map, researchers estimated the frequencies of SNP markers in samples collected from contemporary individuals who identified as white. The researchers called these samples "European American" and used their estimated SNP frequencies as a stand-in for marker frequencies in "ancestral Europeans." Similarly, under the assumption that some ancestors of contemporary African Americans came from West Africa, they collected and genotyped DNA from individuals currently residing in West or sub-Saharan Africa. They then used the marker frequencies estimated from these samples to stand in for "ancestral" African frequencies. In a puzzling twist, for some SNPs they genotyped DNA from contemporary African Americans and then created statistical genetics formulas for computationally estimating "ancestral African" frequencies from these contemporary frequencies. Finally, by comparing the SNP frequencies they had constructed for "ancestral European" and "ancestral African" groups, they selected those markers with large frequency differences between the two "ancestral populations." These markers are now known as AIMs, and they circulate as such among researchers as part of an "admixture map for African Americans." At each SNP in the admixture map, the variant that appears to have a higher frequency in "ancestral West Africans" (by their methods) is thought to be indicative of "African" ancestry, and the other variant specifies "European" ancestry.

Thus, admixture mapping accomplishes both a geographical elision and a generational elision, assuming similarities and differences between groups separated both in time and in space. The researchers assume that SNP frequencies in contemporary "European American" samples can be treated as equivalent to the frequencies in the "ancestral European" peoples that supposedly contributed DNA to contemporary African Americans. Indeed, labels for groups such as "European" and "European American" were sometimes treated as interchangeable by some respondents, even though both of these so-called groups can be considered to be very heterogeneous in themselves. In admixture map publications, researchers' reasoning for their assumptions about groups is often left unstated. For example, why should those identifying as European American among the geneticists' samples be thought of as able to directly represent "an" ancestral population from

Europe that came to America, as if such a static population existed or as if people living in Europe five hundred years ago were genetically isomorphic with people who identify as white in America today? Many peoples from many countries in present-day Europe colonized present-day America. This treatment of ancestral and contemporary "European groups" as indistinguishable, and essentially unchanged during or since encounters with other peoples, implies an assumption about the *fixity of whiteness.*

Similarly, researchers regarded contemporary West African samples as a good approximation of the gene pools of groups in Africa who were brought to the Americas and contributed DNA to present-day African Americans. On the other hand, frequencies calculated in contemporary African Americans were somehow seen as "admixed." They required further transformation (by statistical genetic algorithms) before they could become a good approximation for frequencies in the "ancestral African" population that supposedly contributed DNA to today's African American groups. Again, as with the genetic diversity of Europe described above, these kinds of manipulations collapse the genetic diversity of Africa. They also tell a particular story about how researchers view the relations between and among various groups separated in time and space. The geneticists conceptualized these African American samples as admixtures of both "African" and "European" DNA for the sake of the overall study of disease, but *more* African than European for the sake of making a map. Thus, they used these samples in a circular way to estimate the frequencies of DNA variants in their putative "African" ancestors.

The admixture mapping algorithms include statistical tests to assess how closely the European American and West African "populations" correspond to the "true" ancestral populations of African Americans (Smith et al. 2004). Nevertheless, these algorithms that are used to validate the mapmaking process have themselves been designed based on statistical formulas from population genetics that estimate measures of genetic drift.[6] These measurements are dependent on probabilistic and statistical models that have been developed using only a small number of *contemporary* samples. Thus, the conceptions of ancestral populations in this research collapse many local histories. For example, the variation and diversity of peoples in West Africa five hundred years ago becomes circumscribed by a few markers sampled from a few individuals in the present, and assembled into a "set" of markers that are then mobilized to tell researchers something about what it means (in terms of disease) to have West African ancestry. The admixture map, which contains the AIMs markers that are central to admixture mapping, is thus built by an amalgam of circular logics and assumptions that reinforce a particular story (and thus legitimize each other) at every step. Genetic stories are interwoven with social histories, giving rise to a complex and contingent tapestry of mutual reinforcement, sometimes serving as legitimization for the admixture mapping approach, and sometimes as explanation for the observed.

Finally, we note that biomedical admixture maps include over a thousand AIMs, while commercial ancestry testing protocols use fewer than a hundred.

The AIMs in the biomedical admixture maps are similar to and may overlap with the first AIMs designed by Shriver et al. (1997; 2003). This first set of AIMs are being used in commercially marketed genetic ancestry tests sold by DNAPrint Genomics and other companies, to provide consumers with information about their percentages of ancestry from different continents. Some have pointed out that this use of AIMs to distinguish among continental populations over-simplifies and potentially geneticizes race, by inscribing sociopolitical conceptions of race onto test-takers' DNA (Bolnick et al. 2007; Fullwiley 2008; TallBear 2008). However, our respondents working in biomedical genomics, as opposed to ancestry testing, were careful in their publications to distinguish their marker sets from those of Shriver and others, indicating an unwillingness to use their markers and methods for identifying any specific individual's continental ancestry.

The Practices of Admixture Mapping: How Specific Ancestries Get Linked to Specific Diseases

As discussed above, admixture mapping tools such as the admixture maps construct particular correspondences between groups and markers. Researchers believe a particular map or set of markers is useful only for the particular group it was designed for, such as African Americans, or Latin Americans. We will discuss how the marker maps are used to link groups (and particular "ancestries") to diseases, referring to fieldwork done in a lab that narrowed down a large region of Chromosome 8 as being associated with prostate cancer in African Americans.

Once they have constructed an admixture map of AIMs for use with a particular population, researchers use the map to connect genetic markers to diseases. Researchers genotype DNA samples from disease-affected individuals, determining which variant each individual DNA sample has, at each of the SNP markers in the admixture map. They look for large chunks of the genomes of disease-affected individuals that appear to have an excess of the markers that they have assigned to one of the ancestries—for example, an excess of "African" SNP variants, or an excess of "European" SNP variants. Any regions that exhibit an excess of one of the two sets of "ancestral variants" is selected as a candidate for disease association. They then use statistical methods to assess candidate regions and identify those that appear to be most likely associated with the disease under study.

Put another way, in this step of admixture mapping researchers attempt (as they describe it) to infer continental ancestry at each point in the genome, for each of their samples. There is an analogous process in commercial genetic ancestry testing, whereby companies genotype the DNA of test-takers and generate a summary readout of the percentages of each of their ancestries across their genomes, calculated based on AIMs technology (Fullwiley 2008). However, in the case of admixture mapping in biomedical research, individuals are never told which chunks of their chromosomes are likely to be from which of their ancestries. But in positing that disease arises at least partly from a chunk of DNA inherited from one ancestral group versus another, admixture mapping researchers explicitly connect not just the 'race' of the admixed group to the disease in question, but also indirectly designate a particular continental ancestry as being the "source" of the disease.

For example, our respondents reported that DNA inherited from African ancestors (or what they termed the "African chromosome") was responsible for increasing the risk of prostate cancer in African Americans, compared to the risk in white Americans and other groups. However, one might surmise (according to the logic of admixture mapping) that if genetics plays a role, then West Africans should have a high incidence of prostate cancer as well, because of their continental ancestry. Yet, despite the finding of "risk alleles" for prostate cancer due to "West African" ancestry, it has never been established that peoples in West Africa have a high incidence of prostate cancer. It is likely that environmental factors play a considerable role, and it is possible that they interact with DNA (perhaps even DNA currently thought to be indicative of "non-African ancestry"), leading to variable outcomes in people who live in different parts of the world.

In this way, concepts of continental ancestry and related race categories are embedded within the continuum of practices constituting admixture mapping. They collide and tangle with notions of population (bounded by time and space) that are used to guide the map-making process, and they become central to the (re)constructed histories of various peoples and their diseases, which emerge from interpretations of disease-genetic marker associations. These concepts of continental ancestry are different from concepts of ancestry that are part of the scientific practices of, for example, genome-wide association studies (GWAS). Compared to GWAS, admixture mapping uses different theoretical frameworks and a different interpretation of ancestry, which can be described as "continental ancestry"—that is, they use a model in which ancestors of contemporary group study subjects are believed to have come from different continents. In other words, they try to identify genetic differences across continents. Thus in admixture mapping, the markers, chromosomes, risk alleles and "chunks of DNA" that are linked to disease are explicitly coded with continental and racial labels, and circulate in the literature and in further research with these labels firmly attached.

The Triangulations of Geography, Ancestry, Genetic Histories, and Disease

Within admixture studies, practitioners mix geographical descriptors with their concepts of race and continental ancestry to describe individuals and groups. Where groups (actually present today, or imagined as ancestors) are or were located comes to matter crucially for the links to fit together. But people move, and these histories are rarely straightforward or traceable. Still, genetic history is constructed alongside geographical history, and the two are woven to arrive at present-day "race" groups and their diseases.

This leads to the question, how do notions of continental ancestry differ from notions of race? We argue that the two are different, but often superimposed. Notions of ancestry and stories of geographical and continental origins are frequently interlaced, and even talked of interchangeably. But researchers also relate stories of continental origins to contemporary American race categories. We interviewed members of a leading lab in this area of study who have been using the admixture map described above to identify genetic variants for prostate cancer in African American men. One scientist respondent in our study described what they are doing as "tracking continental origin of lines of descent." This population geneticist asserted that the ancestral populations of African Americans were "very different . . . at a population level, genetically." The use of a whole set of tools and stories (as described in this paper) create the knowledge that leads to such assertions, and such assertions justify the tools and stories, and validate the knowledge. This includes theories about the relative incidence of disease, the contributions of genetics to disease risk, the relationship between continental ancestry and genetics, and the relationship between continental ancestry and race. In triangulating all of these, this population geneticist and colleagues in his discipline have constructed and cast admixture mapping as a reasonable approach to test their belief that genetics might partially explain why prostate cancer appears to be more prevalent in African Americans than in other groups.

In explicitly connecting continental ancestry to race, scientists encode geographical descriptors in the code of the genome. Alleles and even chromosomes are labeled with continental descriptors. For example, in publications scientists have referred to "the African chromosome" to indicate that a particular chunk of MALD markers in the genome appears to be more closely related to the "ancestral African" sequence of SNPs in that region than to the "ancestral European." "African allele" is used to refer to a particular SNP variant that is estimated to be more frequent in African ancestors than European ancestors. Thus, "chunks of DNA"[7] in the genome acquire geographical qualifiers, via a vernacular that pins down their origins to (and collapses the genetic histories and diversity of) entire continents.

As scientists deploy particular genetic, historical, and geographical discourses that cross and intersect, genomic stretches of SNP markers acquire genealogies that are rooted in place. However, in another move, scientists extend the explanatory power of the risk SNPs to people in other groups who have the disease. Even if African American or other supposedly "admixed" samples are used to identify genetic associations for the diseases under study, such associations are considered to be potentially translatable across populations. For example, SNPs in a genomic region of chromosome 8 that were believed to confer elevated risk for prostate cancer in African Americans were subsequently tested in other "ethnic" groups, such as Japanese Americans, Native Hawaiians, Latin Americans, and European Americans, to see if the findings could be replicated in other groups. All of these groups displayed evidence of statistically significant association of variants at this locus to prostate cancer risk (Freedman et al.

2006). What is it about this region of chromosome 8 that makes it "African"? We have described above the methods, assumptions, and practices with which geneticists make such conclusions.

Complexity in Genomic Studies of Common Complex Diseases: Clinical Implications

The diseases under study in these projects are complex and thought to be the result of multiple genetic and environmental factors acting in combination. Reinforcing this idea, the first paper to report the 8q24 region linked to prostate cancer described above did not use admixture mapping; its authors found this region using family linkage analysis in several pedigrees of affected Icelandic males (Amundadottir et al. 2006). Others have identified the same region as associated with increased risk of prostate cancer, in various populations, using genomic-wide association studies.

Such studies have been done in African American men and non-Hispanic white or European men. Each of these studies has reported different SNPs, and even differing variants of SNPs, within the large 8q24 genomic region as being most significantly associated with prostate cancer risk. Therefore different SNPs, SNP variants, genes, or even alleles may be involved in different individuals. Other studies have found SNP alleles in this region to also be involved in colorectal cancer (Haiman et al. 2007b; Tomlinson et al. 2007; Zanke et al. 2007), and urinary bladder cancer (Kiemeney et al. 2008), suggesting that some of these risk variants may be pleiotropic, that is, they have multiple effects on the etiologies of several kinds of cancers, or perhaps even other diseases.

With the level of complexity involved in prostate cancer and other common complex diseases, what are the implications for association studies like admixture mapping to identify causative genetic elements? Because researchers use the technique to focus their attention on very large regions of the genome, and not on genes, or even specific genetic markers, further experimental analysis is necessary to determine if and how 8q24 is involved in prostate cancer, either directly or indirectly.

Given the variety of reports of genomic regions, disease associations and populations studied, it remains unclear how this information can and will be used in clinical settings to shed light on individual or group risk. As the American Society of Human Genetics has stated, "Numerous studies using MALD are underway, but even at its best, MALD is likely to be an effective strategy for only a small fraction of health-related traits, since genetic differences may not be the major cause of observed population differences in disease incidence. These limitations justify caution in the interpretation of data from these studies and in the clinical application of results from the related DTC genetic tests" (ASHG 2008).

Indeed, one respondent admitted that in terms of ancestry and conceiving of admixed populations, "what they are generating is a *model* not the truth" and that some details may be incorrect. In addition certain outliers may not fit the model. One respondent stressed that in practice "it's very important clinically that individuals should be treated as individuals." The genetic findings of admixture studies, however, are based on risk probabilities for groups, not individuals. Indeed, the scientists we studied were quick to point out that they cannot make any claims about individual cases, either in terms of their geographic or ethnic ancestry, or in terms of their disease risk status.

There are many examples of diseases for which genetic explanations emerging from laboratory research became associated with more frequent occurrence in certain socio-historical groups. For example, several diseases are now thought to be most prevalent in Jewish, African, or Caucasian genetic backgrounds, such as Tay-Sachs, sickle-cell anemia, and cystic fibrosis, respectively. Thus some diseases and associated genes come to be described with ethnic or racial qualifiers. Indeed, as part of the standard of care at many clinics, healthcare providers test for each of these diseases specifically in individuals who self-identify with the relevant race or ethnic category.[8] In similar fashion, when regions of the genome that appear to derive from one of two presumed "ancestral populations" harbor SNP variants that become associated with disease in a particular population through admixture mapping studies, they acquire names such as "African risk allele" in the biomedical literature. Such interpretations reinforce the imputed group specificity that motivates these studies in the first place, even though, as described above, the risk alleles are often found in other groups as well.

This is not simply a labeling problem, since the practices used to arrive at such labels shape and reinforce how biomedical scientists think about the relationships between genes, diseases, and certain populations. These practices construct diseases and population groups as interconnected in particular ways. For example, one such assumption about self-identified African Americans is that they are so recently admixed that their ancestry is *predominantly* African, and only in small fraction European. However, many people who self-identify as African American may have had a "more European" ancestor as recently as one generation back, for example, Barack Obama. Another assumption is that those who identify with a particular race or ethnic group are more genetically related to each other than to individuals who do not identify with that group. Relatedly, another assumption is that genetics may be involved in diseases that are reported to occur more often in individuals who identify with the same socio-cultural race or ethnic group. Together, these assumptions stack and imbricate in ways that connect estimates of disease incidence to estimates of African ancestry in an appeal to "common sense" interpretations of which groups are "more" or "less" African, or more or less prone to disease.

In a more applied example, companies offering direct-to-consumer genetic risk tests are channeling the results of admixture mapping studies to individual diagnosis, regardless of scientists' claims that these findings are too premature. Within the field of admixture mapping, a company called Proactive Genomics is developing a test to predict risk for prostate cancer, which is expected to cost about $300 (Kolata 2008). After genotyping DNA from blood or saliva, they will analyze the SNP variants at five different regions of the genome thought to affect susceptibility, each conferring an independent (and therefore additive) risk (Haiman et al. 2007a; Zheng et al. 2008). The more susceptibility variants a person has, the higher that person's estimated disease risk. The availability of Proactive Genomics' test will, according to some clinicians, lead to earlier screening of higher risk groups, including African American males (Kolata 2008).

What is clinically important here is that most prostate cancer cases advance so slowly that they are generally benign if left alone, but unnecessary treatment can result in unwanted side effects like impotence or incontinence. Because doctors cannot predict in advance which tumors will become aggressive, increased screening is likely to result in more decisions to prematurely and unnecessary treat patients, hastening side effects and worsening the overall condition of patients. Many prostate cancer specialists worry about these implications. Like the Prostate-Specific Antigen screening test, which has never been shown to actually reduce the risk of prostate cancer fatality and for which false positives are common, it is unclear if the risk estimates generated by Proactive Genomics' test will actually lead to better health outcomes for individuals or unnecessary invasive surgery and treatment.

Finally, AIMs have also been tailored to the goal of trying to determine individuals' ancestry proportions. At least one company, DNAPrint Genomics, uses AIMs, for example, in consumer tests that purport to be able to distinguish a person's various continental "biogeographical" ancestries, which they claim is the heritable portion of "race" (Bliss 2008; Bolnick et al. 2007; Fullwiley 2008; TallBear 2008). The cautions and limitations of ancestry testing are summarized in Bolnick et al. (2008).

It is not possible for scientists or regulatory bodies to fully control the commercial applications of their findings, regardless of their intended usage. Though our respondents helped to find an association to prostate cancer at one region of the genome, much more work will be required to determine which, if any, of the DNA within that stretch is causative or even indirectly correlated to prostate cancer. Even if genes are found to be statistically associated with prostate cancer, researchers would need to do more analysis to determine their function. The interpretation and application of admixture mapping findings, once disseminated into public domains (including to other practitioners in the sciences, who may or may not be aware of these caveats), becomes difficult to manage. With this degree of uncertainty, it is difficult to imagine what information the commercial test for prostate cancer can actually offer patients, or how they might act on it. Many of our respondents worry about the ramifications of untrained commercial ventures using genetic findings to make broad claims about an individual's risk for certain diseases, particularly because the FDA has not implemented any regulatory oversight or approval process for "homebrew" tests offered directly from a company, rather than through licensed clinical or medical practitioners.

The Future of Admixture: Technical, Public Health, and Policy Implications

Given that other methods exist, such as GWAS, which can potentially avoid the imprecision of race categories in genomics research (Fujimura and Rajagopalan, 2011), why do some researchers choose admixture mapping over GWAS? One rationale our respondents have provided for this choice is that admixture mapping is much smaller in scale and thus cheaper in terms of the technologies. Population geneticists have designed the science of admixture mapping to be more affordable, while still generating statistically significant results. Further, admixture mapping studies are less time-consuming and technology-intensive to conduct than GWAS studies. Admixture mapping studies use fewer DNA samples from disease-affected individuals than GWAS, and only genotype about three thousand AIMs in each DNA sample, as opposed to the hundreds of thousands of markers genotyped per DNA sample in GWAS. Thus some researchers believe that certain diseases may be studied more inexpensively using an admixture mapping approach. However, as one respondent noted, GWAS can be used to generate the same findings as admixture mapping without being restricted to admixed populations, and the admixture mapping approach is thus falling out of favor at some labs, even as it remains in use at others.

Understanding how admixture mapping works, and how it makes connections between populations and diseases, is critical for understanding the limitations of commercial ancestry testing and disease risk testing, whose methods are based in genomic assumptions like those we have described. Many companies have begun to offer both types of tests directly to consumers, for a fee, including DNAPrint for the former and 23AndMe, Navigenics, and deCODEMe for the latter. These tests have received much attention from consumers and the media. They are not simply recreational or for entertainment—many consumers place some degree of trust in the results they receive (Bolnick et al. 2007; Nelson 2008). Significantly, the databases and methods that these tests use (derived from the findings of genomics research like that which we describe) are specifically not designed for individual ancestry or disease risk assessments, according to our respondents. As genomics becomes increasingly integrated into health care in the United States, perhaps even under the Obama administration, recognizing the limitations of such approaches as admixture mapping will be important for informing policy around the potential clinical applications of such methods and their findings.

The choice of groups that scientists study as admixed in this vein of genomic research are particularly indicative of the tenor of debates around race-based medicine in the United States. As Steve Epstein has noted (2008), there has been a regulatory push at the level of the federal funding agencies for the inclusion of minorities in American biomedical research. The rise of admixture mapping research speaks to both this regulatory context and to the desire on the part of some scientists to include their own minority communities in their research programs (Fullwiley 2008).

Indeed, thus far in our reading, individuals who identify as European American or non-Hispanic white have not been the focus of an admixture mapping search for associations between disease and genetics. Why not? Are they considered too admixed, and therefore not amenable because the ancestral populations are too difficult to define? Here, the operative history may be one of the multiple waves of migration from various parts of Europe, a Europe that is differentiated in ways that "west Africa" is not, into national, geographic, linguistic, cultural, and possibly reproductively distinct groups. Alternatively, such groups may be viewed by researchers as not admixed, or not admixed recently enough. The idea that European American groups are not admixed in the way that other groups who encountered Europeans are suggests an "unmarked category" status for European American categories within this science.

Other groups, such as those identifying as African American, become, in a sense, Europeanized by this work, in that European ancestry is imputed regardless of individuals' own genealogical self-understandings. These assumptions gain the authority of science, and stories of geography, history, and genetics stabilize each other in mutually reinforcing ways. Just as socio-cultural histories and human geographies are used to legitimate the inquiry into genetics, the genetic findings and the presumed stability of DNA reaffirm and stabilize historical stories.

Conclusion

In this essay we have begun to untangle the relationships between continental ancestry, geography, history, population, and race in the practices, technologies, research designs, and research analyses/results of some admixture mapping studies in U.S. biomedical research. In admixture mapping, researchers differentiate DNA into chunks by deploying geographical, continental and ancestral labels that buttress certain stories and make them robust. During the research processes, social histories of population origins and migrations thus become embedded in the research philosophy. Geography plays a major role, as these researchers trace groups of peoples across the globe to separate "ancestral" homes delineated by continent, thus shaping concepts of "continental ancestry." Discourses of race and ancestry are deeply entangled in the constitution of genetic histories in contemporary biomedicine, in ways that are contingent and mutually reinforcing. These discourses, as embedded in the technologies of admixture mapping, have consequences for how disease studies, medical practices, public health policies, and popular culture use and interpret genetics to construct categories of difference.

NOTES

1. The quotations indicate that these terms are used by the population geneticists who use admixture mapping.

2. A phenotype is an observable characteristic, attribute, or trait of an organism.

3. Although some of our respondents argue that methods used in GWAS to account for ancestry will supersede/displace/supplant admixture mapping technologies, the latter are still very much in use today.

4. We note here that genetic studies are different from clinical practices, in which self-reported race is a very common heuristic used by clinicians in diagnosis and treatment decisions. Some argue that race is a useful proxy for other kinds of information when dealing with patients, especially in budget-restricted or time-sensitive medical situations, where obtaining genetic or other information is too expensive or could delay treatment and compromise the patient's health. Still, there are debates about the use of race in clinical practice.

5. American research groups have also used this same approach to study disease in other geographical contexts, including Argentina and Mexico. However, our discussion is limited to the American biomedical context and study subjects in the United States.

6. Population geneticists have formulated the theory of genetic drift to describe processes that may cause two groups of people to become more genetically different from each other with each generation. These can include: geographic isolation from each other, different selection pressures, mutation, and bottlenecks (when only a small subset of the group reproduces and contributes genetic material to the next generation).

7. A population geneticist used this nontechnical term with us to help make the point clear. These "chunks of DNA" are more technically described as portions of the genome with significant linkage disequilibrium, or regions that are believed to be relatively unchanged over recent generations. These portions of the genome are assumed to have "traveled" intact through generations with minimal recombination.

8. This is the case at one of our fieldsites.

WORKS CITED

American Society of Human Genetics (ASHG). 2008. Ancestry Testing Statement. Available at: http://www.ashg.org/pdf/ASHGAncestryTestingStatement_Final.pdf.

Amundadottir, L. T., P. Sulem, J. Gudmundsson, A. Helgason, A. Baker, B. A. Agnarsson, A. Sigurdsson, et al. 2006. A common variant associated with prostate cancer in European and African populations. *Nature Genetics* 38 (6) (June):652–658.

Bliss, C. 2008. Mapping race through admixture. *International Journal of Technology, Knowledge and Society* 4 (4):79–83.

Blumenbach, Johann Friedrich. 1795. *De generis humani varietate nativa liber (On the natural variety of mankind)*. Goettingae: Vandenhoek et Ruprecht.

Bolnick, D. A., D. Fullwiley, T. Duster, R. S. Cooper, J. H. Fujimura, J. Kahn, J. S. Kaufman, J. Marks, A. Morning, A. Nelson, P. Ossorio, J. Reardon, S. M. Reverby, and K. TallBear. 2007. Genetics: The science and business of genetic ancestry testing. *Science* 318 (5849) (Oct. 19):399–400.

Burchard, E., E. Ziv, N. Coyle, S. L. Gomez, H. Tang, A. J. Karter, J. L Mountain, E. J. Perez-Stable, D. Sheppard, and N. Risch. 2002. The importance of race and ethnic background in biomedical research and clinical practice. *New England Journal of Medicine* 348 (12):1170–1175.

Cooper, R. S., J. S. Kaufman, and R. Ward. 2003. Race and genomics. *New England Journal of Medicine* 348 (12) (Mar. 20):1166–1170.

Cooper, Richard S., Bamidele Tayo, and Xiaofang Zhu. 2008. Genome-wide association studies: Implications for multiethnic samples. *Human Molecular Genetics* 17 (R2):R151–155.

Duster, Troy. 2003. *Backdoor to eugenics.* New York: Routledge.

Epstein, Steven. 2008. The rise of "recruitmentology": Clinical research, racial knowledge, and the politics of inclusion and difference. *Social Studies of Science* 38(5):803–834.

Feldman, M. 2006. Continental ancestry and human history in the "race" debate. In *Human Biology Symposium VI* (Madison, Wisconsin).

Fujimura, J. H., and R. Rajagopalan. 2011. Different differences: The use of 'genetic ancestry' versus race in biomedical human genetic research. *Social Studies of Science* 41(1):5–30.

Fujimura, J. H., R. Rajagopalan, P. N. Ossorio, and K. A. Doksum. 2010. Race versus ancestry: Operationalizing populations in human genetic variation studies. In *What's the Use of Race*, edited by D. Jones and I. Whitmarsh, 169–186. Cambridge, MA: MIT Press.

Fullwiley, Duana. 2008. The biologistical construction of race: "Admixture" technology and the new genetic medicine. *Social Studies of Science* 38(5):697–737.

Haiman, Christopher A., Nick Patterson, Matthew L. Freedman, Simon R. Myers, et al. 2007a. Multiple regions within 8q24 independently affect risk for prostate cancer. *Nature Genetics* 39(5):579–580.

Haiman, Christopher A., Loïc Le Marchand, Jennifer Yamamato, Daniel O. Stram, et al. 2007b. A common genetic risk factor for colorectal and prostate cancer. *Nature Genetics* 39(8):954–956.

Halder, I., M. Shriver, M. Thomas, J. R. Fernandez, and T. Frudakis. 2008. A panel of ancestry informative markers for estimating individual biogeographical ancestry and admixture from four continents: Utility and applications. *Human Mutation* 29 (5) May):648–658.

Kahn, J. 2006. Genes, race, and population: Avoiding a collision of categories. *American Journal of Health Policy* 96 (11):1965–1970.

Kiemeney, Lambertus A., Steinunn Thorlacius, Patrick Sulem, Frank Geller, et al. 2008. Sequence variant on 8q24 confers susceptibility to urinary bladder cancer. *Nature Genetics* 40 (11):1307–1312.

Kolata, Gina. 2008. $300 to learn risk of prostate cancer. *New York Times*, (Jan. 17). www.nytimes.com/2008/01/17/health/17cancer.html [Accessed June 15 2008].

Marks, Jonathan. 1995. *Human biodiversity: Genes, race, and history.* New York: Aldine de Gruyter.

Morning, Ann. 2007. Everyone knows it's a social construct: Contemporary science and the nature of race. *Sociological Focus* 40 (4):436–454.

Nelson, A. 2008. Bio science: Genetic genealogy testing and the pursuit of African ancestry. *Social Studies of Science* 38 (5) (Oct.):759–783.

Ossorio, Pilar N., and Duster, Troy. 2005. Race and genetics: Controversies in biomedical, behavioral, and forensic sciences. *American Psychologist* 60 (1):115–128.

Sankar, P., and M. K. Cho. 2002. Genetics: Toward a new vocabulary of human genetic variation. *Science* 298 (5597) (Nov. 15):1337–1338.

Shields, Alexandra, Michael Fortun, Evelynn M. Hammonds, Patricia A. King, Caryn Lerman, Rayna Rapp, and Patrick F. Sullivan. 2005. The use of race variables in genetic studies of complex traits and the goal of reducing health disparities. *American Psychologist* 60 (1):77–103.

Shriver, Mark D., Esteban J. Parra, Sonia Dios, Carolina Bonilla, et al. 2003. Skin pigmentation, biogeographical ancestry, and admixture mapping. *Human Genetics* 112 (4):387–399.

Smith, Michael W., Nick Patterson, James A. Lautenberger, Ann L. Truelove, et al. 2004. A high-density admixture map for disease gene discovery in African Americans. *American Journal of Human Genetics* 74 (5):1001–1013.

TallBear, Kimberly. (2008) Native-American-DNA.com: In search of Native American race and tribe. *In Revisiting Race in a Genomic Age*, edited by B. A. Koenig, Sandra Soo-Jin Lee, and S. S. Richardson, 235–252. Stanford, CA: Stanford University Press.

Tomlinson, Ian, Emily Webb, Luis Carvajal-Carmona, Peter Broderick, et al. 2007. A genome-wide association scan of tag SNPs identifies a susceptibility variant for colorectal cancer at 8q24.21. *Nature Genetics* 39 (8):984–988.

Wailoo, Keith, and Stephen Gregory Pemberton. 2006. *The troubled dream of genetic medicine: Ethnicity and innovation in Tay-Sachs, cystic fibrosis, and sickle cell disease.* Baltimore: Johns Hopkins University Press.

Zanke, Brent W., Celia M. T. Greenwood, Jagadish Rangrej, Rafal Kustra, et al. 2007. Genome-wide association scan identifies a colorectal cancer susceptibility locus on chromosome 8q24. *Nature Genetics* 39 (8):989–994.

Zheng, S. Lilly, Jielin Sun, Fredrik Wiklund, Shelly Smith, et al. 2008. Cumulative association of five genetic variants with prostate cancer. *New England Journal of Medicine* 358 (9):910–919.

10

Waiting on the Promise
of Prescribing Precision

Race in the Era of Pharmacogenomics

SANDRA SOO-JIN LEE

Announcing the arrival of a "Brave New Pharmacy" at the turn of the millennium, *Time* magazine forecasted in 2001 a new era of genomic medicine, in which current strategies in drug development would be replaced by "something much more rational and systematic."[1] The article suggests that the significant public investment in human genetics research would result in improved clinical encounters through which, "Doctors will treat diseases like cancer and diabetes before the symptoms even begin, using medications that boost or counteract the effects of individual proteins with exquisite precision, attacking sick cells while leaving healthy cells alone." Forecasting that health professionals "will know right from the start how to select the best medicine to suit each patient," *Time*'s narrative of stealth and precision is emblematic of public misunderstanding of the new genetics in the twenty-first century.

Suggesting that the growing arsenal of human genomic data will answer the question of why certain individuals are at greater risk for disease, and why certain drugs have no effect or, worse, end up making people sicker, reflects not so much the current struggles in genomic research as the iconic power of DNA in the public imagination.

Despite the setbacks in gene therapy during the 1990s, the promise of genomics has refocused on the potential for gene sequencing techniques to bear fruit in differentiated strategies for the prevention of disease at the molecular level and improved health through targeted medicine.[2] Technological developments have fostered the burgeoning field of pharmacogenomics in the study of gene-to-gene interactions through the use of high-throughput abilities of supercomputers and growing storage capabilities of microchips.[3] The hope is that these developments will help scientists to identify drug responses for molecular subgroups through differential diagnosis during the early stages of drug development, which will lead to the creation of "tailored" drugs of greater efficacy.[4] Although the promise of pharmacogenomics, as evidenced in the *Time* article,

164

emphasizes an imminent era of individualized medicine, the reality of the current research landscape is a focus on populations. Building on research that reveals population differences in frequencies of alleles known to be salient for drug response, several pressing questions emerge, particularly related to the ongoing struggle to eliminate health disparities in the United States. These include: Will the identification of molecular subgroups map onto current categories of race and ethnicity? What role do race and ethnicity have on drug specificity? How will pharmacogenomics contribute to a more equitable and rational landscape for genomic medicine?

A review of the pharmacogenomics literature reveals a history within the scientific community of stratifying patient populations by race or ethnicity. This approach dovetails with the well established practice in healthcare of using race as a risk factor in clinical decision-making, and the more recent, but growing, interest among pharmaceutical companies in discovering untapped market niches in anticipation of targeted products as fewer blockbuster drugs come to market.[5] In light of this convergence, many scholars have warned against the use of race as a proxy for genetic relatedness or as an interim strategy of using race as shorthand for variation.[6]

In order to change course, several challenges must be met, including increasing DNA sample sets from diverse populations, improving guidelines for characterizing ancestry of the individuals donating DNA, and greater regulatory oversight of putatively race-based therapeutics by federal agencies. Without major shifts in how researchers approach population differences in research practice, the much heralded brave new world of genomics may give way to a strangely familiar landscape that emboldens notions of racial biologies, oversimplifies understandings of genetic contributions to human health, and could ultimately undermine the hopes for equity in healthcare.[7]

The Alluring Promise of Precision

The shift from "-etics" to "-omics," involves a significant jump in magnitude and scope in the study of possible gene effects. While pharmacogenetics has historically involved the investigation of single gene-to-gene interactions, pharmacogenomics builds on high-throughput technology that makes possible instantaneous comparisons of multiple genes. By identifying these "genetic recipes," researchers hope to discover the molecular basis for differences in drug responses among individuals.

In September of 2003, five months after the fiftieth anniversary of the modeling of DNA by James Watson and Francis Crick, the first international scientific meeting on pharmacogenomics was cosponsored by leading scientific institutions Cold Spring Harbor Laboratories, in the United States, and the Wellcome Trust, an independent charity that provides the largest source of nongovernmental funds for biomedical research in the United Kingdom. The first conference was held in

Hinxton, a small picturesque town near Cambridge University, sixty miles from London and home to the Wellcome Trust Genome Campus. The meeting's co-organizer, David Bentley, director of the Sanger Institute, welcomed the attendees by openly challenging presenters to answer a basic and seemingly facile question. "What," he asked, "is pharmacogenomics?" The response of widespread laughter in the auditorium confirmed just how pertinent and difficult this query is.

Underlying the challenge of defining pharmacogenomics is how to distinguish it from "pharmacogenetics," originally a subfield of pharmacology, recognized in the scientific literature since the early 1950s. Over the past several years, health institutions have attempted to provide some clarity to this terminology, with uneven success. In its 2007 Draft Guidance on Terminology on Pharmacogenomics, the FDA defines *pharmacogenomics* in general terms as "the investigation of variations of DNA and RNA characteristics as related to drug response."[8] The National Institute of General Medical Sciences (NIGMS), which sponsors the NIH Pharmacogenetics Research Network (PGRN), suggests that the two terms, pharmacogenetics and pharmacogenomics, can be used interchangeably and offers a more metaphoric explanation, stating that:

> Just as genes contribute to whether you will be tall or short, black-haired or blond, your genes also determine how you will respond to medicines. Genes are like recipes—they carry instructions for making protein molecules. As medicines travel through your body, they interact with thousands of proteins. Small differences in the composition or quantities of these molecules can affect how medicines do their jobs.[9]

This framing makes plain that pharmacogenomics is the study of how genes influence the way a person responds to a drug, including both positive and negative reactions. Scientists describe drug response as a complex trait that is influenced by many different factors, which include genetic and environmental variables. While acknowledging the interplay of the multitude of contributing factors, scientists working in pharmacogenomics are focused on identifying genes involved in drug response in order to develop genetic tests that could predict a person's response to a particular drug.

Reducing Adverse Drug Reactions

In defiance of conventional wisdom, most drugs do not work on everyone.[10] Drug therapies exhibit wide variability among individuals in their efficacy and toxicity, contributing to an estimated 100,000 patient deaths and 2.2 million injuries annually, as the direct results of adverse drug reactions (ADRs) in the United States. The incidence of serious and fatal cases in hospitalized patients is reported at 6–7 percent, making ADRs the fourth leading cause of death in the United States.[11] Currently, negative effects from medications are monitored only after they are prescribed to patients. On a case-by-case basis, clinicians adjust dosage and treatment type according to the reported reactions of individual patients to initial prescriptions. This trial-and-error approach has been criticized for exposing patients to potentially harmful drug therapies and for taking up costly clinical consultation time. The downstream healthcare cost of drug-related morbidity and mortality is estimated to be $177.4 billion in the United States, as of 2001.[12] Of this total figure, approximately $101 billion is believed to be avoidable. Through the study of human genetic variation, researchers hope to minimize ADRs and improve safety and efficacy by creating genomic-based medications, which they believe will provide individuals with the "right" medication at the outset, as dictated by their unique genetic signatures.[13]

The search for the genetic basis for drug response focuses on identifying the relatively small variations in the nucleotide sequences that make up genes. As discussed earlier, this effort has resulted in a rapidly growing infrastructure of biobanks that catalog these differences in the human genome among global populations. These variations, called single nucleotide polymorphisms, or SNPs are scrutinized by researchers who hope to use them as a diagnostic tool to predict a person's drug response. For SNPs to be used in this way, a person's DNA must be sequenced for the presence of specific SNPs known to be associated with a particular effect. Although traditional gene sequencing technology remains slow and expensive, new approaches involving DNA microarray have allowed the identification of hundreds of thousands of genes in a short period of time. As DNA microarray technology develops further, scientists predict that SNP screening could become common clinical practice in prescribing medications. The question that remains is whether identifying SNPs will translate into a reduction of ADRs and greater drug efficacy, improving health status for individuals.

Until cost effective ubiquitous genotyping emerges, identifying and acting on genetic variation will depend on focusing on groups. Scientists suggest that although individuals share the vast majority of their genome, populations will have different SNPs. Pharmacogenomics may reveal groups of individuals that share similar patterns of SNPs in parts or chunks of their genome, where the general population might be divided into genetic groups based on the presence of SNPs that contribute to a particular drug response. Researchers predict that routine genetic sequencing of the population may result in subgroups that exhibit different SNP profiles, creating genetically based groupings that may have biological implications, but also, some scientists have suggested, may correlate meaningfully with existing social groupings and relationships.[14]

In an industry that invests approximately $24 billion in the research and development of new drug therapies annually,[15] using pharmacogenomic data is viewed as a potentially critical approach to drug development. Some have predicted potential savings of up to 60 percent of current costs, which now average $880 million to bring one drug from bench to market.[16] These savings could be dwarfed by the savings that may result from more efficient drugs in the overall cost of healthcare in the United States.[17] One pharmacogenomic approach taken by the pharmaceutical industry is the screening of individuals for SNPs believed to be associated with a particular drug response before enrolling them in clinical trials. This strategy depends on being able to identify a particular population with the desired SNP profile and excluding those that carry SNPs which may render a drug ineffective or contribute to harmful side effects. Pre-screening human subjects would allow clinical trials to be smaller, faster, and therefore less expensive. Costs of participant recruitment for Phase II and Phase III of clinical trials could be decreased by "enriching" the study population with those having the candidate genotypes. As a result, fewer participants would be needed to achieve the anticipated effect, decreasing the time spent on these stages of drug development. The drug would then be labeled for use by only those with the genotypes in question. However, this method depends on the development and use of genetic tests to identify responders.

A pharmacogenomic success case is the development of Herceptin, a drug that has been shown to be effective in women with metastatic breast cancer who test positive for a specific version of a gene called HER2. Klaus Lindpaintner, global head of genomics at pharmaceutical giant Hoffman-La Roche, which produces Herceptin through its majority ownership of biotechnology company Genentech, notes that, "[Herceptin] has become a major blockbuster. If you have a medicine that may be applicable only to a smaller part of population but is uniquely well applicable, then you tend to actually penetrate that market segment very completely." U.S. sales of Herceptin in 2005 increased 56 percent to $747.2 million from $479.0 million in 2004.[18]

While such approaches may prove to be more effective, the question remains as to whose genotypes will be the foci of interest for these newly tailored therapeutics? In a climate of rising healthcare costs and pressures to keep medical procedures to a minimum, will clinical decisions on the appropriate use of drugs be truly individualized, or will racial profiling be a compromise solution? In addition, who will be included or excluded from clinical trials, and what will be the scientific, economic, and medically relevant issues that will inform such decisions?

There is concern among some scholars that stratifying individuals into patient groups based on a combination of genotypic and phenotypic information by pharmacogenomics would result in smaller markets of "orphan patients," who have rare alleles and may be perceived as unattractive for pharmaceutical investment.[19] Scholars worry that the beneficiaries of pharmacogenomics research will be among populations that are seen to constitute larger, more profitable market share. This concern is exacerbated by the gap in regulatory measures that would counter potential disincentives to develop pharmacogenomic products and services for these potentially small patient populations.[20] These issues highlight the stakes for how drug development in a genomic age will be handled in both the clinical and research settings. Our assumptions about race and biology and answers to the question of what to do about population differences set us on a trajectory that will ultimately create the future landscape of healthcare and affect issues of health disparities, equity, and justice.

The Problem of Interpreting Difference

The central challenge in pharmacogenomics is how to identify the illusive SNPs that influence drug response—the metaphoric needles in the haystack of clinical significance. Understanding the relative frequencies of SNPs in different populations is one strategy for decreasing the size of the haystacks one would be required to inspect. Race is often used as one method of segmenting the populations and may be incorporated into research design and hypothesis building. Many have suggested that this use of race in early studies of potentially important SNPs is merely an interim strategy—a quick proxy of convenience—and that with further development of genetic sequencing technologies race will eventually disappear from the genetic sciences altogether.

However, even a quick review of the pharmacogenetic literature reveals a robust legacy of research that validates race and ethnicity as major demarcations for stratifying drug response. This trend reveals a deeply held framework that begins with a priori assumptions about where meaningful differences among groups are most likely to be found. Race and ethnicity have long been built into research design, and more recently been institutionalized into the research process with the passage of the National Revitalization Act of 1993, which mandates the inclusion of racially identified groups into research.[21] Using race and ethnicity as de facto variables of potential biological difference began well before the genomic turn and is only amplified as race serves as a quick proxy for genetic relatedness.

The most common mechanism for drug elimination is metabolism by the cytochrome (CYP) P450 superfamily of drug metabolizing enzymes, which has been a major focus of pharmacogenetic research over the past fifty years. CYP variants have been associated with a broad range of agents involved in the breakdown of drugs, including the metabolism of warfarin, an anticoagulant active in a many different kinds of medications. Common coding-region CYP variants that affect drug elimination and responses have been shown by scientists to have high variability among racially identified populations. For example, up to 10 percent of white and African American persons are homozygous for loss of activity of a cytochrome P450 genetic isoform, CYP2D6. Persons with this poor-metabolizer genotype are not able to break down medication, including some antidepressants, and the drug accumulates in the body, causing dangerous side effects. In addition, persons who are poor metabolizers do not process codeine to its active metabolite morphine and thus have reduced pain relief. An important implication of the identification of highly variable CYP2D6 activity is that new drug candidates that are eliminated predominantly by this enzyme are often not further developed or brought to market. Given that CYP isoforms differ significantly in frequency for racially identified population, selection of study population becomes an important issue that may have broad implications on which drugs are ultimately developed. For example, one isoform, CYP2C19, is believed to be more common in Asian persons, and persons with this genotype experience higher drug concentrations and a greater cure rate of *Helicobacter pylori* infections during therapy with the CYP2C19 substrate omeprazole.[22] If studies did not include Asians in large enough numbers to detect these differences, such associations would be largely missed.

The problem of replication in genetic ancestry research and the challenges of controlling population stratification are significant in pharmacogenomics. Scientists have argued that non-replication may be the result of poorly defined phenotype, such as racial or ethnic identity attributed to individuals recruited into studies, which make it difficult to identify, with any precision, how underlying genetic substructures among populations may ultimately effect study results.

Although these characteristics may not have a clear causative role at the molecular level for a particular drug response, failing to account for variation within a study population of what is often interchangeably referred to as "black," "African," "African American," or "white," "Caucasian," or "European," can misconstrue findings. Scientists suggest that narrow phenotype definition may be a simple approach to clarifying the genetic architecture of study populations and may increase the chances for the replications of results.[23] This simple suggestion belies the ongoing challenge of defining what race, ancestry, and difference mean in the context of designing genetic association studies. Bioethicists Pamela Sankar and Mildred Cho have shown that the language used by scientists in reporting results of population differences in the biomedical literature is a potpourri of terms that transect different and often incomparable units of analysis. They write:

> Nonequivalent use of labels is illustrated by the common juxtaposition of terms such as "white" with "African-American," where skin color and geographical location are treated as equivalent. Another example is the juxtaposition of "Asian-American" with "Mexican-American," which implies that people of Asian ancestry now living in the United States represent a level of genetic diversity that is equivalent to that of people of Mexican ancestry now living in the United States. Such examples indicate a need for more consistent attention to definition of groups and to the need to explain the rationale for their equivalence.[24]

Scientists struggle in seeking new language to characterize what they understand to be the highly circumscribed search for population differences in genetic ancestry in the context of their specific research questions. Population stratification has long been a controversial issue in human genetic research. One cardiologist whom I interviewed put it simply: "Race is a fast and cheap genetic test, and it can give you a wealth of information in assessing risk." The problem occurs when this "cheap genetic test" suggests that the population under study is assumed to be homogeneous with respect to allele frequencies, but in fact comprises subpopulations that have different allele frequencies for the candidate gene. If these subpopulations vary randomly in their frequencies of specific genes, then subpopulation membership can be a confounder,[25] and an association between the candidate gene and disease may be incorrectly estimated without properly accounting for population structure. A legitimate question is whether the assumptions that accompany dominant views of race as related to genetics obscure important pharmacogenomic differences in drug response and end up creating more complications and ADRs than the current model of adjusting dosages through trial and error on an individual basis.

In addition, the existence of genetic subgroups or substructure in a population may lead to spurious associations if the subgroups are not equally represented in cases and controls. For example, if one subgroup has a higher prevalence of disease, then this subgroup will likely be overrepresented among cases compared to controls. Scientists understand that this may alter their results where any allele that has a higher frequency in that subgroup by chance may appear to be falsely associated with the disease. Theoretically, if cases and controls are matched by their genetic ancestry, then the confounding due to population stratification should be eliminated.[26] This is a problem with not only significant scientific implications but broad social and ethical impact as well. In most cases the relevant population structure may not be known, as DNA samples from many minority groups are limited. The current landscape of DNA samples taken from predominantly European American populations may obscure medically relevant findings where allele frequencies differ as the result of the history of human migration. Characterizing the ancestry of DNA samples in a rigorous and meaningful manner is a critical challenge for progress in pharmacogenomic research.

Guidance Beyond Race

Policy decisions made early in the development of a field create the trajectory on which an area of inquiry unfolds. The categories scientists use to characterize DNA samples inform the range of questions that may be asked. The focus on racial difference fits with practices in clinical medicine where using race as a proxy for biological variables and for disease risk is routine. As such, race has become the first filter through which difference is determined. Nowhere is this more apparent than in the emerging landscape of personalized medicine.[27] Race is not only useful in assessing risk or identifying genetic variants that are associated with drug response, but is also an important demarcation for stratifying potential markets and identifying potential consumers. Increasing interest by the pharmaceutical industry and biotech companies in what one corporate executive described as the "as yet untapped racial market niches" indicates a significant shift. More than merely an academic debate fought on the editorial pages of academic journals, the meaning of race and genes is considered big business—one that has coupled itself to the moral mandate of addressing ongoing health disparities.

The case of BiDil, the antihypertensive drug approved by the FDA in 2005 for use exclusively among African Americans, is illustrative of this shift and has become a flashpoint in debates over the relevance of race for genomic medicine and its potential impact on ongoing health disparities. The company, Nitromed, Inc., that produces and markets BiDil introduces the drug on its website by first explaining the excessive burden of heart failure in the African American community. The company states that not only are blacks 50 percent more likely to develop heart failure compared with white Americans, but that blacks tend to develop heart failure at an earlier age than other Americans.[28] While there is some evidence in the literature that African American patients are more likely to die of heart failure compared with whites,[29] there are many hypotheses being put forward as to why this might be. These include unequal treatment in the clinical encounter, limited access to the most advanced and aggressive treatments, higher risk within the population for contributing diseases including diabetes, hypertension, obesity, and behavioral factors such as limited physical activity and poor diet.[30]

Nitromed focuses on putative biological differences among groups by focusing on a hypothesis of impaired bioavailability of nitric oxide, which is thought to contribute to the structural remodeling of the left ventricle that increases the rate of death or other complications. The company suggests that African American patients may have a disproportionately lower nitric oxide bioavailability. Isosorbide acts as a nitric oxide donor and hydralazine as an antioxidant, and so together the company suggests they might ameliorate the long-term effects of heart failure.[31]

Several scholars have criticized the scientific legitimacy of the data presented by Nitromed in their application for FDA approval, including the two clinical trials in the early 1980s—the Vasodilator Heart Failure Trials (V-HeFT I & II)[32] that fell short of showing convincing evidence of improved outcome among patients. Researchers were only able to *rescue* BiDil when they presented *post hoc* analysis that extracted data only on self-identified black patients and found what looked to be a benefit. This was enough for the FDA to make the unusual decision to approve BiDil, pending similar results from a new clinical trial to be conducted exclusively among self-identified black patients.

The African American Heart Failure Trial (A-HeFT) conducted by Nitromed to validate the efficacy of BiDil included over 1,000 patients, who were randomized to a fixed-dose combination of isosorbide and hydralazine or placebo added to existing standard of care (for the majority, ACE inhibitors for their condition). Although the study was originally planned for eighteen months, it was terminated after six months, because of early results of significant differences in mortality between the case and control groups. Whereas 32 patients died in the group being treated with BiDil, 54 died in the control group, which meant that BiDil provided a 43 percent reduction in risk.[33] Based on these results, the FDA recommended on June 16, 2005, that BiDil be approved specifically for the treatment of heart failure in "self-identified black" patients.

To be clear, BiDil was "rescued" by *post-hoc* analysis when the results of its two earlier trials were rejected by the FDA. The race-based indication for the drug as "self-identified black" was both an artifact and emblem of the institutionalization of race into biomedical research. Human subjects are effectively sorted into racial and ethnic groups, often without careful thought as to how these variables of population difference are to be operationalized within specific research questions. This can lead to "race-based" findings that then develop into "race-based" drugs, without careful consideration of what mechanisms lead to different drug response. Whether the A-HeFT trial legitimized the historical decision to create the first racially label drug approved in the United States is open for debate. As A-HeFT enrolled only African American subjects, the question of whether other patients might also benefit from adding isosorbide dinitrate and hydralazine hydrochloride to their existing drug regimens for congestive failure remains unanswered.[34]

Coupling Racial Biology with Health Disparities

Although genetic data was not presented in the application for approval by the FDA, the case of BiDil has emerged as a critical event in the study of race, genetic variation and health disparity because it reflects the evolving landscape of governance of personalized medicine and the enduring controversy over the relevance of race for genomics. BiDil comes at a critical juncture for pharmacogenomics as the field grapples with how to address meaningful genetic differences among populations. In the recent FDA Guidance on the Collection of Race and Ethnicity Data in Clinical Trials,[35] BiDil is cited as rationale for the adoption of census categories of race and ethnicity issued by the Office of Management and Budget (OMB) to characterize human subjects in clinical trials data. Despite explicit warnings by the OMB that these categories "represent a social-political construct designed for collecting data on the race and ethnicity of broad population groups in this country, and are *not anthropologically or scientifically based*,"[36] the FDA followed NIH's well established policy that requires researchers to sort human subjects into racial and ethnic bins, stating that doing so will "facilitate comparisons across clinical studies analyzed by FDA and data collected by other agencies."[37] As a test case, BiDil further institutionalized racial categorization into drug development and categories intended for social analysis have become more fully integrated as scientific variables. Sociologist Steven Epstein identifies this process as "categorical alignment" through which "bureaucratic and scientific classification come to be treated as functionally equivalent both to one another and to the categories of everyday life."[38]

Another reason for BiDil's prominence in the discourse on pharmacogenomics and health disparities is the explicit framing of the approval BiDil as a matter of social justice by its advocates in the FDA, Nitromed and African American communities. These narratives describe BiDil as more than a drug involved in the reduction of hypertension, but as a test case toward redressing historical inequities in biomedical research. Responding to those critical of the FDA for setting a precedent for race-based therapeutics, FDA Advisory Committee Chairman Stephen Nissen defended the administration's decision to approve BiDil by commending those at Nitromed for their courage. "First of all, I think this was a courageous thing to do, to try to develop a drug for this population which seems to have a disproportionate burden of disease . . . yes, the road to hell is paved with biological plausibility but here is a biological plausible explanation" (transcript from the FDA Hearing on the Approval of BiDil, 6/25/05). In valorizing Nitromed for developing a drug for the African American population, Nissen lends support to the fundamental and implicit assumption of a biological basis for why the drug may work better in African Americans. Nissen's statement suggests that the disproportionate burden of heart disease suffered by African Americans justifies whatever costs may be associated with accepting putative claims of racial biology.

The persistence of health disparities as moral justification for the approval of BiDil was echoed by several individuals at the FDA hearing speaking on behalf of African Americans and other organizations that have publicly endorsed FDA approval of the drug. In an impassioned speech, Donna Christensen, chair of the Congressional Black Caucus, stated,

> I want to say to you that today, ladies and gentlemen, you have before you an unprecedented opportunity to significantly reduce one of the major health disparities in the African American community and, in doing so, to begin a process that will bring some degree of equity and justice to the American healthcare system. . . . Addressing these in eliminating the disparities that exist in all aspects of our lives is our highest priority until those gaps are closed. Their continued existence despite our best efforts must not be used to deny treatment to those for whom treatment has been denied and deferred for 400 years. Today this panel is being asked to reverse that history. (Testimony at FDA Hearing on BiDil, 6/25/05)

The stakes are made plain in Chistensen's framing of BiDil's approval as a matter of racial justice in biomedicine. Saddled with the weight of a long history of racism and unequal treatment, the approval of BiDil is recast as act of moral redemption for a legacy of excluding and exploiting African Americans in biomedical research. However, what has been less amplified in the media and in public statements made by individuals like Christensen are the somewhat paradoxical views within the African American community on BiDil's implication of inherent biological differences among so-called races. Many hold a seemingly incongruous dual position from which they simultaneously maintain that the approval of BiDil represents an important step towards social justice yet, at the same time, vigorously disavow ideas of a distinctive racial biology. A member of the Association of Black Cardiologists, an organization that offered strong public endorsement for the approval of the drug, reveals this paradox. He explained,

> The reality is that the health of blacks in this country has always been a terribly neglected issue. It has and always will be a struggle over resources and frankly, a result of a long legacy of racism in this country. Do I support BiDil? Sure, I do. Do I think that it is a drug that will only work on blacks? No,

I don't. I suspect that race, or at least conventional ideas about race, has little to do with why it works. There are probably a lot of other folks who could benefit from the drug, but am I going to discourage the FDA from approving it? No way. If they want to make drugs that work on black people, then I say that's one win out of a long line of setbacks towards just health-care in this country. (July 15, 2005, personal interview)

The hope for a "win" towards social justice obscures the strong rejection of BiDil as a "black drug" by this supporter. However, the current landscape leaves little room for a dual position—that BiDil must be made available to African Americans as a matter of social justice, but is not evidence of racial differences in biology. Such a position has no place in how BiDil is perceived in the wider public imagination. Race-based therapeutics further entrenches the notion of a racial biology. In her essay, "Medicine's Race Problem," American Enterprise Institute Fellow Sally Satel cites BiDil as the "smoking gun" to questions over a biological basis for race. Referring to Jay Cohn, the principal investigator whose research resulted in BiDil, Satel suggests that the "ultimate purpose of work like Cohn's and other biological realists is to identify factors that may be genetic in origin." She criticizes those who warn of the dangers inherent in practicing race-based medicine, as "wanting it both ways" arguing that one cannot use race to "root out social injustices in medicine" without accepting that race is "mediated by physiology."[39]

The case of BiDil provides a useful illustration of the need for gatekeepers, such as the FDA, to provide institutional guidance when race-based findings are asserted in applications for therapeutics. In its review and ultimate approval of BiDil, the FDA advisory committee made two seemingly contradictory arguments. The first was the claim that the approval of BiDil is a moral imperative due to significant health disparities among African Americans. The second was that race is an interim solution as the "best available proxy," suggesting that the use of race is acceptable only until further research reveals the biological mechanisms that explain differential drug response. As such, race is justified as merely a way station on the road towards personalized medicine.

The juxtaposition of these two claims reveals a recurrent paradox in discussions of race and pharmacogenomics, and biomedicine more generally. The first claim suggests that some drugs are effective only in certain racially identified populations, due to biological differences, and that these differences may also contribute to health disparities. The argument simultaneously frames both race and health disparities as having primarily biological bases. However, the second claim asserts that race will be rendered obsolete once underlying variables are identified. The paradox emerges when the use of race is justified in the first instance by a model of racial biology and yet, in the second instance as a temporary solution, ultimately having little explanatory power.

What is most disturbing about the paradoxical use of race is the effect it may have on the trajectory of ongoing human genetic variation research. By making the moral argument that race-based therapeutics address injustice in healthcare and at the same time, maintaining that genetics research will ultimately eliminate the need for racial categories; racialization is allowed to proceed, unchallenged by inherently contradictory claims that race is both biologically meaningful and meaningless. Rather, than a "way station," the use of race is allowed to become more fully embedded in the production of scientific knowledge and medical practice.

The Call for Clarity on Race

In the same year that BiDil was approved as the first racially labeled medication, the pharmaceutical company AstraZeneca announced that it would voluntarily withdraw its drug, Iressa (gefitinib), despite promising initial clinical trial results. Iressa was intended to treat patients with non-small cell lung cancer (NSCLC), which accounts for 80 percent of all lung cancer and an estimated 800,000 deaths a year. Since there are few therapeutic options, initial findings that Iressa contributed to significant tumor shrinkage and might be effective against NSCLC looked promising. However, phase III clinical trial data failed to show improved survival rates for patients treated with the drug as compared to those on placebo. Similarly to the case of BiDil, researchers conducted *post hoc* analysis that resulted in a "race-specific finding" that indicated benefit for a subset of patients identified as East Asian. Tom McKillop, chief executive officer of AstraZeneca, reported at the annual meeting of shareholders that, despite this finding, the company would cut back on their investment in select markets. He stated:

> As a responsible company, we have voluntarily withdrawn promotion of the product in the US market while we work with the FDA to ensure that Iressa is only taken by patients who are deriving benefit. *The dilemma we all face is that many people clearly benefit from Iressa, but it is currently difficult to determine exactly which are the patients most likely to do so* [emphasis added]. The advantages in patients of Asian origin demonstrated in our clinical trials and their experience to date has led the Advisory Committee of the Japanese Ministry of Health to recommend the continued availability of Iressa and has led to approval for the marketing of Iressa in China and other Asian markets.[40]

McKillop's confusion over who might best benefit from Iressa is curious in light of the company's own findings that self-identified East Asians patients improved with the drug. Clearly, the company's decision to increase marketing efforts in Japan, South Korea, and China and to withdraw its drug applications in Europe reflect a sense of who Iressa's beneficiaries might be. A pressing question is why did *post hoc* analysis that indicated a race-based benefit result in the rescue of BiDil and yet, for Iressa, yielded the gloomy headline, "Iressa Casts Cloud over Anti-Cancer Class."[41] Opting not to invest more funds in researching the underlying biological and/or genetic basis for their differential findings, AstraZeneca treated Iressa as a de facto racial drug, however, it chose not to apply for a race-specific patent as did Nitromed.

The difference may be in the differing expectations and resources placed in the respective drugs. AstraZeneca had expected Iressa to emerge as a blockbuster anti-cancer drug, commanding a sizable market share. Having shown efficacy in a relatively small percentage of the general U.S. population, it seems that the drug has been viewed largely as a failure by the industry despite its reported benefits for patients identified as East Asian.

The other reason for the difference between BiDil and Iressa may be how comfortable companies are in incorporating racial labeling into corporate strategy. According to Lindpaintner, of multinational pharmaceutical company Hoffman-La Roche, kin, color, and self-confessed ethnicity are nothing but cheap surrogates for some underlying genetic variant that is more common in African Americans than in Caucasians. As a result, Lindpainter insists that Hoffman-La Roche would likely never market a drug exclusively for one racially identified group unless it were lifesaving, worked exclusively for that ethnic group, and an underlying genetic cause could not be found. The first two of these conditions were allegedly fulfilled in the cases of BiDil and Iressa. However, neither Nitromed nor AstraZeneca were forced to satisfy the last condition of finding a genetic cause. Lack of regulatory guidance on this issue is a critical stumbling block in moving beyond race as a mere way station on the road to personalized medicine. Without such leadership, the two options illustrated by BiDil and Iressa are limited to accepting the limitations of race as a crude proxy for biological difference or simply not having a drug available to patients who might potentially benefit from it.

Political leadership is necessary to create institutional changes that will clarify how population differences, race and genes, should be approached in drug development. Institutional guidance is needed to look past race to the specific variables that cause differential findings among groups. The FDA should require investigators, and their companies, that attribute differential drug response to race to pursue additional research that further explicates the underlying mechanisms of these findings. At a minimum, research data used to justify race-based findings should be made available to enable others to determine the basis for findings of difference among groups.

The meaning of race is never given, but produced through structures of beliefs, practices, and values. This infrastructure constrains the trajectory of human genetic variation research where genes are often uncritically mapped onto social categories of race as used in the United States, focusing the search on new "racially inscribed" market niches. The danger is that the convergence of these processes may well derail a genetic revolution that many envisioned would counter notions of distinct racial biologies and bring into full view a broader spectrum of factors that contribute to ongoing health disparities. Early signals from the emerging field of pharmacogenomics suggest that, too often, race as an undefined proxy is allowed to remain the only explanatory tool for interpreting these differences.

ACKNOWLEDGMENTS

This chapter is a modified version of Dr. Lee's article "Pharmacogenomics and the Challenge of the Health Disparities," published in *Public Health Genomics* 12 (2009):170–179. This work was supported by NIH Grant #K01 HL72465.

NOTES

1. "Brave New Pharmacy," *Time* (Jan. 15, 2001).

2. G. S. Ginsburg and J. J. McCarthy, "Personalized Medicine: Revolutionizing Drug Discovery and Patient Care," *Trends in Biotechnology* 19, no. 12 (2001):491–496.

3. D. B. Goldstein, S. K. Tate, and S. M. Sisodya, "Pharmacogenetics Goes Genomic," *Nature Reviews* 4 (2003):937–947. The distinction between pharmacogenetics and pharmacogenomics is not clear; while some have argued that differences of scale and focus distinguish the fields, this article uses the term, pharmacogenomics, to mean the broad scope of research on inherited variation in drug response.

4. K. Lindpaintner, "Pharmacogenetics and the Future of Medical Practice," *Journal of Molecular Medicine* 81, no. 3 (2003):141–153.

5. R. E. Taylor, "Pharmacological and Cultural Considerations in Alcohol Treatment Clinical Trials: Issues in Clinical Research Related to Race and Ethnicity," *Alcoholism Clinical and Experimental Research* 27, no. 8 (2003):1345–1348.

6. S. S. J. Lee, "Race, Distributive Justice and the Promise of Pharmacogenomics: Ethical Considerations," *American Journal of PharmacoGenomics* 3, no. 6 (2003):385–392; R. S. Cooper, J. S. Kaufman, and R. Ward, "Race and Genomics," *New England Journal of Medicine* 348, no. 12 (Mar. 20, 2003):1166–1170; P. Sankar, "MEDLINE Definitions of Race and Ethnicity and Their Application to Genetic Research," *Nature Genetics* 34, no. 2 (June 2003):119, discussion 120.

7. E. Mordini, "Ethical Considerations on Pharmacogenomics," *Pharmacological Research* 49, no. 4 (2004):375–379; W. Kalow, "Pharmacogenetics and Personalised Medicine," *Fundamental Clinical Pharmacology* 16, no. 5 (2002):337–342; P. Lipton, "Pharmacogenetics: The Ethical Issues," *Pharmacogenomics Journal* 3, no. 1 (2003):14–16.

8. Center for Biologics Evaluation and Research, "E15 Draft Guidance Terminology on Pharmacogenomics," Food and Drug Administration (2007):4

9. www.nigms.nih.gov/Initiatives/PGRN/Background/pgrn_faq.htm.

10. S. Conner, "Glaxo Chief: Our Drugs Do Not Work on Most Patients," *Independent* [UK] (December 8, 2003).

11. J. Lazarou, B. H. Pomeranz, and P. N. Corey, "Incidence of Adverse Reactions on Hospitalized Patients: A Meta-Analysis of Prospective Studies," *JAMA* 279 (1998):1200–1205.

12. F. R. Ernst and A. J. Grizzle, "Drug-Related Morbidity and Mortality: Updating the Cost-of-Illness Model," *Journal of the American Pharmacists Association* 41 (2001):192–199.

13. R. March et al., "Pharmacogenomics—Legal, Ethical, and Regulatory Considerations," *Pharmacogenomics* 2, no. 4 (2001):317–327; D. Veenstra et al., "Assessing the Cost-Effectiveness of Pharmacogenomics," *AAPS PharmScience* 2, no 3 (2002):29.

14. N. Risch et al., "Categorization of Humans in Biomedical Research: Genes, Race, and Disease," *Genome Biology* 3, no. 7 (2002):2.

15. B. Mehl, and J. Santell, "Projecting Future Drug Expenditures—2000," *American Journal of Health System Pharmacy* 57, no. 2:129–138.

16. P. Tollyma, P. Guy et al., *A Revolution in R&D* (Boston: Boston Consulting Group, 2001).

17. J. A. Johnson and J. L. Bootman, "Drug-Related Morbidity and Mortality: A Cost of Illness Model," *Archives of Internal Medicine* 155 (1995):1949–1956.

18. Genentech, "Genentech Announces Full Year and Fourth Quarter 2005 Results," Press Release (2006).

19. D. C. Wertz, "Ethical, Social, and Legal Issues in Pharmacogenomics," *Pharmacogenomics Journal* 3, no. 4 (2003):194; A. M. Issa, "Ethical Perspectives on Pharmacogenomic Profiling in the Drug Development Process," *Nature Reviews, Drug Discovery* 1, no. 4 (2002):300–308; A. Webster, P. Martin, G. Lewis, and A. Smart, "Integrating Pharmacogenetics into Society: In Search of a Model, *Nature Genetics* 5 (2004):663–669; K. I. Morley and W. D. Hall, "Using Pharmacogenetics and Pharmacogenomics in the Treatment of Psychiatric Disorders: Some Ethical and Economic Considerations," *Journal of Molecular Medicine* 82, no. 1 (2004):21–30.

20. G. Emilien, M. Ponchon, C. Caldas, O. Isacson, and J. M. Maloteaux, "Impact of Genomics on Drug Discovery and Clinical Medicine," *Quarterly Journal of Medicine* 93, no. 7 (2000):391–423; A. K. Rai, "Pharmacogenomic Interventions, Orphan Drugs, and Distributive Justice: The Role of Cost-Benefit Analysis," *Social Philosophy and Policy* 19, no. 2 (2002):246–270.

21. S. Lee et al., "The Meanings of Race in the New Genomics: Implications for Health Disparities Research," *Yale Journal of Health Policy, Law and Ethics* 1 (Spring 2001):33–75; S. Epstein, *Inclusion: The Politics of Difference in Medical Research* (Chicago: University of Chicago Press, 2007).

22. D. M. Roden et al., "Pharmacogenomics: Challenges and Opportunities," *Annals of Internal Medicine* 145, no. 10 (2006):749–757.

23. M. J. Sillanpaa and K. Auranen, "Replication in Genetic Studies of Complex Traits," *Annals of Human Genetics* 68 (2004):646–657.

24. P. Sankar and M. Cho, "Toward a New Vocabulary of Human Genetic Variation," *Science* 298 (2002):1337–1338.

25. D. G. Kleinbaum, L. L. Kupper, and H. Morgenstern, *Epidemiologic research: Principles and Quantitative Methods* (New York: Van Nostrand Reinhold, 1982).

26. L. R. Cardon and L. J. Palmer, "Population Stratification and Spurious Allelic Association," *Lancet* 361, no. 9357 (2003):598–604.

27. J. F. Solus et al., "Genetic Variation in Eleven Phase I Drug Metabolism Genes in an Ethnically Diverse Population," *Pharmacogenomics* 7 (2004):895–931; U. Yasar, E. Aklillu, R. Canaparo, M. Sandberg, J. Sayi, H. K. Roh, and A. Wennerholm, "Analysis of CYP2C9*5 in Caucasian, Oriental and Black-African Populations," *European Journal of Clinical Pharmacology* 58, no. 8 (2002):555–558. Epub 2002 Nov 1; J. Blaisdell, L. F. Jorge-Nebert, S. Coulter, S.S. Ferguson, S. J. Lee, B. Chanas, T. Xi, H. Mohrenweiser, B. Ghanayem, and J. A. Goldstein, "Discovery of New Potentially Defective Alleles of Human CYP2C9," *Pharmacogenetics* 8 (2004):527–537.

28. www.nitromed.com/bidil/index.asp [Accessed July 11, 2007].

29. B. Smedley, A. Stith, and A. Nelson, *Unequal Treatment: Confronting Racial and Ethnic Disparities in Health Care* (Washington, DC: *Institute of Medicine*, 2003).

30. J. N. Cohn, G. Johnson, S. Ziesche et al., "A Comparison of Enalapril with Hydralazine-Isosorbide Dinitrate in the Treatment of Chronic Congestive Heart Failure," *New England Journal of Medicine* 325 (1991):303–310.

31. A. L. Taylor, S. Ziesche, C. Yancy et al., "Combination of Isosorbide Dinitrate and Hydralazine in Blacks with Heart Failure," *New England Journal of Medicine* 351 (2004):2049–2057.

32. J. Kahn, "How a Drug Becomes 'Ethnic': Law, Commerce, and the Production of Racial Categories in Medicine," *Yale Journal of Health Policy, Law, and Ethics* 4, no. 1 (2004):1–46; P. Sankar and J. Kahn, "BiDil: Race Medicine or Race Marketing?" *Health Affairs* W5 (2004):455–463.

33. R. Lapu-Bula et al., "The 894T Allele of Endothelial Nitric Oxide Synthase Gene Is Related to Left Ventricular Mass in African Americans with High-Normal Blood Pressure," *Journal of the National Medical Association* 97, no. 2 (2005):197–205; Taylor et al., "Combination of Isosorbide Dinitrate and Hydralazine in Blacks with Heart Failure."

34. M. G. Bloche, "Race-Based Therapeutics," *New England Journal of Medicine* 351 (2004): 2035–2037.

35. Food and Drug Administration, *FDA Guidance on the Collection of Race and Ethnicity Data in Clinical Trials* (2005).

36. minorityhealth.hhs.gov/templates/browse.aspx?lvl=2&lvlID=172

37. Food and Drug Administration (2005).

38. Epstein, *Inclusion.*

39. S. Satel, "Medicine's Race Problem," *Policy Review* 110 (2002). www.policyreview.org/DEC01/satel.html

40. T. McKillop, AstraZeneca, *Annual Meeting Shareholders Report* (2005).

41. Sandra Soo-Jin Lee, "Pharmacogenomics and the Challenge of the Health Disparities," *Public Health Genomics* 12 (2009):170–179.

PART THREE

Stories Told in Blood

11

French Families, Paper Facts

Genetics, Nation, and Explanation

NINA KOHLI-LAVEN

Within the human and natural sciences, the genealogical diagram has long been the dominant mode for theorizing relatedness, whether of people, plants, languages, or genetic alleles, from biblical ethnology to comparative linguistics, social anthropology, and contemporary biology (Alter 1999; Bouquet 1996; Trautman 2006). In Quebec, for example, genealogical trees are shaping how people explain bodies in pain and predict prevalence rates for disease. At two demography institutes, researchers are using archived church records to generate multigenerational family trees for medical genetic research. Medical researchers are using these family trees to map the intergenerational transmission of genetic traits in the past, predict future risk, and target local health outreach and education. People both within and beyond the purview of health and medical institutions often articulate the causes of complex diseases such as asthma, breast cancer, and hypertension in relation to these family trees.

In this article, I explore how genealogies in Quebec genetics are animating a certain history and logic of racial difference. In particular, I focus on how Quebec medical researchers are using genealogies to draw boundaries between French Canadian and North American aboriginal groups. These two groups formed families, lived, and worshipped together across early North America. Yet, genetics and demography researchers and clinicians in Quebec are producing genealogies that presume French Canadians and aboriginal tribes were separate and almost always "married-in." Here, I unearth the exigencies—from colonial French Church writing strictures to medical database infrastructures—of how medical research and diagnoses are remaking parameters of ethnic and regional belonging vis-à-vis these family trees. In doing so, I engage a broader set of questions about how racial and nationalist ideologies should be posed (or not) in relationship to genetic practice.[1]

Population and genealogies are two modes of representation that are intimately inter-related. What is a population in genetics? Early geneticists proposed that individuals can be amalgamated and divided into groups based on shared common biological characteristics that are due to mating and genealogical ties.[2]

The population idea incorporates a particular set of genealogical understandings about families, relatedness, and belonging: the idea that people reproduce within the bounds of delineated groups over series of generations and the idea that people pass on traits to their descendants, maintaining the distinctive qualities of the group. In fact, these genealogical relations are what make—what constitute—a "population."

Genealogies define the parameters and fix the boundaries of the population unit. This is especially the case in Quebec. By assuming such a clearly delineated population, medical genetic researchers investigating diseases in the "French Canadian population" are implicitly postulating that multigenerational in-group genealogical ties among French immigrants to Canada exist. They are also explicitly using a database of digitized French Canadian family genealogies to generate and validate population parameters. This is why Quebec offers a unique entry-point into the study of how genealogical ideas figure in population and medical research, precisely how contemporary science and society are dividing the world into "population" groups, and with what kinds of consequences.

The basic premise of population-thinking in health and medical research is that meaningful inferences about the causes of disease can be drawn from the study of whom is affected by certain diseases and what the shared characteristics of these individuals are, when taken as a group. The social epidemiologist Geoffrey Rose wrote in 1985 of the importance of studying rates of disease incidence across groups: "I find it increasingly helpful to distinguish two kinds of aetiological question. The first seeks the causes of cases, and the second seeks the causes of incidence. 'Why do some individuals have hypertension?' is a quite different question from 'Why do some populations have much hypertension, whilst in others it is rare?'" (Rose 2001) Rose's insight became the bedrock of entire fields of health research that continue to investigate the broad environmental, biological, and psycho-social contexts that lead to the prevalence of disorders in certain places and "populations" (for example, colorectal cancer in males, lung cancer in smokers). Though some scholars have criticized the analytics underlying this type of population-thinking (the focus on frequencies, the practice of drawing inferences about groups from samples, and the focus on proportional relationships between variables), the problems I seek to highlight are not with these premises (Le Bras et al. 2000; Hacking 1976; Hacking 2001:47–54, 105–114). In this essay, I am concerned with how scientists are drawing lines that define populations *according to ancestral ethnic and racial logics* (Lemon 2002). How are Quebec health and medical researchers defining French Canadian and aboriginal "populations"? In doing so, what kinds of genealogical evidence are they marshalling and with what effects?

Genealogical Evidence and a Medical Genetic
Population Database in Quebec

In 1967, the directors of the demography department at the Université de Montréal began a multimillion-dollar initiative to consolidate North American

French Catholic Church registers into a digital family history database. The Church registers are a compendium of all of the births, marriages, and burials performed by four centuries of priests in French North America. In the seventeenth and eighteenth centuries, that included not only current-day Quebec, but parts of the Great Lakes, Louisiana, and central Canada. The directors had found they could piece together entire families across this geographic expanse, going back as much as five hundred years, by tracking the inscriptions on Church birth and marriage records that indicated presiding relatives, such as parents, cousins, aunts, and uncles, at the time of an event. They held that collecting these reassembled lineages in a computerized family history archive would arm social and natural scientists with the tools to study past shifts in marital patterns, residence, birth rate, and other population-wide behavior. They argued the data could also aid geneticists in the search for origins of hereditary disease (Charbonneau and Légaré 1967). In 1993, the database was brought under the umbrella of a genetic epidemiology research institute at the Université de Québec à Chicoutimi called BALSAC.[3] Chicoutimi researchers made the genealogies available to a continental network of medical researchers and clinicians. These researchers and clinicians now correlate the genealogies with people's medical data to infer the distribution, origin, and location of specific alleles within contemporary Canada, to plan regional health outreach programs, and to explain genetic risk to medical patients. In 2006, the database was formally incorporated into the first population-wide DNA databank and the largest public population genomics research project in North America, CartaGENE.

In constructing large-scale family histories, historical demographers rely on church records in particular, for several reasons. Historical demography, a discipline that developed and was standardized and then globally diffused from a small group of Paris research centers, entrenched the parish record as its main historical source in the 1950s. Church registers often have the best time-depth—sometimes going as far back as the eleventh century—to support multigenerational genealogical reconstructions (Hollingsworth 1969). In Quebec, a French colony founded in the seventeenth century and deeply influenced by Catholic authorities until the 1950s, this is especially the case. Parish-based vital records registration systems were established in the French mainland and informally spread to North America over the course of the seventeenth and eighteenth centuries via colonial priests (Goulbert 1965). In 1678, French North American colonial authorities formally established a Church-administered records system, and the Canadian Archdiocese later published guidelines for recording names and dates at Catholic baptisms, burials, and marriages. The records from that period are incomplete for the first decade after 1678, but thereafter become highly detailed for most regions and towns. It was evident in Quebec that demographers interpreted this encyclopedic appearance of the records as evidence that the information contained within them is the unambiguous, statistical reporting of an omniscient ecclesiastical power. The level of detail in Church registers is also

why the BALSAC family history database is especially appealing to medical geneticists who want to study the relationship between heredity and disease. Medical
geneticists in the United States and Canada often promote Quebec as home to
the most comprehensive historical demographic resources in North America
(Secko 2008).

BALSAC and the Université de Montréal demography departments emerged
in the 1960s in vibrant connection with French Canadian nationalist movements.
As in many places around the globe with self-determination movements waged by
struggling minorities, demography is important to the French Canadian (now
often called Québécois) national project. Immigration and reproduction are
touchstones of the self-determination agenda—the first being posed as a threat
and the second as a salve. Between 1960 and 1966, Quebec nationalists established
a large, professional, multi-departmental, state bureaucracy that included a new
network of public colleges and universities, public health planning bodies, and
cultural ministries.

The most controversial of these ministries was the Ministry for Cultural
Affairs. The ministry embarked on an ambitious program of cultural planning
intended to resurrect and strengthen French-language and Francophone culture.
The minister proposed the cultural and political exclusion of "outsiders" in order
to preserve Quebec as a French enclave. Provincial politicians and legislators
have discussed "problems" with Québécois fertility since the 1960s, when the
birth rate precipitously declined (Gevrais and Gauvreau 2003). In the 1970s and
1980s, provincial leaders encouraged a higher birthrate as a guarantee against
assimilation into an increasingly multicultural, multi-language, immigrant society, calling for a "Revenge of the Cradle" (Fenwick 1981). In the late 1970s, the government established an institute to coordinate long-term research on the "cultural
development" of the province (Handler 1987). The institute distributed funds for
research on the history, demography, sociology, and folklore of early North
American settlers from France, enabling new specialized demographic research
centers—such as the Université de Montréal Program for Historical Demography—
to become powerful brokers in the production of knowledge about Quebec.

The widespread idea within Quebec demography that contemporary white,
French Canadians are "pure Québécois" descendants of the first settlers from
France, "the founders," mirrors the historiography these French nationalist movements. Early Quebecers, the story goes, lived in idyllic cultural isolation until British
Conquest in the 1760s, reproducing the charm, grit, and intimacy of everyday village life in France in the North American wilderness. Lionel Groulx, a nationalist
historian and politician, declared at a 1938 conference on French Canadian folklore, "What is constant for us is our peasant roots. We were born and we became
people in the country . . . as a French and a Catholic peasantry, tillers of the earth
and pastoral tenders" (Velay-Vallantin 1997, 294). Folklorists, linguists, and
museum and tourism workers have all since elaborated romantic visions of this
French Canadian past: homogenous agricultural collectives that were bastions of

Gemeinschaft, which British Conquest and modern commerce eroded. Quebec language, architecture, and folklore conservation groups depict the founders and their immediate descendants as marooned in isolated clusters on a vast and empty Canadian frontier.

Names, Biology, Ancestry, and Reading Race in the Records

In the historical demography office at the Université de Montréal where the Church records were first punched onto cards and then transferred into digital software, graduate students sat on two sides of a small room before computer screens. The students modulated between two monitors as they entered data into files. They had empty forms that constituted a "family file" open on one monitor screen and digitized scans of the original handwritten parish records on another (fig. 2). Each family file contains the digitized names of one set of parents, their children, and their children's spouses. All of the married children also have their own separate files, or "familes," listing the names of their children and children's spouses. By searching the names of a successive string of parents in the database, a researcher can bring up multiple files that, when assimilated, represent one overarching multigenerational list of relatives. Programmers at BALSAC have developed software that displays the names and families from these lists in a branching-tree diagram that geneticists use to study disease transmission.

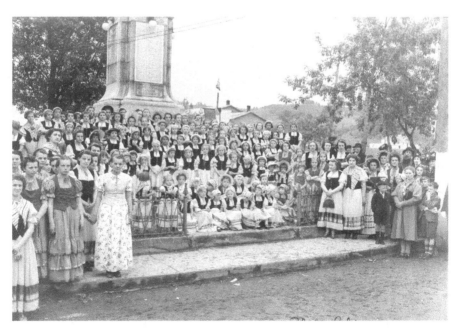

FIGURE 2 "Homage to Sageunayen Founders" [Homage aux fondateurs saguenayennes], 1938 Centennial Celebrations, Saguenay-Lac-Saint-Jean.

Archives Nationales du Québec, Chicoutimi, Phototècque, SHS-P2-S7 Album No. 5, p. 19.

I sat with a data-enterer named Aimée, who was looking at the digitized church burial record of a child named Joseph Belanger. The boy died at age seven, in 1743, in a village near Quebec City. The record is in the official mission register for the Huron Reserve at Loretteville. The name appears in the register under the heading, "whites" (National Archives of Quebec). The Jesuits established the Lorette mission around 1667. Loretteville is now a small residential suburb of 13,000 people located ten miles from downtown Quebec City. I asked Aimée, "Why are there non-natives in the Lorette mission register?" and she replied, "There were French settlements close by." Until the late 1800s, natives and non-natives worshipped together in the same congregation at Loretteville (Bélanger 1990; Village des Hurons, Wedake, undated). The Quebec government and clerical authorities then established a separate Church and municipality with its own register for the Hurons in 1904. In 1986, the Government of Canada incorporated land on which the Huron settlement was located into an Indian Reserve named Wendake. Many people today believe that the two groups—French settlers and natives—were always separate. European tourists now visit the reserve in the summer, eating braised buffalo meat at the Wendake Grill and purchasing native arts and crafts at stands next to the chapel. Tribal guides describe how Hurons subsisted through centuries on the cultivation of squash and corn, surviving against a distant backdrop of French then British invasions. The now separate Indian spaces and structures that inhabit the reserve make it seem like the category "Indian" must have always existed. Looking to the cemetery headstones half-submerged in earth next to the original chapel, a woman at Wendake once told me, "Our ancestors are buried there." "Are there any French?" I asked. "No," she laughed. "*Our* ancestors." In Montreal at a 2006 conference convened to discuss aboriginal rights in Quebec, a Université de Montréal doctoral researcher presenting her new study of Wendake implied that the Hurons there had only recently come into contact with French Canadians (Iankova 2006).

In fact, data from a broad spectrum of sources suggests Loretteville was the site of an integrated, mixed French-Huron community before the twentieth century. Most notably, in 2003, a genealogist in St. Foy, Quebec, named Serge Goudreau did a study of the Hurons of Lorette. From a 1754 land sale contract, Goudreau found that the chief, Ondiarate, was the son of a Huron man and a French woman named Geneviève Andhechonniak, who had been adopted by the Hurons in the 1730s. A Jesuit missionary married Ondiarate to a French-Huron woman named Veronique Tehonatsenhong, his cousin, in 1767. Ondiarate had a brother from the same parents named Sebastien Sarenhes, who married a mixed French-Huron woman. Tracking back and forth between Church, civil, and private records, it is then possible to make a series of connections over the succeeding century between Ondiarate's extended family, ten neighboring French clans, and an Anglican-born Catholic convert named Zacharie Hotesse (née Otis). Many people had double names, one French and one native, depending on the type of record (church, civil, notarial), suggesting that the settlement residents interacted on both sides of the supposed aboriginal-French divide. Pierre Tehoronhiong and Louise Aouendaes were elsewhere Pierre Romain and Louise Duchesneau. François-Xavier Otsistaru was François Simon. Augustin Hokandoron was Augustin Picard. Nicolas Hannenhoutata was Nicolas Jacques. Simon Teennontaxen was Simone Hélène (Goudreau, 2003).

Loretteville exemplifies a widespread problem for current renderings of Quebec and Canadian history. The categories that are supposed to identify someone—as French, native, Catholic, Indian, aboriginal—have shifted over time, in ways that render the task of reading records for straightforward facts about ancestry a particular vexing pursuit. Archival work like Goudreau's suggests a highly mixed society of French and native interaction. Catholic records, in contrast, describe a society where "whites" existed alongside but separately from Hurons. Complicating things further, after the incorporation of Wendake and diffusion of the new official category of "Indian" into bureaucratic parlance and writing, there were yet new definitions of who was native and who was not (based on residence on the reserve or official legal Indian status under new acts passed in the 1870s) (Lawrence 2003). At the Université de Montréal demography department, I asked Aimée, "How do you know a native?" and she replied, "They look native." By this, she explained she meant skin and facial features were the key signs when she sees someone on the street. But who counts as a native in the past? I asked Aimée, "How do you know a native in the records? You can't see them," and she replied, "You know one by his name." That was how she knew that young Joseph Belanger, seized by death at seven, was French and that the priest at Lorette in 1743 had placed his burial record in the right list—the list for "whites." In her reading of the early Church records, she assumed a correlation between names and ancestry.

Names, Baptism, and Racial Difference in the Colony

Part of the reason the Church registers divided natives and "whites" is the racial and religious politics of the colonial French civilizing mission in North America. In fact, these categories did not mean what they might conventionally mean today. Priests in New France often viewed holistically what many people took for granted in the twentieth century as self-contained categories of "culture," "religion," "biology," "mind," "spirit," and "body." They apprehended human difference as something cutting across intellectual, physical, and spiritual planes. They distinguished natives, not just as biological others, but as different according to a cumulative sum of differences in all of these domains.

This logic led colonial authorities in New France to try to assimilate and "civilize" natives by altering their religious, moral, spiritual, and physical ties and practices—through education, marriage, and religious conversion. Like elsewhere in the French empire, priests and colonial administrators approached missionary evangelization, in particular, as a way of educating aboriginals in moral, intimate, and sentimental norms, in addition to religious rites. There were proper ways of speaking, dressing, farming, and singing. The priests in New France used baptism and religious education to enact and formalize these civilizational conversions, giving new French names and identities to natives who had learned to behave, interact, and work like French Catholics.

Successive royal intendants, administrators, and church leaders in the French North American colonies argued that, through changes in comportment and "values," in addition to education in prayer, liturgical chants, and scripture, natives would fully convert—not just to Catholicism but to "civilization" and, specifically, into Frenchmen and Frenchwomen. They called natives "savages."[4] The French naturalist Georges-Louis Leclerc, Comte de Buffon, wrote of "the Amerindian" in 1788: "having neither conquered the seas nor directed the course of rivers, nor cultivated the soil, he was in himself only an animal" (quoted in Jaenen 1982:47). Jesuit priests wrote often about the strange temperament and desires of natives. The nineteenth-century missionary Abbé Raynal alleged that the inhabitants of the New World were strangely indifferent to sex, possessing "a sort of impotence that reveals clearly how new the continent is" (Jaenen 1982:51). Working in Acadia, a former French region of central Canada, in the early seventeenth century, Father Pierre Biard found natives "ignorant, lawless, and rude" (Thwaites 1898–1901:147). The majority of priests put forward baptism, which involved renaming with a French identity, as the main way to "de-barbarize" North American aboriginals. From their perspective, baptism could assimilate natives not just into the Catholic faith but on these moral, national, and religious planes. Baptism was the culmination of a process of conversion that tethered natives to, not just a new faith, but a new way of life.

The archbishop of Quebec ordered priests in New France to give out the revered names of French saints "in order that the [baptized] might imitate their virtue" (Musée de la civilization). Priests working in the colonial mission, mostly from the Jesuit order, gave natives French Catholic names.[5] In their letters and official reports to the Society of Jesus in Paris, the Jesuits wrote often and in detail of baptism, specifically, as a way of bringing natives into "the French family." In the minutes of a meeting held between four Mohawk leaders and British forces near Montreal in 1755, converted Mohawks are reported as saying of baptism, "the French and we are one blood." When a priest at the first French native reserve, Sillery, baptized a Montagnais leader named Nenaskoumat, renaming him François Xavier, one of the tribe members was reported to have said that he was at that point "related to the French," having "received their belief" (quoted in McLeod 1996). Baptism and renaming seem to have forged family ties in both directions: There are reports that mission priests also took native names in the villages of native converts to whom they ministered (Rapport de l'Archiviste de Québec 1926–1927:283).

Priests also baptized native women who married French settlers with French first names and surnames (Van-Kirk 1980). Priests and administrators focused on these marital unions between native women and French men as particularly effective means of hastening the civilizing process. From 1667 to the 1680s, the French government sent money for native women's dowries to colonial governors. The French colonist and explorer Samuel de Champlain reportedly announced to a native group "our young men will marry your daughters and we shall be one people" (quoted in Aubert 2004:476n27). Champlain specifically mentioned mixing with Indian women as a possible route to civilizational order and the betterment of native tribes. In 1639, the Jesuit Order in Quebec convinced the royal supervisor of the colonies to promise free cleared land to any native woman who married and settled with a Frenchman. The founders of Montreal, nuns and priests of the Society of Notre Dame, wrote that they expected intermarriages between native and French to result in mass conversions, leading to an expansion of the colonial population and political and social stability. They recruited native girls into Jesuit schools and later married many of them to French settlers (Giry 1687:98–99).

The rhetoric of French and Catholic conversion—often referred to as "francification"—was a key part of the French North American clerical and civil regime's stated ideology about native groups. Cardinal Richelieu wrote in the charter for the colonial merchant Company of New France in 1627 that "the Savages who will be led to the faith and to profess it will be considered natural Frenchmen." Louis XIV later requested that native children be raised "after the French manner of life, in order to civilize them, bit by bit" (*Jesuit Relations* 53:205). His minister of the marine, Jean-Baptiste Colbert, became a major force behind the founding of native schools, writing that "through the instruction of [savages] in our religion and our customs they can join with the [French] habitants of Canada to become one people" (Jaenen 1976:n37). Much later, in an undated early nineteenth-century letter back to a colleague in Paris, the bishop of Quebec wrote with pleasure that young native women in a recently established mission school were learning how to dress, speak, and live like the French. "Some of them have learned under us how to be tailors, other have become cobblers, and yet others are masons who have already built by their own hands little European-style houses" (Mandements, Lettres Pastorales, et Circulaires:209–211).

The actual practices of priests and colonial administrators may have been exclusionary when it came to natives, but the Church records, as a public genre of colonial and Church discourse, were mediated by this official rhetoric of inclusion. There were three main kinds of public writing that colonial Church administrators, in particular, engaged in while in New France: the *Jesuit Relations*, annual reports sent back from the head of the mission in New France to France; letters sent from the bishops of Quebec to parish priests and the bishops of France; and the Church registers. In the *Relations* and letters, both written in detailed and extensive narrative form, priests regularly drew connections, implicit and explicit, between blood, baptism, the Christianization of native names, and the francification of native manners. Countless references to the mission baptism of Amerindians conveyed an image of the complete transformation of Indian bodies, souls, and in one case, specifically, "blood" through baptism. Through baptism, the Indians were said to have "broke[n] from [their] cruel and filthy culture." Another missionary wrote in the *Relations*: "they believe that to be good Christians they have also to do everything like the French."

There were precedents from mainland France for the French North American colonial and clerical equation of racial categories with cultural and moral competence. In both the mainstream and at the margins, French philosophers had forwarded the idea that the "racial" or "national" or "special" composition of a society would determine its civilizational fate. In the seventeenth century, most of these public discussions focused on the issue of noble blood. Representatives of the French nobility insisted on their natural superiority to officers who had purchased royal status, arguing that noble status was only bestowed by birth. It was said that nobles transmitted through their blood "seeds of valor and virtue" (Aubert 2004:444). Many nobles wrote that "mixed marriages" between people of different social rank could threaten their blood purity and, in turn, the stability of the social order.

They also wrote, as a caveat, that lower ranking women could transmit the blood and qualities of their husbands to their children and were thus easier to assimilate. As a result, the logic went, noblemen could take plebeian women as wives without jeopardizing their blood. Philosophers, jurists, and politicians used this equation of blood with rank and aptitude to apprehend the various physically and socially different people who inhabited new African and American colonies (Peabody 1996).

French North American Church records, with their emphasis on representing successive lists of French names—of individuals baptized into French Christian identities—might be viewed, rather than as authoritative documents of "bare facts," as part of an overall project to represent and enact the spread of colonial Church power through the control and conversion of such religious/racial/national/moral comportment and selves. Demographers in Quebec, by interpreting names in the Church records as proof of biological ancestry, are foreclosing the possible presence of natives in French Catholic records and colonial families, especially native women who were "made French." The contemporary demographic reconstruction of genealogies at Montreal and BALSAC, by linking people into families according to church-recorded names, is reanimating the early modern colonial French racial logic of the records, this time with a biological lens: interpreting French names in the records as indicators of, not just French social, moral, and religious status, but of "French biology." The multigenerational family trees they are constructing using these records evince a genealogical past in which families married for decades within the French settler group, one French Canadian to another. The genealogies represent a mixed frontier society as biologically pure.

The Founder Effect

In the 1980s in Quebec, geneticists began to incorporate the genealogies from the Université de Montréal and BALSAC—and the visions of ancestry, family belonging, and ethnicity embedded within them—into epidemiological studies of both rare and common diseases. New laboratory equipment, advances in medical detection technologies, and the expansion of health services to more rural and distant inhabitants of the provincial territory had led local paediatricians to detect clusters of cases of six rare childhood diseases in northern Quebec.

Some medical researchers began to focus on these newly detected diseases and the regional sub-populations where they had been found. At the time, the field of genetics was changing on a global scale, turning toward population history in order to find patterns in the way diseases spread and traveled from one generation to the next (Adams 1990). Provincial researchers followed this trend. Many turned to the genealogies at BALSAC for demographic data on historic Canadian marriage patterns. They began to use BALSAC genealogies to anchor theories about the French origins of a wide range of biogenetic markers related to these childhood diseases and, gradually, to other more common conditions like breast cancer, asthma, and hypertension. The consensus of all of these strands of research is that the origin of numerous diseases and conditions in Quebec's white French-speaking population is the result of a "founder effect."

The evolutionary biologist Ernst Mayr developed the founder effect concept in 1952 to describe the ecology of islands. He hypothesized that, as a result of the loss of genetic variation in a large population, a subset population that migrates to an island may be genetically and physically different from the parent population. Mayr proposed that, in extreme cases, reproduction, isolation, and inbreeding within the founder population could lead to the evolution of a new species (Mayr 1952). In Quebec, numerous geneticists and demo-geneticists hold that "the French Canadian population arose from a small . . . sample of the French population," that migrated to New France from the Atlantic seaports of Normandy and Brittany and the outskirts of Paris in the seventeenth century. Geneticists both within and outside Quebec say that Quebec is a good candidate for application of the founder effect theory because, though not a physical island, the French Canadian population constitutes a cultural and biological island in North America. Geneticists and genealogists agree that there were about 2,600 founders. They argue the founders settled in the fertile valleys flanking the St. Lawrence River, farmed, and intermarried for nine generations. "Linguistic and religious barriers discouraged admixture of French Canadians." Effectively, geneticists are dividing both past and present Quebec into French (labeled "French speaking," "French Canadian," or "French originating") and non-French (everyone else). They are calling many diseases that affect people in these regions where the founders and first settlers lived "French Canadian" or "French" (Heyer and Gagnon 2001; Gradie and Gavreau 1987; Hamet et al. 2005).

Most often, contemporary genetic studies of disease in Quebec focus on tracing back through the Church records to find the founding French settlers who are believed to have brought a particular disease to North America. In a 2005 article on breast cancer in *Human Genetics*, a group of Chicoutimi-based genetic researchers led by a BALSAC demographer discussed the role of the founder effect in the spread through generations of a particular genetic mutation they believe is linked to breast and ovarian cancer (Laberge, Jomphe et al. 2005). They located a single founder couple from seventeenth-century western France that they believed to be the point of diffusion for the mutation by correlating medical histories and DNA profiles of seventy-two people with genealogies in the BALSAC database. The founder couple appeared in genealogies for all eighteen of the Quebec carriers of the allele who participated in their study but only twenty-six out of fifty-four control genealogies. They wrote, "We believe our combination of molecular, haplotypic, and genealogical approaches for the study of a specific mutation has allowed us to perform one of the most in-depth studies of this type conducted so far. Although the identification of the founders who introduced the mutation will always remain probabilistic we are confident that our method, based on the use of control groups and criteria of frequency and specificity to select ancestors, gives us a very high probability of having pinpointed the right couple."

Some genetic researchers in Quebec have addressed native-French mixing in only a limited manner. In an article in *Clinical Genetics* in 1995, five Montreal-based medical geneticists took care to address admixture involving the French population. Admixture is a term that is used within population genetics to describe reproductive mixing between different populations. The researchers mentioned the well-documented intermarriage between French Catholic settlers and Irish Catholic migrants who came to Quebec between 1846 and 1851, after the Great Potato Famine. They then touched on the French expansions west: "In the eighteenth and early nineteenth centuries, French Canadian explorers penetrated the heart of North America, followed by [further French Canadians] engaged in the fur trade. Some mingled with native populations. In the late nineteenth and early twentieth centuries, between 500,000 and 900,000 French Canadians emigrated to New England in search of employment. The 2000 U.S. census estimates that over 2.3 million Americans report having French Canadian ancestry." (Laberge, Michaud et al. 2005:289.) The geneticists argued that French settlers exported their genetics to populations beyond Quebec but remained biologically homogenous in New France. They ruled out the possibility of French-native admixture (instead of or in addition to a founder effect). "Despite increasing . . . urbanization, mobility, and immigration . . . [the original founders] remain a vital . . . component of medical genetics in Quebec."

Population, Genealogy, Blame, and the Links to BALSAC

How have these institutional and scientific processes at BALSAC and in demography and genetics projects affected clinical and everyday understandings in Quebec of relatedness, illness, and human difference? Conversely, are everyday understandings of relatedness, illness, and human difference in Quebec the animus for the genealogical logic at BALSAC and in Quebec demography and genetics?

There are clear affinities between how healthcare workers, physicians, and ordinary people in Quebec are characterizing diseases as French and how researchers at BALSAC are drawing lines around a bounded entity they call the French Canadian population.

In their everyday lives, people both within and outside of the purview of health and medical institutions talk about individual risk for disease only insofar as the person can be viewed through the lens of his or her population. People regularly refer to the "French Canadian population" as a descriptor, model, and mode of explanation for a broad range of physiological conditions, from asthma to hormonal imbalances. Throughout my fieldwork in Quebec, people often said "it came from the founders" or "it came from France" as they strove to explain the reasons for illnesses in their families, clinics, and neighborhoods.

"When you tell a patient his child is sick, the first question they ask is 'Why do we have it?' " Dr. Lucien Laberge, a pediatrician treating children with a fatal recessive disorder in the Saguenay-Lac-Saint-Jean region told me in 2008 at his clinic. "And that is when we explain the founder effect." Laberge has been diagnosing the disorder he specializes in since 1985 and is partnering with a local patient association to establish a government-funded genetic screening program in Chicoutimi. "You see," Laberge continued, "we have not mixed. Multiculturalism in Quebec is changing that, particularly in Montreal, and this dilution is medically good. We will have less disease. But, for centuries, French Canadians only married each other." Like BALSAC geneticists, Laberge was affirming historiographic hypotheses about the way French families used to live on the frontier by enfolding medical explanations in familiar historical refrains. In a gymnasium south of Montreal a year prior, I had interviewed research subjects who were donating DNA for a genetic study of a sensory neuropathic disorder by a Montreal neurologist. A woman said two of her brothers, both in their fifties, had the disorder. She had pointed to the family tree form she was filling to hand in with her DNA: "They came from Charolles." Charolles is a village in the Bourgougne region in central France that many genealogists have posed as the ancestral origin of several French Canadian names. "They are the ones who brought it. The Gagnons." Like Laberge, she enfolded a familiar story about the French Canadian past in her explanation of an illness. "When they became ill, I knew we must have been marrying only among ourselves," she continued. She was also, in reverse, using illness to infer that familiar story.

One day in Chicoutimi, in January 2007, I accompanied Geneviève Turncotte, a coordinator from the regional hospital's community education wing, on an outreach session at a local college. "Every population globally is affected by hereditary disease. In [our region], the frequency of certain defective genes and inherited illnesses is elevated because of the founder effect," Geneviève said to the group of fifteen students, pointing to a drawing of a group of people from western France. "Many people are carriers of a recessive copy of a disease and don't know it. Though they are not sick, they maintain the risk of transmitting illness." Pointing to western France on the map, she began to tell the familiar story of the French Canadian frontier. Geneviève's implication for everyone in the room was that the insides of their bodies were walking museums—capsules of a frontier history that lingered on in every cell. The map of France, genetic carriers, and founder effect were all part of a seamless link she was posing between geography, genealogy, and biology—a link stitched together in the biochemical matter within cells that constituted each students' genotype. Here, there are answers to questions of location: where is human difference and belonging being located in contemporary genomics? People are moving difference deep inside the body to the inner workings of cells (Nelson 2008). There are also answers to questions of mechanism: How is race being remade in contemporary genomics? People within and beyond medicine are turning enzymes and nucleotides into signs of race. They are also connecting these cellular processes to geographies and genealogies with astounding specificity—to particular towns in countries far away and to certain people in those towns, all through written records. By linking and layering the genealogical trajectories of these people—tracking lines from each ancestor in France to a descendant in Quebec one-by-one—Geneviève, like Laberge and the woman at the gymnasium research recruitment drive, was using the founder effect explanation in ways that turned medical conditions into "French Canadian diseases."

Had BALSAC caused them to reframe their medical explanations using the French Canadian rubric? Did they already have preformed ideas that led them to believe illnesses were the result of intermarriage in Quebec before BALSAC's explanations became public and widespread? Did BALSAC simply reanimate these ideas? Did their ideas, in fact, predate and originally animate the work at BALSAC? One day in Chicoutimi, I met Christine Tremblay, the founder of a smaller, early patient advocacy association for parents of children with one of several recessive metabolic disorders that exist in high prevalence in Quebec. In 1981, a local physician diagnosed her son with the disorder. "At that time, I was ashamed, because we had a feeling that we had done something wrong, that there was something wrong about *us*." She continued on to say that her family thought their ancestors may have been consanguineous and that this was the reason for her son's diagnosis. "We were relieved when we found out it was not us but the founder effect from [one of the BALSAC scientists]. That diminished our sense of genetic blame. All of a sudden we knew it was not us but our population as a whole. We never took an interest in genealogy after that." In Tremblay's case, it seemed that the founder effect explanation disseminated by BALSAC had led her to reframe the illness as "French Canadian" but that she had always understood the illness to be the result of in-marriage. In other words, she had a preexisting notion that her ancestors had "married-in" but BALSAC had led her to revise her notion of how to link those ancestors to illness. For Tremblay now, genealogies are not an end or an explanation in themselves. They are a route, through finding connections to a founder, to proving belonging in a population and explaining pain as an effect of that belonging.

How to Link Racial Logics to Genetic Practice?

The affinities between the ways people in the world of medicine and genetics are drawing population boundaries and the way Quebec nationalists have forwarded their historiographic and political agendas are striking. Are genetic renderings of "populations" such as those in Chicoutimi and at BALSAC simply laboratory and clinical effects of more broadly accepted social norms for dividing people into races, such as the Quebec nationalist classifications of Quebeckers into "immigrant" and "pure French?" Everywhere I turned during and after fieldwork—from professional meetings to casual lunches with friends—people threw about the word *nationalism* as if it contained a flawless intelligibility that could fruitfully be brought to bear on the question of genetics and race in Quebec.

Two respected historians of Canada once told me they believed the Montreal and BALSAC databases and the genetic genealogies based on them embodied the exclusionary stance of Quebec nationalism perfectly (Nash 2007). Nation-building projects were indeed the context within which the demographers at the Université de Montréal originally developed their database. Does that mean nationalism is the explanation for all of the racial categories, forms of interpretation, and stances toward illness and race that followed? This is a question with relevance beyond nationalism studies. Many critics explain exclusionary practices of genetic science by reference to broader contemporaneous social ideologies about race. Just how should we or can we empirically link the laboratory to these ideas at large?

What seemed important to me in spending time at demography and genetics laboratories in Quebec was that people approached the elements of their daily work—transcribing and converting church records into genealogies for genetics—with specific stances toward how to read and interpret a document. Absent those stances, the Quebec genealogies would look entirely different, nationalist movement or not. Demographers' stance toward church documents and the politics of documentary history shaped their demo-genetic productions: They accorded certain types of legal documents (church documents) a privileged authenticity, based on perceptions about the trustworthiness of past Catholic bureaucracies. They read the documents for race in ways that overlooked the way those documents had been produced; the old documents themselves are products of institutional actors who sought to promote certain missionary evangelist familial taxonomies. These evidentiary, reading, and credibility norms pose a specific causal relationship between collective agency and subjectivity. In this relationship, shared attitudes toward documents, writing, and bureaucracy as well as the very written documents themselves, the racial typologies they incorporate, and the forms of social transformation (native assimilation) that they effected in early North America, mediate genealogical and genetic practices surrounding race, ancestry, and relatedness.

This raises even further questions. Did these credibility and reading norms arise independently of genetics, medicine, or people's beliefs about illness? Can they be posed as a primary cause that led demographers and geneticists to act as they did? During fieldwork with genealogists with no links to the world of health and medical institutions I met Germain Desjardins, a retiree who was researching his family genealogy at the national archives in Montreal. Desjardins told me after many conversations that he had first set out to do genealogies because he wanted to explain his wife's illness. Like most genealogists, he had worked mainly with parish records to produce a multi-generational family tree. Showing me his wife's genealogy chart, he pointed to the line that he said led back to Catherine de Baillon, a supposed descendant of Charlemagne who came to New France in 1669. A French Canadian priest published a book on de Baillon in 1991 that used parish records to trace her lineage through French noble houses in the Middle Ages to contemporary French Canadian family names (Jetté 1991). Desjardins then pointed on the chart to the places where his wife's maternal and paternal line had shared ancestors: great-great-great-aunts and uncles who had married into both her mother's and father's family. "That was inbreeding." For him, the link to de Baillon was a proof of the French provenance of his wife's ancestors—for not only were they French, they were, as he told it, part of the very core of early modern French society in Europe. He had then connected these three points—his wife's illness, the lines of consanguinity he had found in her family tree, and the links to French royals. He treated the consanguinity and royals as explanations for the illness. He treated the illness, conversely, as suggestive of the consanguinity and French royals. Outside of the purview of scientific research institutions and formal medical diagnoses people like Desjardins were using a perceived endogamous French Canadian past and connection to early modern France to explain disease.

In Montreal, I interviewed a member of my basketball team, Alexandre Boivin, whose brother has a rare metabolic disorder. "I will never marry a Quebecker," he said. "I'll never have kids." He explained that he thought he was permanently tainted and that his family, for being French in Canada and for marrying within French Canadian families, was to blame. Like Christine Tremblay and Geneviève Turncotte, he was using a population frame to explain a family illness. He shared with them a sense of the parameters of French society in North America: French Canadians come from France and French founders; they maintained cultural unity for centuries, evidenced by their successive in-marriage; and these two facts have culminated in illnesses by which they are now beset. Were these "folk" etiologies effects, antecedents, parallel to, or intersecting with demographic research at the Université de Montréal and BALSAC? Were the norms for reading and trusting parish records and for connecting stories about the French Canadian frontier to illness part of the social context within which BALSAC developed? Were they instances of scientific knowledge and practice at BALSAC filtering, indirectly, over years and across webs of social groups and institutions, into daily life? Were they simply suggestive of a shared repertoire of reading styles, medical explanation, and historiographic practice throughout Quebec, both within and outside of medical science?

Scholars specifically studying Quebec genetics have argued that the tendency to represent French Canadians as homogenous and endogamous, whether in science or society at large, is a symptom of the dominance of the nationalist mood (Bibeau 2004; Nash 2007; Lloyd 2001). They suggest that BALSAC genealogies are a surface for the projection of preformed human needs and desires about the nation, belonging, and history in Quebec. Their argument follows the logic of familiar nationalism theories such as Benedict Anderson's. It implies that genealogists, geneticists, and everyday people have self-abstracted themselves into individual instances of the "French Canadian collectivity." They conceive of themselves as connected across time and space to other similarly abstracted individuals with whom they are linked by virtue of that collectivity. They imagine that this collective indexes shared blood and shared history, creating fictional boundaries between insiders and outsiders. The argument further implies that they are generating various artifacts that represent this, such as genealogies, and acting on that imaginary in exclusionary ways. This explanation depends on the view that people have an idea in their heads of exactly what they want to do before they start to interact in the world. I was never sure whether the demographers and genealogists I observed were working with some coherent French nationalist inclination lodged in their heads as they did their daily work. This mode of explanation also leaves no room to bring the parish records, how people read them, write them, and the genealogical world they evince into my explanation of how diseases became "French Canadian" in Quebec.

The records and norms for trusting, reading, and gleaning information from them play a major role in the way Quebec demographers, geneticists, and genealogists pose family and regional history in relation to biology. Demography was not a place where they projected preformed ideologies about the collective. It was a form of knowledge-making that required evidentiary procedures, rules, and standards for determining proof, and, to a certain extent, a mixture of opportunistic, pragmatic, and culturally/academically conditioned choices about which evidence to trust. They used and trusted Church records. Their everyday conversations about how to structure genealogies were about how to use the records to validate facts. A major problem was that their focus was only on validating, and not situating facts. The questions they were concerned with were whether various ways of distinguishing cases from controls or how various periodizations and geographic divisions of Church record data would affect the validity of conclusions.

The argument from the article I quoted earlier—that researchers are confident in their method because it is "based on the use of control groups and criteria of frequency and specificity to select ancestors"—captures this stance toward scientific experimentation well. The nation-building programs of the Quebec government in the 1960s and 70s set the parameters of the original genealogical database on which their conclusions depended—the database was supposed to be for the study of French Canadians, conceived of as a bounded and homogenous group. There may have been widespread beliefs within the communities that BALSAC scientists lived in that French Canadians always married-in—beliefs that shaped their predispositions to certain kinds of explanations and interpretations of evidence. However, regional stances toward reading records, local histories of the production of records, and professional demographic and quantitative experimental norms also mitigated toward the homogenized, racialized genealogies at BALSAC.

BALSAC's journey from records to evidence to fact—its crafting of demographic and genetic conclusions—sheds light on how material artifacts and evidentiary norms interact with forces that produce collective belonging and the dynamics of scientific institutions to explain bodies in pain. The case of BALSAC suggests that, in looking at how ideas about race, nation, and belonging are being brought to bear on genetics in contemporary society, we should not overlook the material forms that scientific inquiry takes: the types of evidence scientists choose, the ideas about credibility and counterfeit that factor into these choices, and the mechanics of how evidence is converted into scientific models and conclusions. In Quebec, a discussion between a doctor and patient about a seizure can invoke visions of the past and create a sense of belonging and place. That logic has emerged in the purview of specific cultures of French colonial ecclesiastical writing, certain stances toward the credibility of written records, and widespread evidentiary norms within European and North American historical demography.

NOTES

1. I conducted twenty months of ethnographic fieldwork at hospitals, medical research centers, genealogical societies, and with patient advocacy organizations in Montreal and the Saguenay-Lac-Saint-Jean region of northern Quebec. I have changed the names and some other identifying details of all of the individuals and some of the organizations I mention in this article.

2. Evolutionary biologist Ernst Mayr characterized populations: "Under ideal conditions a population consists of a small group of individuals clearly separated from other individuals of the species by a physical barrier. Examples of such isolated populations would be those on islands in the sea, or in the oases of the desert, or on mountain tops, and the like."

3. BALSAC is not an acronym.

4. In French, "sauvages," or "sauvagesses" for women.

5. Looking at French colonial authorities in turn-of-the-century Indochine, Ann Stoler has noted how officials there also used names to categorize the cultural affiliation, racial identity, and legal rights of colonial subjects (Stoler 1992:522).

WORKS CITED

Adams, Julian. 1990. Introduction: Genetics and demography and historical information. In *Convergent issues in genetics and demography*, edited by Julian Adams, David A. Lam, Albert I. Hermalin, and Peter E. Smouse, 3–13. New York: Oxford University Press.

Alter, Stephen G. 1999. *Darwinism and the linguistic image: Language, race, and natural theology in the nineteenth century*. Baltimore: Johns Hopkins University Press.

Aubert, Guillaume. 2004. "Purity of blood": Race and purity of blood in the French Atlantic world. *William and Mary Quarterly* 61 (3):3.

Bélanger, Pauline. 1990. *Inventaire des registres paroissiaux catholiques du Quebec 1621–1876*. Université de Montréal/Programme de Recherche en Démographie Historique.

Bibeau, Gilles. 2004. Le Québec transgénique: Science, marché, humanité (Transgenic Quebec: Science, market, humanity). Boréal: Montreal.

Bookstein, Fred L. 1995. *Utopian Skeletons in the biometric closet*. Series of occasional papers. Ann Arbor: University of Michigan, Institute for the Humanities.

Bouchard, Gérard, and André LaRose. 1976. La réglementation des actes de baptême, mariage, sépulture au Québec, des origines à nos jours (The regulation of baptism, marriage, and burial acts in Quebec from the beginning to the present). *Revue d'Histoire de l'Amerique Française* (French American History Review) 30 (64):67–84.

Bouquet, Mary. 1996. Family trees and their affinities: The visual imperative of the genealogical diagram. *Journal of the Royal Anthropological Institute* 2:43–66.

Le Bras, Hervé and Sandrine Bertieaux, eds. 2000. *L'invention des populations*. Paris: Odile Jacob.

Charbonneau, Hubert and Jacques Légaré. 1967. La Démographie Historique au Canada. *Recherches Sociographiques* (Sociological Research) Series, Vol. 8, No. 2. Quebec: Laval University Press.

La Chaire de Recherche du Canada Sur La Question Territoriale. *Authochtone lettre d'information*. Université du Québec à Montréal, 1 (3):2.

Lettre de Mnsgr. L'Evêque de Québec, ou il rend compte à un de ses amis de son premier voyage de Canada, et de l'état ou il a laissé l'église et de la colonie (Letter from the Bishop of Quebec, where he recounts to one of his friends his first trip to Canada and the state in which he has left the Church and colony). *Nd. Mandements, Lettres Pastorales, et Circulaires des Évêques de Québec (Mandements, Pastoral Letters, and Circulars of the Bishops of Quebec)*. Québec: Imprimerie Général A. Coté et Cie. 209–211.

Fenwick, Rudy. 1981. Social change and ethnic nationalism: An historical analysis of the separatist movement in Québec. *Comparative Studies in Society and History* 23 (1):212.

Fontaine, Louise. 1995. Immigration and cultural policies: A bone of contention between the Province of Québec and the Canadian federal government. *International Migration Review* 29:1044.

Fullwiley, Duana. 2007. The molecularization of race: Institutionalizing racial difference in pharmacogenetics practice. *Science as Culture* 16:1–30.

Gevrais, Diane, and Danielle Gauvreau. 2003. Women, priests, and physicians: Family limitation in Québec, 1940–1970. *Journal of Interdisciplinary History* 34 (2):294–314.

Giry, François. 1687. *La vie de M. Jean Jacques Olier, prêtre, fondateur et premier Supérieur du Séminaire de Saint-Sulpice*. (The life of Monsieur Jean Jacques Olier, priest, founder, and first Superior of the Seminary of Saint-Sulpice). Pais: SI.

Goudreau, Serge. 2003. Un chef Huron du Village du Lorette. (A Huron Chief of the Village of Lorette). *Memoires de la Société Généalogique Canadienne-Française (Memos of the French-Canadian Genealogical Society)* 54(4):269–288.

Goulbert, Pierre. 1965. Registres paroissiaux et démographie dans la France du XVIe Siècle (Parish registers and demography in 16th-century France). *Annales de Démographie Historique* (Annals of Historical Demography) 2:43–48.

Gradie, Margaret and Danielle Gauvreau. 1987. Migration and hereditary disease in the Saguenay population of Eastern Québec. *International Migration Review* 21:592–608.

Hacking, Ian. 1976. *The logic of statistical inference*. Cambridge: Cambridge University Press.

Hacking, Ian. 1991. *The taming of chance*. Cambridge: Cambridge University Press.

Hamet, P., E. Merlo, O. Seda, et al. 2005. Quantitiative founder-effect analysis of French Canadian families identifies specific loci contributing to metabolic phenotypes of hypertension. *American Journal of Human Genetics* 76:815–832.

Handler, Richard. 1987. Holistic culture, bureaucratic fragmentation: Government administration of culture in Québec. *Anthropology Today* 3:6–8.

Heyer, Evelyn and Alain Gagnon. 2001. Intergenerational correlation of effective family size in early Québec. *Human Biology* 13:645–659.

Hollingsworth, T. H. 1969. *Historical demography: The sources of history.* Studies in the Uses of Historical Evidence Series. London: The Sources of History Ltd in collaboration with Hodder and Stoughton Ltd.

Iankova, Katia. 2006. La territorialité urbaine de Wendake, née du choc du cultures (Wendake's urban territoriality, born of culture clash). Paper Presented at Université de Québec à Montréal colloquium "Le Territoire et Les Autochtones." September 21.

Jaenen, Cornelius. 1976. *Role of the Church in New France.* Toronto: McGraw Hill/Ryerson.

Jaenen, Cornelius. 1982. "Les sauvages Ameriquains": Persistence into the 18th century of traditional French concepts and constructs for apprehending Amerindians. *Ethnohistory* 29 (1):47.

Jesuit Relations (1669–1670), Vol. 53, 205.

Jetté, René. 1991. *Traité de généalogie* (Genealogical treaty, *lit.*). Montréal: Les Presses de l'Université de Montréal, 112–114, 593–598.

Kahn, Susan. 2005. Are genes Jewish?: Conceptual ambiguities in a new genetic age. Paper presented at Reproductive Disruptions Conference. University of Michigan, Ann Arbor.

Laberge, A. M., J. Michaud, A. Richter, E. Lemyre, M. Lambert, B. Brais, and G. A. Mitchell. 2005. Population history and its impact on medical genetics in Quebec. *Clinical Genetics* 68:287–301.

Laberge, A. M., M. Jomphe, L. Houde, H. Vezina, M. Tremblay, B. Desjardins, D. Labuda, M. St.-Hilaire, C. Macmillan, E.A. Shoubridge, and B. Brais. 2005. A "fille du roy" introduced the T14484C Leber's hereditary optic neuropathy mutation in French Canadians. *American Journal of Human Genetics* 77 (2):313–317.

Lawrence, Bonita. 2003. Gender, race, and the regulation of Native identity in Canada and the United States: An overview. *Hypatia* 18:3–31.

Lemon, Alaina. 2002. Without a "concept"?: Race as discursive practice." *Slavic Review* 61:54–61.

Lloyd, Stephanie Jean. 2001. Genetic states: Collective identity and genetic nationalism in Iceland and Quebec. Ph.D. dissertation, Department of Anthropology, McGill University.

Mandements, lettres pastorales, et circulaires des évêques de Québec (Mandements, pastoral letters, and circulars of the bishops of Quebec). Québec: Imprimerie Général A. Coté et Cie. 209–211.

M'Charek, Amade. 2005. *The human genome diversity project: An ethnography of scientific practice.* Cambridge: Cambridge University Press.

Macleod, D. Peter. 1996. Catholicism, alliances, and Amerindian evangelists. *Catholic Church Historical Association Historical Studies* 62:69.

Mayr, Ernst. 1942. *Systematics and the origin of species.* New York: Columbia University Press, 27.

Mayr, Ernst. 1952. *Populations, species, and evolution: An abridgment of animal species and evolution.* Cambridge, MA: Belknap Press.

Nash, Alice. c. 2007. Amerindians in the PRDH. Unpublished ms.

Nelson, Alondra 2008. Bio science: Genetic ancestry testing and the pursuit of African ancestry. *Social Studies of Science* 38 (5):759–783.

Pálsson, Gísli, and Kristín E. Hardardóttir. 2002. For whom the cell tolls: Debates about biomedicine. *Current Anthropology* 43:271–301.

Parish Registers, XVII–XIX Century, National Archives of Quebec, Montreal. (Registre de Hurons de Loretteville, Roll #4604). Original: "blancs."

Rapport de l'Archiviste de Québec, Vol. 1926–1927, Lettres de Père Alneau Collection.

Peabody, Sue. 1996. *"There are no slaves in France": The political culture of race and slavery in the Ancien Régime*. Oxford: Oxford University Press.

Rose, Geoffrey. 2001. Sick individuals and sick populations. *International Journal of Epidemiology* 30:427–432.

Rituel du Diocèse de Québec (Rites of the Diocese of Quebec), 1703, Musée de la civilisation, Bibliothèque du Séminaire de Québec.

Secko, David. 2008. Why Quebec is a gift to geneticists: Rare history, common disease. *The Scientist* 22 (7):38–45.

Simpson, Bob. 2000. Imagined genetic communities: Ethnicity and essentialism in the twenty-first century. *Anthropology Today* 16:3–6.

Stoler, Ann. 1992. Sexual affronts and racial frontiers: European identities and the cultural politics of exclusions in Colonial Southeast Asia. *Comparative Studies in Society and History* 34:522.

Taussig, Karen Sue, Rayna Rapp, and Deborah Heath. 2003. Flexible eugenics: technologies of the self in the age of genetics. In *Genetic nature/culture: Anthropology and science beyond the two-culture divide*, edited by A. Goodman, D. Heath and M. S. Lindee, 58–76. Berkeley: University of California Press.

Thwaites, Ruben Gold, ed. 1898–1901. *The Jesuit relations and allied documents: Travel and explorations of the Jesuit missionaries in New France 1610–1791*. 73 vols. Cleveland, OH: Burrows Publishing. Vol. 6 (1634).

Trautmann, Thomas R. 2006. *Languages and nations: The Dravidian proof in colonial Madras*. Berkeley: University of California Press, 1–41.

Van-Kirk, Sylvia. 1980. Many tender ties: Women in fur-trade society, 1670–1870. Ph.D. Dissertation, Department of History, University of London.

Velay-Vallantin, Catherine. 1997. Usages de la tradition du folklore en France et au Québec (1937–1950) (Uses of the folklore tradition in France and Quebec): l'Investiture du politique. In *Une langue, deux cultures: Rites et symboles en France et au Québec* (One Language, Two Cultures: Rites and Symbols in France and Quebec), edited by Gerard Bouchard and Martine Segalen, 273–301. Quebec: Les Presses de l'Université Laval.

Village des Hurons, Wedake. Undated. Canadian-U.S. International Boundary Commission Report (Legal Surveys Division, Historical Review). 74.125.93.104/search?q=cache: yA4PnABb9aQJ:internationalboundarycommission.org/data/fh/village_des_hurons_ang .pdf+Wendake,+Legal+Surveys+Division,+Historical+Review&cd=1&hl=en&ct=clnk& gl=ca, [Accessed on June 10, 2007].

12

∞∞

Categorization, Census, and Multiculturalism

Molecular Politics and the Material of Nation

AMY HINTERBERGER

In the early twentieth century there was a vociferous debate in the Canadian press on whether the category *Canadian* should be available as a choice on the census. A census-taker could tick a range of "ethnic identifiers" such as English, French, Chinese, or German, but not Canadian. A 1921 newspaper article weighing in on the debate pondered: "Who and what are we? Is there such a person as a Canadian? The Government of Canada says there is not" (Ruppert 2007:24). Another article, this time supporting the government's discouragement of *Canadian* as a census category, argued that "no matter how far back a man can trace his Canadian source, he is of foreign origin, unless he happens to be an Indian, or the child of an Indian mother" (Ruppert 2007:24). It was not until 1996 that *Canadian* was officially added to the list of available options for choosing one's ethnic origins in the Canadian census (Boyd, et al. 2000). Up until that point, *Canadian* as a census category did not officially exist.

Why was including *Canadian* on the census so contentious? What made it so different from English or French? According to Evelyn Ruppert, census participants had referred to themselves as "Canadian" since 1871 on the census, but this was often scratched out by compliers, and individuals were then recategorized on the basis of surname (Ruppert 2007:24). Fundamentally, it was an issue of what was called "ethnic stock." In other words, it was about knowing just what kinds of people were "making up" Canada. Concerns over the accurate monitoring of ethnic stock led government authorities to discourage the use of the category *Canadian*. According to Ruppert, during the early twentieth century the Dominion statistician (a bureaucratic position now titled chief statistician) argued that no fewer than seven questions were related to the determination of who was a "Canadian": nationality, year of immigration, year of naturalization, birthplace, mother and father birthplace, language spoken, and racial origin (Ruppert 2007:26). Nationality, the Dominion statistician argued, was a necessary but insufficient condition for being Canadian, as it did not provide the state with practical knowledge about things such as the nation's "basic ethnic stock" (Ruppert 2007:26).

Though terms such as *ethnic stock* may have fallen into disuse, population classification in the census continues to shape the identification, monitoring, and inclusion of the kinds of people that make up Canada. What has significantly changed is the rhetoric of population classification. Governmental authorities measure populations along ethnic, cultural, linguistic, and ancestral lines, but no longer in the name of ethnic stock. Rather, they do so in order to monitor who makes up Canada's "rich cultural mosaic" (Statistics Canada 2010).

In this chapter, I explore how processes of classification, relating to race, ethnicity, and ancestry, are gaining salience in the large-scale study of human DNA for health and disease in Canada. Over the last ten years, there has been increasing investment and acceleration of population genomics research for health in Canada. This is a pivotal arena, where vexed questions of how difference comes to matter are negotiated. In this chapter, I emphasize the need to look towards the past to remember that the structures, borders (real and imagined) and peoples that populate the nation of Canada did not always exist as they do now. Though it may seem an obvious point, the formation of the nation was itself a historical process. As a result, the colonial histories, census categories and population genealogies of Canada are not only part of the unsettled past, they are inextricably bound up in the unsettled futures of human genome science. For example, in this chapter I will show how Canada's national rhetorics of multiculturalism are becoming increasingly relevant to understanding the relationship between the corporeal body and molecular politics in genomics-based biomedicine. In other words, examination of the national and institutional aspects of Canada's multicultural policy—how bodies are counted up, what value they are attributed, and what resources they are seen to add—is central to exploring the groups emerging under the auspices of genomics and health in Canada.

The central guiding question of this chapter is: How are human groups in Canada made up in order to be included within emerging biopolitical contexts, where human genome science and public health meet? Answering this question requires engaging with the ways populations are constituted as the subjects, publics, groups, communities and beneficiaries of scientific research. This chapter examines in detail the classificatory logics of institutionalized multiculturalism in the Canadian census, as the census offers an explicit site where human groups are made up in order to be included. The chapter thus considers how particular legacies of classification and standardization of difference in settler colonies are intermeshed with contemporary politics of biomedicine and health in genomics research. In particular, the chapter explores constructions of populations, such as the category of *visible minority* and *Aboriginal persons*[1] to demonstrate that the already constructed can shape social and scientific practice in multiple ways.

Contemporary politics of classification in Canada are firmly entrenched within the political logics of Canada's institutionalized multiculturalism. In fact, what sets Canada apart from many other nations is that governmental authorities and agencies have dealt with difference by multiplying measures and categories of group difference, rather than by suppressing them as in France or Israel (Goldscheider 2002:81). When it comes to the census, Canada is referred to as a "complicated case" (Goldscheider 2002:79), and others have explored how Statistics Canada, the body that oversees the census, has experienced considerable difficulty and debate regarding measures related to race, ethnicity, and population (Boyd et al. 2000).

The institutionalization of multicultural difference in the census constructs populations recognized by diverse governmental agencies and adjacent institutions, and also contributes to the capacity of subjects to recognize themselves as members of a social group and population. This chapter seeks not only to set out in detail how people are classified and counted, but also to begin linking these classificatory processes to broader biopolitical contexts that indicate who can count (Epstein 2006:330). Policy-makers, funders, ethicists, and scientific researchers conducting large-scale population genomics on human health are increasingly brought under the kinds of monitoring, measuring, and reporting that overlap with multicultural classification in Canada. In seeking public legitimation, then, population genomics projects often draw on already constructed categories offered through official channels such as the census.

Genomics and Health for the Public Good

The goal of health, or promise of health, has become a kind of meta-value in liberal democracies. As Monica Greco argues, "speaking in the name of health is one of the most powerful rhetorical devices" (2004:1). Genomics research offers significant insight into the prevention and surveillance of diseases, consequently illuminating the field of public health. The impact, then, of what has been called "public health genomics" is said to have significant consequences for the future of public health (Burke et al. 2006).

The promises of health offered by public health genomics are often combined with an emphasis on social justice and the ending of health inequalities between groups. For example, a recently published paper on genomics and public health in Canada concludes that addressing the needs to Canada's indigenous peoples and recent immigrants, who are more likely to experience health inequalities, is a central task of genomic medicine (Little et al. 2009:117). When combined with the promises of genomic medicine, support for large-scale genomics research forms a powerful narrative. By curing the ills of certain populations, genomic research will also cure the ills of an unjust society.

Public health genomics has gained salience in Canada particularly in relation to long-term and large-scale investment in human genome science, as well as the creation of resources and infrastructure to support these technologies, such as large-scale biobanks. Public health genomics is a strategic priority area for investment by Canada's Public Health Agency, and Genome Canada has invested substantially in a range of projects addressing genomics and public health, such as the biobank CARTaGENE.[2] Canada has a federal body in charge of funding health research and setting guidelines for research. It is the Canadian Institutes of Health Research (CIHR). The CIHR was established in 2000 in order to "excel in the creation of new knowledge and its translation into improved health for Canadians and to strengthen Canadian health care system from the study of molecules, to research on health policy and populations" (CIHR 2004:1). Canada does not have a specific public health genomics research strategy. However, human health genomics is a research priority area that has been aggressively funded in the last ten years. The landscape of large-scale genomics funding in Canada is dominated by those who set policy for funding (such as the Prime Minister's Office), the federal departments that receive funding for genomics research and development (like Industry Canada), and the funding providers such as Genome Canada and the CIHR to which researchers apply and compete for funds.

How exactly has public health genomics been described? In 2005, a meeting was convened in Bellagio, Italy, with a multidisciplinary group of eighteen experts from Canada, France, Germany, the United Kingdom, and the United States. The group defined public health genomics as "the responsible and effective translation of genome-based knowledge for the benefit of population health" (Report: Genome-based research and population health 2005:4–5). Genome-based knowledge refers to the findings of genetic and molecular science (for example, the Human Genome Project) and how these combine with new technologies and applications for healthcare. Public health genomics thus includes:

> Better characterisation of disease at the molecular and cellular level; genetic testing for diagnosis of inherited disorders; therapeutic advances such as pharmacogenetics; and new approaches to drug design and development. It draws from what might be called the population sciences. It combines epidemiology and other population sciences like cohort studies (biobanks) as well as the meta-analysis of genetic association studies. (Report: Genome-based research and population health 2005:11)

Public health genomics then runs the gamut from the "low-tech" recruitment of participants into cohort studies and biobanks, to the newest genomic techniques such as genome-wide association studies. The technologies encompassed in a public health genomics approach are thus diverse, and range from getting genotype information and biological specimens, to recording environmental information, to collecting demographic information on populations.

One of the goals of public health genomics, then, is to develop large databases of genetic variation in different population groups. Advocates of public health genomics argue that it is largely through understanding human genomic diversity within and between populations who inhabit different environments that the insights needed for genomic medicine will emerge (Khoury et al. 2000). However, these large-scale studies require large-scale funding. The creation of Genome Canada, for example, has been key to making these funds available in order to design and implement population genomics research on a large-scale in Canada. As a term, public health genomics, has an international remit and is used by organisations such as the Foundation for Genomics and Population Health (UK) and research networks like the Public Health Genomics European Network (EU), and is the focus of research papers published in a range of journals (Segiun et al. 2008; Avard et al. 2009). Similar to other "genomic terms," such as genomic medicine, *public health genomics* operates as a buzzword that represents the imagined futures of genomic research, rather than its current reality.

Categorical Alignment in Public Health Genomics

A central goal of public health genomics is something called *knowledge integration* (Report: Genome-based research and population health 2005:16). This involves the selection, storage, collation, analysis, and dissemination of information about populations across a variety of fields and sites, such as epidemiology, biostatistics, computer software design, and ethics review boards in hospitals and universities. However, this emphasis on knowledge integration means that public health genomics is highly susceptible to what Steven Epstein calls "categorical alignment" (Epstein 2007:91). This is where "common-sense" group differences (such as those naturalized in the census and used by governmental agencies) take on an increased prominence in biomedical research. Bodies already linked to constructed social identities become increasingly medically significant: "Characteristic of this way of thinking is the assumption that social identities correspond to relatively distinct kinds of bodies—female bodies, Asian bodies, elderly Hispanic male bodies, and so on—and that these various embodied states are medically incommensurable" (Epstein 2007:2).

Epstein's concern about this common-sense approach to difference is that it promotes a kind of uncritical inclusion and measurement of difference that can have an effect exactly the opposite of its desired aims. He outlines a series of unintended consequences of attaching biomedical significance to socially significant identities. These include ignoring the ways health risks are distributed across society, valorizing some forms of identity and concealing others from view, and potentially obscuring individual-level differences by focusing on groups (Epstein 2007:11).

While the ideas and goals of public health genomics are of significant importance in the process of translating genomics research into health interventions, the emphasis on knowledge integration requires specific attention. This is because there is increasing overlap between the classification practices of the nation-state (like the census), the naming practices of identity-based social movements (like multiculturalism), and the new population techniques of human genome science. Indeed, the adoption and use of census categories in publicly funded genomic health research is increasingly common. For example, Andrew Smart et al. found that the majority of U.K. scientists they interviewed reported that they adopted census classification for practical reasons in biobanking research (Smart, 2008, 407). However, the unreflective use or routine adoption of census classifications can result in the naturalization of population groups whose relationship to genetic research is often contradictory and unclear (Smart et al. 2008:417–418).

According to public health experts, genetic researchers, and policy-makers, Canada is well placed to develop population-based genomics health research. In 2001 the CIHR held a workshop in Quebec on human population genetics that was jointly sponsored by Genome Canada. The workshop reviewed the status of population genetics research in Canada, and made the case that Canada was well placed to develop the area of population genomics for health in the following ways:

> Canadian scientists have already developed significant scientific expertise in this area. A large-scale Canadian cohort study in human population genetics/genomics research could be established, based on a combination of existing data sets, augmented by targeted new data acquisition to address gaps among the databases . . . The entire Canadian population is "well-defined" due to the existence of individual clinical records of significant depth and duration in all provinces and territories. These records are accessible through the existence of unique identifiers for all citizens already attached to clinical health records. (CIHR 2001:2)

Canada has a universal publicly funded health care system, provided by provincial and territorial health insurance plans. Each province has its own public health legislation, although the age and content of these vary considerably. Most public health activities are resourced at provincial or territorial levels, with strategic coordination from national bodies.

Observations about the well-defined nature of Canadian populations due to the public health system are echoed in other reports. A 2006 proceedings report from a Genome Canada national retreat held in Ottawa discussed the trends in genomics research and the future of Canada's stake in this research. The report noted that: "Canada's diverse population—as well as its genetically unique human populations—offers opportunities to pursue cohort studies. . . . Canada's centralized health care system also provides effective and accessible data collection" (Genome Canada 2006:5). This remark raises some basic questions as to who makes up Canada's diverse populations. Who is genetically unique? How are understandings of these diverse and unique populations linked to wider discourses of diversity and difference in Canada?

A recent article on public health genomics in Canada answers some of these questions by drawing on census data to describe the population history and present make-up of Canada, including visible minorities, "whose rates are growing at a much faster rate than the total population" (Little et al. 2009:113), the current Quebec population, "who are descended from a homogenous sub-population of founders" Little (2009:113), and First Nations, Inuit, and Métis Peoples and new immigrant populations, "whose potential needs for genetic services require further consideration" (Little 2009:117).

Although Canada does not have an official public health genomics strategy, the political logics of multicultural classification are becoming an indelible feature undergirding discourses of public health and genomics in Canada. Drawing on these specific constructions and categories of the populations relevant to public health genomics, in what follows I examine how these classifications have become part of the everyday knowledge and understandings of who makes up Canada. I specifically examine the classification practices in the census that have emerged from the institutionalization of multiculturalism. After examining population classification in detail through the census, I will return at the end of the chapter to how these classifications are increasingly intersecting and informing the design and conduct of population genomics research for health in Canada.

From Monitoring Ethnic Stock to Framing Diversity as a Resource

The census is one of the most important means by which states statistically depict collective identities (Kertzer and Arel 2002:3). The practices of census-taking and the categorization of populations have been particularly important for scholars interested in the legitimating narratives of national, colonial, and "New World" states such as Canada. However, there is a need for further consideration of how particular legacies of classification and the standardization of differences in settler colonies have shaped contemporary politics in relation to biomedicine and health research as it is expressed in genomics research. Census categories are increasingly used in large-scale population genomics research for health as a basis for legitimate and publicly accepted taxonomies for medical or population projects (Epstein 2007; Smart et al. 2008).

The creation of federal Canada in 1867 brought about new attempts at classifying and categorizing populations, particularly in relation to categories of race and ethnicity (Hall 2006, 460). Though these categories have developed specifically within Canada, formulas of classification were heavily shaped by histories of empire. As a colony, Canada inherited systems of classification through a merging of European (natural) history and North American social science, particularly in regard to racial and ethnic categories as the way to count populations (Day 2000:116). Historians point out that, even though Canada's specific national characteristics of census design and analysis make it different from other nations, the development of the census was part of a wider transatlantic network of intellectuals, politicians, and state servants who, during the time of "New World" settlement, were attempting to standardize and manage an assortment of technologies, including languages, weights, and measures (Curtis 2001:18).

Like most countries, Canada "went statistical" between the late eighteenth and mid-nineteenth centuries (Curtis 2001:4–5). Canadian historians have explored how the census was a central mechanism for governmental authorities to monitor undesirable groups. For example, during the interwar period there was a high level of immigration into Canada by people from southern and eastern Europe. This pushed the limits of the liberal elite notion that Canada was mainly populated by people of English and French descent. The ethnic origins question on the census, which I referred to in the beginning of this chapter, was a key indicator to measure the degree to which non-English and non-French peoples were settling in Canada. The tracking of these "non English" and "non-French" populations, and the analysis of immigration statistics, were developed in part due to the influence exerted by those who supported eugenic policies (Beaud and Prevost 1996:1).[3]

The political logics of institutionalized multiculturalism, however, are based on a different approach to population monitoring. There is not an explicit rhetoric to monitor and classify undesirable populations, but precisely the opposite. Multiculturalism is narrated through the idea that different population groups add value to Canadian society. The Department of Heritage, responsible for administering multicultural programs and tracking the size and number of multicultural groups in conjunction with Statistics Canada, defines multiculturalism in the following way:

> Canadian multiculturalism is fundamental to our belief that all citizens are equal. Multiculturalism ensures that all citizens can keep their identities, can take pride in their ancestry, and have a sense of belonging. Acceptance gives Canadians a feeling of security and self-confidence, making them more open to, and accepting of, diverse cultures. The Canadian experience has shown that multiculturalism encourages racial and ethnic harmony and cross-cultural understanding, and discourages ghettoization, hatred, discrimination, and violence. (Dept of Heritage 2008)

Groups, as they are categorized through the logics of multicultural classification, need to be monitored in order to ensure they are being valued and included, not excluded. The Multiculturalism Act further extends these ideas, arguing that multiculturalism is part of Canadian identity and a resource for Canada's future: Multiculturalism "is a fundamental characteristic of Canadian heritage and identity and it provides an invaluable resource in the shaping of Canada's future."[4] In 1982, an official policy of multiculturalism was written into Canada's constitution, with an article in the Charter of Rights and Freedoms specifying that the Charter must be interpreted "in a manner consistent with the multicultural heritage of Canadians" (Art 27 of Charter of Rights and Freedom cited in Ley 2007:4). Which exactly are the groups that "count" toward multiculturalism? And what kinds of groups are seen as a diversity resource?

The Creation of "Visible Minority" Populations

The category *visible minority* is an example of the political logic of multicultural classification. In committing to the inclusion of "diverse groups," governmental agencies faced a dilemma: "how to effectively prevent discrimination without statistically distinguishing the people most likely to be discriminated against" (Kertzer and Arel 2002:13). The response to this dilemma was the creation of the distinctively Canadian category *visible minority*. The term is used in many domains of research and policy, and has a general currency in Canada (Kinsella 2007). It was established as part of the judicial lexicon when in 1986 the Canadian government passed the Employment Equity Act, which required federal employers to report annually on the make-up of their workforce in regard to the number of women, persons with disabilities, Aboriginal peoples, and visible minorities they employed. Visible minorities, it was argued, needed to be counted in order for employers to demonstrate that they were hiring diverse groups. In order to track the correlation between just how many visible minorities there were in Canada and how many were represented in the federal workforce, Statistics Canada added what it called "the visible minority group variable" to the census. Officially defined, the category *visible minority* applies "to persons who are identified according to the Employment Equity Act as being non-Caucasian in race or non-white in colour. Under the Act, Aboriginal persons are not considered to be members of visible minority groups" (Statistics Canada 2008a). Despite its good intentions, the invention of *visible minority* is an example of what Sara Ahmed calls "institutional whiteness," where persons visibly "non-white" become hyper-visible within organizations (Ahmed et al. 2006:8). The creation of the visible minority category does not just distinguish between white/Caucasian and non-white/non-Caucasian, but is explicit that Aboriginal persons in Canada are not considered visible minorities. This is not because government classification schemes approach "Aboriginal persons" as part of the invisible white majority. Rather, it is about counting certain kinds of people (this will be addressed in more detail shortly). People counted as "Aboriginal persons" by the Canadian state are not like any other persons who are counted. Canadians who may be classified as "visible minorities" have in principle, the same sets of rights as other Canadians. Those classified as "Aboriginal persons" fall under a different set of rights in the Canadian judicial, legal, and legislative system.

The person being counted as a visible minority requires a particular pheno-type that is visibly different than the imagined phenotype of "Caucasian" or "white in color." The category is firmly placed in what Linda Alcoff has called "the domain of the visible" (Alcoff 1999:10). The definition takes whiteness as a standard, with white people invisible and non-whites visible. It keeps intact a particular kind of normalcy about who is different, and who needs to be counted and monitored. It is one of the bluntest examples of institutionalized Canadian multiculturalism, which reinforces a normalizing center of whiteness by counting other groups as diversity resources which revolve around this centre (Dyer 1997; Frankenberg 1997).

What constitutes a classification as "white" or "Caucasian," however, can often be rearranged by adding or subtracting criteria. Melbourne Tapper refers to these adding and subtracting processes as "the floating lines of demarcation of the white body" (Tapper 1999:27). Whiteness, then, is notoriously shifty. Who is Caucasian and white enough to not be a visible minority? Assignments of whiteness are decided along a complex array of considerations. The quote below is from the reference guide which Statistics Canada publishes to explain how the visible minority population variable classifies. The guide highlights these classificatory mazes of whiteness, or "floating lines" as Tapper calls them. It would appear that any identification with Europeanness (through language, for example) works to whiten phenotypes:

> In accordance with employment equity definitions, persons who reported "Latin American" and "White," "Arab" and "White," or "West Asian" and "White" have been excluded from the visible minority population. Likewise, persons who reported "Latin American," "Arab" or "West Asian" and who provided a European write-in response such as "French" have been excluded from the visible minority population as well. These persons are included in the "Not a visible minority" category. However, persons who reported "Latin American," "Arab" or "West Asian" and a non-European write-in response are included in the visible minority population. For example, respondents who checked "Latin American" and wrote in "Peruvian" are included in the "Latin American" count. Respondents who reported "Arab" and wrote in "Lebanese" are included in the "Arab" count. Respondents who reported "West Asian" and wrote in "Afghan" were included in the "West Asian" count. (Statistics Canada 2008a)

This quotation is emblematic of the classification practices of the nation-state in all their specificity—someone, or more likely a group of people, had to spend time in meetings sorting out that "Arabs" who reported themselves as French were more likely to be "Caucasian" and "white in colour" than "Arabs" who spoke Lebanese. One can only imagine the type of phenotype-debating that ensues from what constitutes (in)visibility in the micro-decisions of who is and is not a visible minority. The multicultural logic of the visible minority population classification mirrors "classical" models of racial classification based on skin color, despite the abandonment of the term *race* in the Canadian census. These classical or traditional ideas of race as tied to phenotype (skin color most specifically) are deeply entrenched in understandings of continental differences and distances between groups. The classification of visible minority is, as Alcoff argues, similar to the category race, emphasizing distance, with little regard to spatial proximity (Alcoff 1999:386).

Calculations of Canada's visible minority population play a major role in determining who is making up Canada, who is (and is not) Canadian, and who can lay claim to this identity in terms of citizenship and belonging. Statistics Canada has projected that by 2031, one in three Canadians will be a visible minority (Statistics Canada 2010). This made headlines in many Canadian newspapers: "'Visible Minority' Will Mean 'White' by 2031" (Javed 2010); "The Changing Face of

Canada: Booming Minority Populations by 2031" (Friesen 2010); and "Has the Term Visible Minority Become Totally Obsolete?" (Todd 2010). Tensions and anxieties about just who is making up Canada are reflected in these newspaper headlines. These anxieties about the cultural composition of Canada are also attached to larger discourses of ancestry and belonging. For example, in her discussion of lay or popular understandings of genealogy, genetics, and identity, Catherine Nash explains how some of her research respondents, who were Canadian, sought to trace and track their Irish identity as a result increasing numbers of non-white immigrants living in Canada (Nash 2008:50).

In 2007, the United Nations Committee on the Elimination of Racial Discrimination told Canadian government representatives that the use of the term *visible minority* to identify people it considers susceptible to racial discrimination was potentially "racist" and may contravene the international treaty aimed at combating racism, which Canada has signed (Edwards 2007). Specifically, the report stated: "The Committee notes that the term [*visible minority*] is widely used in official documents of the State party, including the census. The Committee is concerned that the use of the term visible minorities may not be in accordance with the aims and objectives of the Convention (art. 1)" (CERD 2007a:3).

The committee then urged the Canadian government to "reflect" on the use of the term. A report from the meeting between the U.N. Committee and the Canadian representatives is particularity instructive about the deep binds which institutionalized forms of classification pose for those who are accountable for the counting practices within nation-states. The Canadian representatives argued that the U.N. Committee had "misunderstood" the use of the term *visible minority* (CERD 2007b). The term *visible minority*, they argued, was specific to the Employment Equity Act and "is part of a particular program relating to employment only" (2007b:4). Like most masterful bureaucratic-speak, this is both true and not true. The term was created specifically under an act of legislation addressing employment. However, like many classification systems meant to address one specific sphere, it has bled out slowly into other domains preoccupied with counting forms of difference. After all, in their own reference guide on the term, Statistics Canada explicitly states that the data generated by the *visible minority* variable is used not only by governments, but also by community groups, healthcare providers and businesses (Statistics Canada 2008a). There are, however, two "non-visible minority" categories, according to the logics of multicultural classification in Canada: white/Caucasian and Aboriginal persons. If those categorized as Aboriginal persons are not visible minorities, how have they been brought into the multicultural logics of population classification?

"How Statistics Canada Identifies Aboriginal Peoples"

"How Statistics Canada Identifies Aboriginal Peoples" is the title of an eighteen-page document published by Statistics Canada that sets out exactly what the title says (Statistics Canada 2007). There is no other published report that explains how a particular group in Canada is identified (though there are shorter reference guides on all population variables used by Statistics Canada). The need for this guide is a testament to some of the most complex forms of population classification embedded in multiple systems of colonial administration. The report explains that, over time, Statistics Canada has collected data on Aboriginal peoples differently. Currently, however, information on Aboriginal people is collected in keeping with the constitutional definition: Aboriginal peoples of Canada include Indian, Inuit, and Métis people of Canada. In this regard, the report further explains that the census collects a variety of information on Aboriginal populations relating to the constitutional definition, including North American Indian, Inuit, Métis, Registered, and non-Registered Indians, and members of an Indian Band or First Nation. Statistics Canada explains:

> There is no single or "correct" definition of Aboriginal populations. The choice of a definition depends on the purpose for which the information is to be used. Different definitions are used depending on the focus and requirements of the user. Each question will yield Aboriginal populations with different counts and characteristics. (Statistics Canada 2007:7)

There is thus a significant number of subcategories within this classification system. Consequently, there is also more than one question on the census used to identify Aboriginal peoples. There are four questions: ethnic origin (including Aboriginal ancestries); Aboriginal identity; Registered or Treaty Indian; and member of an Indian Band or First Nation (Statistics Canada 2007:7). The question on Aboriginal identity offers three main choices for identification. These are North American Indian, Métis, and Inuit, as per the constitutional definition: Innu (northern Canada), Métis (a "mix" of French and Aboriginal), and First Nations. First Nations are under a separate set of legal structures called the Indian Act. The Indian Act is Canada's oldest piece of legislation that governs over Indian reserves and sets out who is and is not an "Indian," along with what rights and legal provisions this entails.

The governmental counting and administration of "Aboriginal persons" in multiple forms are key dimensions of the multicultural logics of classification. Through regulatory systems such as Canada's Indian Act, if one is a "registered Indian" or "status Indian," one is accorded very different rights and resources than those deemed "non-status Indians." Until 1983, under the Indian Act, an Indian woman marrying a white man was dispossessed of her Indian status under the Act (as were her children); however, if a white woman married an Indian man, she gained state-recognized Indian status, and the rights and resources that went with that. Despite the fact that these divisions and regulations were imposed and created in an artificial manner, these markers of identity and citizenship have become very real in experiences of nativeness (Lawrence 2003, 12). Moreover, these administrative distinctions in the census between status and non-status

Indians, as well as among Indian, Métis, and Inuit have exerted an enormous impact on the ways groups are governed, and on how individuals identify themselves as members of a community.

From Nation to Population

The census does not just capture and classify through already-created governmental categories, but also produces populations to whom funding, recognition and status can be claimed. In the five years between 1996 and 2001, Canada's Métis population increased over 43 percent, from 204,000 to 292,000 (Anderson 2008:347). This almost 50 percent rise in the Métis population was not attributed by Statistics Canada to high birth rates, but rather to the fact that more people were identifying themselves as Métis in surveys such as the census (Anonymous 2008). In response to the dramatic rise, Métis organizations argued that people were now more comfortable identifying with and claiming Aboriginal ancestry. Commenting on the sharp rise, the vice president of the Métis Nation of Alberta stated: "I hope the government will sit up and take notice and see that our people are not someone to ignore" (Trevor Gladue quoted in Anonymous 2008).

Métis struggles for recognition from the government of Canada (or the Crown, as it is called in Canadian debates) reach back to the 1869 Red River Resistance and the famous campaigner for Métis rights and land, Louis Riel, who was hanged for treason. The Métis National Council in Canada describes the formation of the Métis nation as a merging of two distinct groups to form a new nation of Aboriginal people:

> Prior to Canada's crystallization as a nation in west central North America, the Métis people emerged out of the relations of Indian women and European men. While the initial offspring of these Indian and European unions were individuals who possessed mixed ancestry, the gradual establishment of distinct Métis communities, outside of Indian and European cultures and settlements, as well as, the subsequent intermarriages between Métis women and Métis men, resulted in the genesis of a new Aboriginal people—the Métis. (Metis National Council 2010)

In this regard, mixedness has been a central differentiating factor in the governmental categorization of Métis people. It is this mixedness that marks Métis identity as distinct from other Aboriginal peoples in governmental classificatory systems. For example, persons classified as "Indians" under the Indian Act were wards of the state, could not own property, and were required to live in Indian reserves, whereas Métis peoples were classified as full citizens under the law (Anderson 2008:357). In contrast to its treatment of Indians, whose movements, cultural practices and identity were heavily regulated under the Indian Act, the federal government dealt with Métis people largely by ignoring them. This argument was used by Métis lawyers in a recent landmark case where the Supreme

Court of Canada ruled that Métis people were an Aboriginal group with a right to hunt and pursue their historical practices (*R. v Powley* 2003). Lawyers representing Métis groups in the case argued that the Métis were strict in assessing who qualifies to be a member of their community—and that, had successive governments not virtually willed them out of existence, Métis genealogical records would be just as complete as those of Indian bands (Makin 2003).

However, the explosion of growth of the Métis population documented in the 2001 census has been met with skepticism by some Aboriginal scholars in Canada. Chris Anderson argues that while this increase in numbers can further political recognition and economic investments in Métis organizations and specific social programs, it does so by constructing Métis people as a distinct population in Canada (Anderson 2008). The census thus works to turn a historic national identity (being Métis) into a racialized population through multicultural classification. According to Anderson, not everyone who has Aboriginal and European ancestry is Métis. If that would be the case, almost everyone in Canada would be Métis. Métis identity, he argues, should rather be based on a connection to the historic homeland of Métis people in Western Canada, and census questions should potentially be altered to include a national identification with being Métis, as opposed to the more ambiguous framings of ethnicity or ancestry (Anderson 2008:362).

In making his argument, Anderson identifies one of the central tensions in Canada's classification systems—that it renders Aboriginal peoples as belonging to racial, ethnic, or cultural groups, rather than as members of sovereign indigenous nations with inherent rights to territory and place. The most pressing and significant political issues relating to genomics research in settler societies such as Canada revolve around questions of nationalism, sovereignty, and rights with regard to the indigenous peoples who live in Canada. Historically, however, the recognition of the distinct status of Aboriginal peoples at national levels has led to inscribing social inferiority and biological pathology onto the bodies and communities of First Nations, Métis, and Inuit people (Kunitz 1994; Kelm 1998; Smith 2005; Anderson 2006). However, in 2007 new national guidelines on conducting biomedical and genetic research in collaboration with Aboriginal peoples have been issued in Canada for any researcher who receives federal funding from research councils.

Some of the guidelines, such as those created in 2007 by the Canadian Institutes of Health Research, set out the distinct status of DNA samples derived from Aboriginal peoples in Canada, which should be considered "on loan" to the researcher. Through concepts such as "DNA on loan" the guidelines seek to "promote culturally competent research" and "enable health research in keeping with Aboriginal values and traditions" (CIHR 2007). Though there is not room in this chapter to discuss these guidelines in detail, it is important to note that, while the guidelines are a significant achievement for the governance of genomics by Aboriginal peoples in Canada, concepts such as "DNA on loan" may present

serious conflicts with the realities of large-scale human health genomics and its
practices of data-sharing.

Molecular Multiculturalisms

We might approach the above examples through the idea of emergent *molecular
multiculturalisms*, which incorporates the political logics of institutionalized multiculturalism as part of legitimizing and framing human genomics research and its
promises for biomedicine. The political logics of institutionalized multiculturalism are based on the notion that differences need to be counted, because certain
differences matter in society, and that, in order to be responsive to these differences, one needs to monitor them. For example, these logics underpinned the
creation of the *visible minority* category in federal legislation. In turn, these logics
are translated into bureaucratic practices of inclusion and ethical conduct, where
demonstrating a high number of visible minority employees means that employers are being accountable, inclusive, and fair. As human genomics research
becomes increasingly associated with public health discourses, scientists, project
designers, and sponsoring institutions face similar requirements. In relation to
the emergence of public health genomics in Canada, policy-makers, funders,
ethicists, and scientific researchers conducting large-scale population genomics
on human health are increasingly brought under the kinds monitoring, measuring, and reporting that require the use of forms of multicultural political classification. In seeking public legitimacy, then, population genomics projects often
draw on already constructed categories offered through official channels, such as
Canada's census.

As with the classificatory logics and rhetorics of inclusion in Canadian
multiculturalism, contemporary large-scale population genomics research is not
unreflective of or unresponsive to concerns about the stigmatization and discrimination of groups. Rather, these concerns are consciously and deliberately coun-
tered through a range of inclusionary techniques: incorporating vulnerable
groups or stakeholders, public dialogue and engagement, as well as community
and group consultation strategies. As Jennifer Reardon notes, "these days, many in
the arena of human genomic variation research require little convincing that the
ideas and practices of this domain of research raise complex and vexed questions
about how to order and value human beings in society" (Reardon 2007:239). In a
social and political context such as Canada, where diversity is rendered a strategic
resource, it is no surprise that large-scale public projects incorporate forms of
multicultural inclusion as a way of gaining public legitimacy. After all, the recent
successes and failures of large-scale population genomics projects (such as the
Human Genome Diversity project) demonstrate that these projects require, not
only funds, but also, to some extent, public faith and conviction.

The incorporation of census classification is increasingly common in the
design, conduct and regulation of human genomics research. An example of this

can be found in an article recently published in the journal *Public Understanding of Science*. Entitled "Ethnocultural Community Leaders' Views and Perceptions on Biobanks and Population Specific Genomic Research: A Qualitative Study," the article argues that ethnocultural community members in Canada are both sponsors and beneficiaries of biobanks, and that, therefore, their views and perceptions should be included (Godard et al. 2009). Noting the substantial investments Canada is making in population-based biobanks, and that the success of biobanks relies on "community support and participation," the article draws on interviews with "ethnocultural community leaders" about their perspectives on population research (Godard et al. 2009:1). The identification of the groups who made up "ethnocultural communities" included individuals who self-identified "with one of nine census populations in the greater Montreal area: Aboriginal, Chinese, Greek, Haitian, Hispanic-Canadian, Indo-Pakistani, Italian, Jewish, and Moroccan" (Godard et al. 2009:3).

In their section on methods and study design, the authors explain that "the section of the study sample, which reflects some of the racial categories often used in biomedical research, has been done according to the ethnocultural portrait from the 2001 census by Statistics Canada" (Godard et al. 2009:3). This research explicitly uses Canadian census data as a kind of taxonomy of difference relevant to population genomics research. It is true that sometimes genetically different or distinct populations do correlate to social groupings, but this correlation cannot be assumed in the case of ethnocultural communities, as it easily presents culturally identified groups as biomedically significant. It is interesting that one Canadian subgroup known to express numerous rare genetic illnesses, that of some French Canadian families (see Kohli-Laven, chapter 11 in this volume), is not included. French Canadians are also the largest population group in Montreal, according to the census. Framing the research through "ethnocultural communities" keeps the political logics of multiculturalism intact by viewing culture and ethnicity as something that "other" groups have and that needs to be brought into the design and conduct of biobanks, not only for ethical reasons, but also for reasons of biomedical significance.

However, the ethical and political stakes of emergent molecular multiculturalisms are often framed as contests to avoid. The report on public health genomics from the expert workshop held in Bellagio, discussed at the beginning of this chapter, exemplifies this kind of approach: "A potential problem with 'genomics' is that it is a term not well recognised or understood by non-scientists, but this might paradoxically be an advantage, as it is unencumbered by negative historical connotations and may enable a fresh start in dialogue with the public" (Report: Genome-based research and population health 2005:6). This chapter argues precisely the opposite. Genomics should not be unencumbered by the history of population classification (and its negative historical connotations), because it continues to draw on these already constructed groups.

The increasing emphasis on knowledge integration between disciplines in genomics, as well as the way specific social categories come to be aligned in genomic practice, requires critical attention. This is especially the case as health risks and disease susceptibilities are increasingly formulated through links to categories of continental ancestry and cultural and ethnic background, all of which are central to the politics of multicultural classification. Particular forms of population politics, such as those of the national census, have been central in tying the formation of subjects who can act and participate in society to institutionalized forms of control, subjection, and classification in liberal democracies. Jennifer Reardon notes that large-scale human genomics research has the potential to transform the very concepts upon which western liberal democratic thinking is founded: "individuals, communities, people, participation and inclusion" (Reardon 2007:241). As a result, it is no longer possible to turn to practices of group inclusion as if they existed in a separate domain from scientific research. Given this, Reardon (2007), along with other scholars of biomedicine, such as Steven Epstein (2007) argue that we need to engage in the more subdued task of analyzing how inclusion happens, what logics underlie it, and what practices it makes up. This chapter has contributed to this task by examining the national and institutional aspects of Canada's multicultural policy; how bodies are counted up, what value they are attributed, and what resources they are seen to add toward under the auspices of genomics and health.

Conclusion

The solution to the dilemmas raised by the unsettled histories of group classification and their increasing entanglement with the futures of genomic medicine is not to stop using categories of difference. This is as unrealistic as it is misguided. As Troy Duster has argued in relation to the United States: "To throw out the concept of race is to take the official approach to race and ethnicity pioneered and celebrated by the French government: 'We do not collect data on that topic. Therefore, it does not exist!'" (Duster quoted in Epstein 2007:301). Canada sought to counter the problem of difference by multiplying categories on which differences between groups and people could be made. It is thus not a solution to argue that governmental and non-governmental bodies should stop using or collecting data on census categories, or on other forms of segmented identities examined in this chapter. For example, it would be difficult to measure any reduction in health disparities without monitoring and recording the health of various populations, and that means continuing to make use of categories by which inequality is made meaningful in a given society (Epstein 2007:301). Moreover, population statistics can be vital for the political mobilization of certain groups. In Canada for example, First Nations require better and more comprehensive access to data that is collected on their own populations, which is, all too often, only held by federal or provincial authorities (First Nations Health Council 2010). Given these concerns, this chapter has not set out to develop a scheme for proper or ethical use of group categories. Rather it has sought to contribute to developing a different kind of approach, one that takes aim at the multiple registers, such as the census, where differences between groups are operationalized and brought into meaning and relevance.

Human genomics research has taken on a new urgency and force in public discussion, because of its promises for unlocking the biological basis of illness and disease. This chapter detailed how Canada contends with the legacy and continuing aspects of its colonial histories as a condition of its transition to a postcolonial or multicultural society where governing is increasingly becoming linked to the life sciences. The systems of population classification and political logics of categorization in Canada may have impacts not only, at the level of recruitment, on clinical and genetic studies, but they may also have an impact on who gets to count as a legitimate group in the design, conduct, and regulation of population genomics research. As groups are incorporated into the logics of multicultural classification, they become readily available to policy-makers and researchers in many domains, including those involved the governance of human genomics research for health. These processes of inclusion are not a one-way street, but rather involve complex relationships between governmental agencies and the self-naming practices of groups themselves. The logics of multicultural classification explored in detail (specifically the categories *visible minority* and *Aboriginal persons*) offer a glimpse into how human groups are made up in order to be included. Consequently, it is these systems of classification and of counting up different kinds of bodies, which act as broader indicators of who counts and what differences matter in processes of inclusion.

The increasing intersections between genomics and biomedical research have revitalized particular histories of human difference, ancestry, and origin, as well as contemporary articulations of the settler, native, national, and multicultural subject in Canada. Considering the futures of genomics research thus requires excavating histories of populations in the New World, along with contemporary political logics of institutionalized multiculturalism, in order to consider the criteria by which progress in human health genomics research is assessed.

NOTES

1. The Canadian Constitution uses the term Aboriginal to refer to three groups of indigenous peoples in Canada, Innu (northern Canada), Métis (French and Aboriginal), and First Nations (who are under a separate set of legal structures, called the Indian Act). These broad terms, along with the term Aboriginal, do little to capture the geopolitical differences between the people(s) who have been grouped within Canada's borders and who identify with the terms Indigenous or Aboriginal. The employment and use of these terms are reflections of political contexts, aims, and positions, as well as complex historical intersections of colonial law, national sovereignty, and identity, which there is not space to address adequately in this chapter.

2. Genome Canada is Canada's main genomics research funding body. For a brief review of the emergence of Genome Canada and its funding priorities, including the biobank, CARTaGENE, see Hinterberger 2010. For further specific discussions of the biobank CARTaGENE see Bibeau 2004; Pallson 2007; Lock 2010.

3. The Canadian eugenics movement gained support in the early twentieth century. Both the provinces of Alberta and British Columbia had Sexual Sterilisation Acts in the 1920s and 1930s, which provided for the sterilization of "mentally deficient" or "feeble minded" individuals. For a history of eugenics in Canada that explains the widespread use of eugenic ideas across governmental and health agencies in Canada, see McLaren 1990 and Grekul, Krahn et al. 2004.

4. *Canadian Multiculturalism Act* (section 3b) R.S., 1985, c. 24, 4th Supp.

WORKS CITED

Ahmed, S., S. Hunter, S. Kilic, et al. 2006. *Final report: Race, diversity and leadership in the learning and skills sector.* www.gold.ac.uk/media/finaldiversityreport.pdf [Accessed June, 2010].

Alcoff, L. 1999. Towards a phenomenology of racial embodiment. *Radical Philosophy* 95:8–14.

Anderson, W. 2006. States of hygiene: Race, "improvement" and biomedical citizenship in Australia and the colonial Philippines. In *Haunted by empire: Geographies of intimacy in North American history*, edited by A. L. Stoler. Durham, NC: Duke University Press.

Anderson, C. 2008. From nation to population: The racialisation of "Metis" in the Canadian census. *Nations and Nationalism* 14(2):347–386.

Anonymous 2008. Métis pride grows with population. *Edmonton Journal.* Edmonton, Canwest. www.canada.com/edmontonjournal/news/story.html?id=64a68347–7fd9–4220-b677–834cad6248bb

Avard, D., L. M. Bacci, M. M. Burgess et al. 2009. Public health genomics (PHG) and public participation: Points to consider. *Journal of Public Deliberation* 5(1):1–21.

Beaud, J.-P., and J.-G. Prevost. 1996. Immigration, statistics and eugenics: Measuring racial origins in Canada. *Canadian Ethnic Studies* 28(2):1–24.

Bibeau, G. 2004. *Le Quebec transgenique: Science, marche, humanité.* Montreal: Boreal Presse.

Boyd, M., G. Goldman, and P. White. 2000. Race in the Canadian census. In *race and racism: Canada's challenge*, edited by L. E. Driedger and S.S.E. Halli. Montreal: McGill-Queen's University Press.

Burke, W., M. Khoury, A. Stewart, et al. 2006. The path from genome-based research to population health: Development of an international public health genomics network. *Genetics in Medicine* 8:451–458.

CERD 2007a. Consideration of reports submitted by state parties under Article 9 of the Convention: *Concluding observations of the Committee on the Elimination of Racial Discrimination (CERD).* Seventieth Session, United Nations.

———. 2007b. Committee on Elimination of Racial Discrimination (CERD) Considers Report of Canada. *The United Nations.* www.galdu.org/web/index.php?odas=1876&giella1=eng [Accessed June 7, 2010].

Canadian Institute of Healkth Research. 2001. Report from Proceedings. *Canadian Institutes of Health Research, Human Population Genetics/Genomics Workshop.* Aylmer, Québec.

———. 2004. Strategic Plan 2004–2009. *Institute of Genetics.* Ottawa, Government of Canada.

———. 2007. CIHR Guidelines for Health Research Involving Aboriginal People. *Canadian Institutes for Health Research.* www.cihr-irsc.gc.ca/e/29134.html [Accessed October 10, 2008].

Curtis, B. 2001. *The politics of population: State formation, statistics and the census of Canada, 1840–1875.* Toronto: University of Toronto Press.

Day, R.J.F. 2000. *Multiculturalism and the history of Canadian diversity.* Toronto: University of Toronto Press.

Department of Heritage. 2008. What is Canadian multiculturalism? *Department of Heritage, Government of Canada.* [Accessed September 8, 2008].

Dyer, R. 1997. *White.* London and New York: Routledge.

Edwards, S. 2007. UN calls Canada racist for "visible minorities" tag. *CanWest News Service,* CanWest News Service.

Epstein, S. 2006. Institutionalizing the new politics of difference in U.S. biomedical research: Thinking across the science/state/society divides. In *The new political sociology of science,* edited by S. Frickel and K. Moore. Madison: University of Wisconsin Press.

——. 2007. *Inclusion: The politics of difference in medical research.* Chicago: University of Chicago Press.

Frankenberg, R. 1997. *Displacing whiteness: Essays in social and cultural criticism.* Durham, NC: Duke University Press.

Friesen, J. 2010. The changing face of canada: Booming minority populations by 2031. *Globe and Mail.* Toronto, CTV Publishing Inc.

Godard, B., V. Ozdemir, M. Fortin, et al. 2009. Ethnocultural community leaders' views and perceptions on biobanks and population-specific Genomic research: A qualitative research study. *Public Understanding of Science.* Online First, published on June 12, 2009: doi:10.1177/0963662509104721

Goldscheider, C. 2002. Ethnic categorization in censuses: Comparative observations from Israel, Canada, and the United States. In *Census and identity: The politics of race, ethnicity, and language in national censuses,* edited by D. I. Kertzer and D. Arel. Cambridge: Cambridge University Press.

Greco, M. 2004. The politics of indeterminacy and the right to health. *Theory, Culture and Society* 21(6):1–22.

Grekul, J., A. Krahn and D. Odynak. 2004. Sterilizing the "feeble-minded": eugenics in Alberta, Canada, 1929–1972. *Journal of Historical Sociology* 17(4):358–384.

Hall, C. 2006. Commentary. *Haunted by empire: Geographies of intimacy in North American history,* edited by A. L. Stoler. Durham, NC: Duke University Press.

Hinterberger, A. 2010. The genomics of difference and the politics of race in Canada. In *What's the use of race: Modern governance and the biology of difference,* edited by I. Whitmarsh and D. Jones. Cambridge, MA: MIT Press.

Javed, N. 2010. "Visible minority" will mean "white" by 2031. *Toronto Star.* Toronto, Toronto Star Newspapers Ltd.

Kelm, M.-E. 1998. *Colonizing bodies: Aboriginal health and healing in British Columbia, 1900–50.* Vancouver: UBC Press.

Kertzer, D. I., and D. Arel. 2002. *Census and identity: The politics of race, ethnicity, and language in national censuses.* Cambridge: Cambridge University Press.

Khoury, M. J., W. Burke, E. Thompson et al. 2000. *Genetics and public health in the 21st century: Using genetic information to improve health and prevent disease.* Oxford: Oxford University Press.

Kinsella, N. A. 2007. Sober second thought: The United Nations and the phrase "visible minority. GLOBUS Conference June 8, 2007. www.sen.parl.gc.ca/nkinsella/PDF/Speeches/SoberSecondThought-e.pdf {Accessed July 5, 2008].

Kunitz, S. J. 1994. *Disease and social diversity: The European impact on the health of non-Europeans.* Oxford: Oxford University Press.

Lawrence, B. 2003. Gender, race and the regulation of native identity in Canada and the United States: An overview. *Hypatia* 18(2):3–31.

Ley, D. 2007. Multiculturalism: A Canadian defence. *Working Paper: No. 07–04 Research on Immigration and Integration in the Metropolis.* Vancouver, B.C.

Little, J., B. Potter, J. Allanson et al. 2009. Canada: Public health genomics. *Public Health Genomics* 12(2):112–120.

Lock, M. M., and V.-K. Nguyen. 2010. *An anthropology of biomedicine*. Oxford: Wiley-Blackwell.

McLaren, A. 1990. *Our own master race: Eugenics in Canada 1885–1945*. Toronto and Oxford: Oxford University Press.

Makin, K. 2003. Métis win Supreme Court recognition. *Globe and Mail*. Toronto.

Metis National Council. 2010. Who are the Metis? www.metisnation.ca/who/index.html [Accessed June 6, 2010].

Nash, C. 2005. Geographies of relatedness. *Transactions of the Institute of British Geographers* 30(4):449–462.

Pallsson, G. 2007. *Anthropology and the new genetics*. Cambridge: Cambridge University Press.

Reardon, J. 2007. Democratic mis-haps: The problem of democratization in a time of bio-politics. *BioSocieties* 2:239–256.

Report: Genome-based research and population health. (2005, 14–20 April 2005). Report of an expert workshop held at the Rockefeller Foundation Study and Conference Centre. dceg.cancer.gov/files/genomicscourse/bellagio-011807.pdf [Accessed June 10, 2010].

Ruppert, E. S. 2007. Producing population. *Centre for Research on Socio-Cultural Change (CRESC) Working Papers* (Open University: Working Paper No. 37): 1–13.

R. v. Powley, 2003. 2 S.C.R. 207, 2003 Supreme Court of Canada 43.

Segiun, B., B.-J. Hardy, P. A. Singer, et al. 2008. Human genomic variation initiatives in emerging economies and developing countries. *Nature Reviews (Genetics)*:s3–s4.

Smart, A., R. Tutton, P. Martin et al. 2008. The standardization of race and ethnicity in biomedical science: Editorials and U.K biobanks. *Social Science of Medicine* 38(3):407–423.

Smith, A. 2005. *Conquest: Sexual violence and American Indian genocide*. Cambridge, MA: South End Press.

Statistics Canada 1995. *75 Years and counting: A history of Statistics Canada*. Ottawa: Government of Canada.

———. 2007. How Statistics Canada identifies aboriginal peoples. *Government of Canada, Catalogue no. 12–592-XIE*. Ottawa.

———. 2008a. Visible minority population and population group reference guide, 2006 census. *Statistics Canada* www12.statcan.ca/english/census06/reference/reportsandguides/visible-minorities.cfm [Accessed June 7, 2008].

———. 2008b. 2006 Census: Ethnic origin, visible minorities, place of work and mode of transportation. *The Daily* www.statcan.ca/Daily/English/080402/d080402a.htm [Accessed November 10 2008].

———. 2008c. Canada's ethnocultural mosaic, 2006 Census: Canada's major census metropolitan areas. *Government of Canada*. www12.statcan.ca/english/census06/analysis/ethnicorigin/montreal.cfm [Accessed April 14, 2009].

———. 2010. Canada's ethnocultural portrait: The changing mosaic. www12.statcan.ca/english/census01/products/analytic/companion/etoimm/canada.cfm [Accessed June 6, 2010].

Tapper, M. 1999. *In the blood: Sickle cell anemia and the politics of race*. Philadelphia: University of Pennsylvania Press.

Todd, D. 2010. Has the term visible minority become totally obsolete? *Vancouver Sun*. Vancouver, CanWest.

13

"It's a Living History, Told by the Real Survivors of the Times—DNA"

Anthropological Genetics in the Tradition of
Biology as Applied History

MARIANNE SOMMER

The term *applied history* refers to genres of history that are located outside academic institutions and that are intended for a larger public and oriented toward markets and entertainment. But *applied* may also refer to the attempt of meeting the intellectual and practical needs of a society. Applied history encompasses a mixture of history for the people, history about people, and history by the people. Examples are historical novels and mythos-films, TV-documentaries and (picture) books about history, historical exhibitions, memorials, historical festivals and enactments, history parks, historical PC-games, and history marketing. An expert use of old and new media is central for an applied history that is often characterized by its multimedia properties, not least because media such as the internet allow for new forms of interactive history.[1]

The current apex in historical interest and in media and esthetic realizations from the cultural heritage may be seen as related to processes of globalization, such as the dissolution of traditional nation states, the increase in mobility and connectedness of people, and the perceived acceleration of social and technological change that necessitates a constant reevaluation of the past. These processes foster fragmentation and disorientation with regard to origins, identity, and belonging. In contrast, the appropriation of knowledge about history is considered formative of identity and meaning, legitimating and orienting the subject within societal structures.[2] A market-led kind of history cultivates this niche and incites concerns within academic circles about the ethical and qualitative standards, as well as about the legitimacy of the discipline.[3]

In this chapter I bring into focus an aspect that has escaped the cultural-studies lenses through which the history boom is analyzed: the applications of a biologically founded and scientifically reconstructed history. Geneticists of the twenty-first century are successfully challenging the historian's position as provider of identity-forming origin narratives. If applied history is characterized by its instrumentalization of age-old human needs that have become accentuated through recent developments, then the life sciences are particularly apt in this "business." They claim access to the fundamental truth about who we are, where we come from, and who we might become. Genetics in particular offers unambiguous answers and objective knowledge with regard to basic human concerns. It promises future possibilities of intervention in the areas of beauty, health, and life itself. But there is also a retrospective promise in the technologies of genomics. Human population genetics (anthropological genetics, genetic/molecular anthropology— these terms are insufficiently differentiated) reconstructs the histories of clans, tribes, populations, ethnicities, races, nations, and humankind. Its commercialization in the genetic ancestry tracing business has brought about what has been called a revolution in identity through its sexy and seductive technologies.[4]

There are many ethical and political issues associated with projects and applications in human population genetics from questions regarding research agendas, sampling strategies, and consent, to concerns about biocolonialism and a genetic determinism related to neo-nationalism and neo-racism. These have been at the center of most studies so far and will be touched on in this paper where relevant for an understanding of the claim for a genetic reconstruction of history.

For this claim the conceptions of the human gene pool as world heritage and of the gene as historical document seem important, and I set out with a short discussion of these within the context of the history of molecular anthropology and human population genetics. The concepts have been relevant in the positioning of the new molecular methods vis-à-vis other—humanistic and natural scientific— approaches to historical reconstruction. In the second part of the paper, I engage in more detail with the question of what kind of history we are confronted with. I argue that the practices and discourses of current projects and commercialization of human population genetics are best characterized as applied history, that is, what I call *applied genetic history*. Both are marked by novel kinds of mediazation, commercialization, and personalization of historical knowledge as products. Using the example of the English geneticist Bryan Sykes, I analyze how applied genetic history works, what its particularities and problems in the sense of history writing are, and how the identities of scientists and customers may be reconfigured in its generation.

Applied genetic history is not an entirely new phenomenon. Human, racial, and national histories have been approached through the study of exterior bodily characteristics, bones, and molecules before, and they might have been applied in the above sense. I therefore set out with an example to probe this point. The choice of H. G. Wells as an entry into the topic also makes clear that there are several possible historical trajectories of *applied biological history*, because towards the end of the paper, an alternative tradition that goes back to racial anthropology will suggest itself. With the example of Wells in the early twentieth century, I argue that the genealogies of applied humanistic and natural scientific history are part of larger developments within the historical discipline and the (perceived) public demand for history for Mr. Everyman. The roots of the above mentioned history boom can be traced further back than the 1970s, and it has been related to progress in media technologies, to the expansion of general education, and to particular historical experiences.

Applied History on a Biological Basis: An Entry

In the preface to *The Outline of History* of 1931, H. G. Wells laments that academic history has left the ordinary citizen alone with his everyday problems. While the discipline was producing detailed scholarly studies, the dramatic rupture caused by the First World War made a history accessible to the layman more pressing than ever. Wells meant to fill this blank with *The Outline of History*—a project he began in 1918. The synthesis of the adventure of human history was aimed at rendering obvious to his readers the urgency of human solidarity and at opening up the hopeful perspective of a federal world-state. In writing a history addressed at laymen, Wells considered his distance from the history guild an advantage: As a popular writer he was close to the needs of Mr. Everyman.[5]

One may expect that Wells's polemics met with antagonism from historians of his times. And such there was. But Wells's statement in favor of a history for everyday life preached to the converted in the case of those inspired by the new history, as coined by the American historian James Harvey Robinson.[6] Wells's *The Outline of History* was reviewed approvingly by Robinson and his student Carl Becker, generally considered one of the founders of American *public history*. Similarly to Wells, Robinson and Becker saw the task of history in the production of applicable explanations of the present and in the orientation toward a particular future: "It may be that Mr. Wells has read the past too close to the desire of his heart. But there are worse things. We may hope at least that the future will be as he thinks. If it should turn out so, Mr. Wells's book will have been more than a history, even if it is not history; it will have been an action that has helped to make history."[7]

Although Becker did not grant Wells's master narrative the status of historical scholarship, for the new and public historian, the end justified the means: Applied history as Becker understood it—and as I will use the term—does not only aim at the writing of history, it aims at the making of history. In line with Robinson's ideas of two decades earlier, in 1931 Becker defined the living history he wanted to create as memory in the wider sense of an interpenetration of the experienced with the mediated past: "History is the artificial extension of the social memory."[8] Appropriated by Mr. Everyman, it shapes his self-perception and his actions in the world.

But of what kind is the living history that Wells regarded of such great use to the common man but was no longer provided by the disciplined historian? In this context, it seems relevant that Wells had studied biology at today's Imperial College in London under T. H. Huxley and made his bachelor in zoology in 1890. This seems to

have influenced his view that an understanding of the present presupposes knowledge of the history of humankind in the sense of the history of life on earth per se.

The beginnings of mankind were still perceptible in modern human life, its
political, religious, and social aspects. Wells, who subtitled the work *Being a Plain
History of Life and Mankind*, even ventured as far as to attribute second rank to the
reconstruction of history on the basis of written sources. Those "documents" that
the geologist, paleontologist, embryologist, and natural historian contributed to
the project of a world history were ontologically superior: "The bookish historian
now accepts, reluctantly and ungraciously enough, his place as a mere contributor
of doubtful documents to the broad ensemble."[9]

Thus, in *The Outline of History* Wells leads his readers through millions of years
into their specific present. He was well aware that everyone already has his private
outline of history, and that the one offered by an author would be examined for
agreement and differences. In fact, Wells interacted with his academic and non-
academic readers in the production of *The Outline* when he took their letters and
comments into account in the process of revising for successive editions. The sales
success and influence of the book therefore testify to his skill in negotiating an outline of history in line with the historical consciousness of his time. The new dimension of a general readership—the publication reached the three-million sales mark
as early as 1931—seemed to bring Wells closer to the aim of history making. Since in
the mass appropriation and application his history developed its performative
force: "This display [that is, this outline of history] ends in a tremendous note of
interrogation. The writer is just a guide who brings his reader at last to the present
edge, the advancing edge of things, and stops and whispers beside him: 'This is our
inheritance.'"[10] It is this understanding of a historical inheritance—that explicitly
includes the biological aspects of human history and the appropriation of which is
deemed necessary for a meaningful life—that will be my concern in the remainder
of this essay.

Wells turned to this inheritance in more detail in 1928 in *The Science of Life*—a
work on which he collaborated with his son and Julian Huxley and that is considered the first modern textbook of biology. In *The Science of Life*, evolution is
elevated to the grand organizing principle of the cosmos. But Wells was also aware
of the problems entailed in biological history writing. In *The Science of Life* (1929–30),
he declared the attempts at reconstructing national and/or racial histories by means
of anthropometric surveys of living humans to have failed. He insisted that, while it
may be that 10,000 years ago the human races had been clearly differentiated,
successively migrations and intermixture had turned this order into chaos impossible to disentangle. At the same time, Wells demonstrated his prognostic talent
when he suggested that it might nonetheless be possible in the future to determine
the various racial contributions to the genetic inheritance of an individual.[11] In *The
Outline of History*, Wells further meditates about those most authentic records for
historical reconstruction that would for example be at the command of the paleo-
anthropologist of the future in the form of fossil skulls.[12] But it is a new kind of

epistemic object that in the aftermath promised the fulfillment of the anthropological dream, and which is of concern here: the DNA-sequence.

Big Anthropology, the Genetic Heritage, and the Gene as Historical Document

Current projects in human population genetics aim at reconstructing the history of humankind and of human groups prior to modern migrations and intermixture. Furthermore, Wells's argument that the organic relics are the more reliable historical documents are part of the discourse that positions genetic vis-à-vis other methods of historical reconstruction. Most of all, I am interested in human population genetics as applied history in the sense developed above: Biologically based identity and history are skillfully mediaized and commercialized; and the possibility for public participation that is sometimes given turns the genetic histories into personalized products and enhances their impression of liveliness.

"Big anthropology" that aims at the reconstruction of histories of humanity and human groups on the basis of large-scale comparative analyses of the genetic variation between living populations may be traced to the call for the Human Genome Diversity Project (HGDP) in *Genomics* of 1991.[13] One of its initiators, the Italian population geneticist Luca Cavalli-Sforza, belongs to the pioneers of the human population genetic approach. Beginning in the 1960s, he studied the relationships between migration patterns and blood-group distributions, and was involved in the development of techniques for the construction of phylogenetic trees.[14] But it was only in the second half of the 1980s that the technologies for large-scale statistical analyses of the genetic variability in humankind were in place.

Reaching back to the discourse of "salvage anthropology" of the previous century, the call for the HGDP presented the sampling and preserving of genetic material as an urgent issue. This opened up the paradox that it was the globalization of science that had rendered such an ambitious endeavor as the HGDP possible in the first place, but that easier and faster transport and communication at the same time threatened what the scientists perceived as the original traces of migration patterns and kinship. Those populations that were thought of as carrying the most informative historical records in their genes, the aboriginal and insular peoples, and ethnic minorities, or the isolation of those populations, were considered under threat.

At a time when public awareness of issues surrounding cultural heritage was at a peak and the field of cultural heritage studies began to emerge,[15] the initiators of the HGDP introduced a *heritage* term that analogized the human gene pool to human languages and archeological and historical legacies. The turn toward the past in Western publics as well as in cultural studies, which began in the 1970s and culminated in the 1990s, is explained by a similar set of reasons that, according to Cavalli-Sforza and colleagues, put the human genetic heritage located in these so called isolated populations into jeopardy: The (perceived) acceleration of technological and social change; mass migration; and genocide.[16] Therefore, introducing a notion of heritage close to Wells's inheritance, the HGDP initiators called: "We must act now to preserve our common heritage"![17]

Even before the project became a public affair, its practical implications for the present and future of humanity in the sense of dealing with a human heritage were taken into account, if somewhat cryptically: "By an intense scrutiny of human diversity, we will make enormous leaps in our grasp of human origins, evolution, prehistory, and potential."[18] Like any "heritageization" process,[19] this one had implications about what it means to be human and to belong to a particular subgroup of humankind. However, recent scholarship in heritage studies warns against an understanding of world heritage as a fund of objects and events to which a historical meaning is inherent. The archeologist Laurajane Smith, for example, argues that relics from our cultural heritage only attain meaning through the role they play in the negotiation and performance of identities. Despite the growing attention that material objects have received, in parallel to the increased attention paid to the past by the public as well as in cultural studies, heritage would always be of an immaterial nature.[20]

In accordance with this understanding of objects from the cultural heritage as sites of negotiation and performance of identities, arguments with regard to primate phylogeny have been, and still are, carried on over the use of DNA as arbiter. Furthermore, as I have argued elsewhere, the notion of the gene as historical document played an important role in the establishment of an identity for the new field of molecular anthropology, a term introduced in 1962 for the application of molecular techniques to primate phylogeny and evolution. At a time when phylogenies were still established on the basis of comparisons of proteins as DNA-substitutes, biochemists and physical chemists increasingly appealed to the supposedly most fundamental and authentic nature of the DNA-sequence in historical reconstruction. The scientists were also attracted to the greater objectivity of the quantitative and technology-mediated approaches vis-à-vis what was sometimes portrayed as a notoriously biased physical anthropology. Therefore, the understanding of genes as historical documents that are superior to traditional historical sources does not originate in big anthropology. Rather, this conception predates the practice of DNA-sequencing. I here only mention the article by Emile Zuckerkandl and Linus Pauling of 1965, "Molecules as Documents of Evolutionary History." They identified the DNA-sequence as the most fundamental and informational *semantide*: "[In the semantide] there is more history in the making and more history preserved than at any other level of biological integration."[21]

The ontological privileging of biological relics, as already done by Wells, is particularly remarkable in popular science. The anthropological geneticist John Relethford, for example, explains in his book *Reflections of Our Past: How Human History Is Revealed in Our Genes* (2003) that, in contrast to the incomplete archives of conventional historical documents and an oral history that is just as limited in time, our genes contain authentic traces of a much older past.[22] Thus, population genetic approaches to history are not only differentiated from traditional anthropological methods, but also, and again on the assumption of the superiority of their "documents" and the greater accuracy of their methods, from humanistic history writing.

It was this putative objectivity that turned the well-meant HGDP into a vampire project—an expression of racist and colonialist exploitation—in the eyes of indigenous groups. As Jenny Reardon has shown, the associated ignorance concerning the fact that population genetic studies always co-produce the social and the natural order contributed to this impression on the part of indigenous groups.

Their cooperation in the design of the project was not intended, so that First Nation Peoples feared for their autonomy. Their fear that was not exactly abated by the fact that they were conceptualized as stuck in the past. The project did not seem to be aimed at their future welfare, but only at benefiting Western science and economy.[23]

We may return to Relethford for another reason. He begins his praise of anthropological genetics by stating the frustrating incompleteness of our knowledge about our ancestors. Then he introduces genetics as the method to fill these voids. Thereby, the reader is led from thinking about his or her grandparents and great grandparents to the evolutionary history of populations, their migrations, and structural developments.[24] The knowledge generated through population genetics is presented as a seamless extension of personal memories and family stories into humanity's deep past. What is sold is a personalized prehistory that is meant as a prosthetic memory of the consumer's very own past to contribute to his or her cultural identity.

This linking of an abstract and anonymous population history to the concrete and personally experienced past is also part of the smaller and larger projects that have followed in the footsteps of the HGDP, such as the Genographic, African Ancestry, and Irish Origins projects that reconstruct ethnic or national genealogy and history.[25] This aspect is particularly relevant in cases where the opportunity for public participation is given.

The Genographic Project, for example, combines a sampling project with the marketing of genetic genealogy. The project, which is supported by the National Geographic Society, IBM, and the Waitt Family Foundation, samples DNA from indigenous, so-called isolated, populations in order to reconstruct human history through comparative genetic analysis. But it is simultaneously connected to a commercial enterprise, and appeals to people of the Western public to have their DNA analyzed for money and the data added to the pool of the larger project.[26] Therefore, while in this case the genetic heritage of humankind is also mainly located in the bodies of indigenous peoples, Western citizens are offered to participate in its reconstruction.

The company Family Tree DNA, which is associated with the Genographic Project, is not the only provider of commercialized human population genetics.

The services offered by DNAPrint Genomics, Genelex, GeneTree, and Relative Genetics™ offer information on genetic genealogy and/or ethnic identity. For money and a cheek swab, the customer might learn whether and in what percentage she is Native American, or whether he descends from the Cohanim. DNA-segments of an African American might be tested for matches with current African populations. Tests may also be suggested for the establishment of membership to a particular Native American tribe that has rights to self-determination and access to resources.[27] The market for these tests builds (on) diasporic feelings of fragmentation and discontinuity. The rhetoric that genetics fills voids within the historical record, finally linking people to their pasts, is quite common in this context. The founder and scientific director of African Ancestry Inc., for example, states that "[s]cience and technology now provides a bridge to the past. Technological advances in DNA technology now open up new and unprecedented opportunities for African Americans to fill centuries-old voids in knowledge of their family history."[28]

In the remainder of the paper, I look more closely at population genetics as a new form of applied history. I am interested in how the relationship to other historical methods, natural scientific as well as humanistic, is negotiated, and in the role that the DNA-sequence as historical document might play in the process. The entanglements of academic research, commercialized history, multimedia distribution, and public participation that are typical of applied history will be traced through the work and business of the British geneticist Bryan Sykes. It consists of popular books, websites, and the services of his genetic ancestry tracing company.

Applied History on a Genetic Basis: An Example

Bryan Sykes is professor of genetics at the Institute of Molecular Medicine, Oxford University, Great Britain. Even though he set out on a career in medical research, he has advanced to become a well-known population geneticist. Most famously, he has expanded to European populations the study by Allan Wilson, Rebecca Cann, and Mark Stoneking of the 1980s, which led to the African Eve model of modern human origins.[29] The African, or mitochondrial, Eve theory is based on the comparative analysis of mitochondrial DNA sequences from about 150 people who were referred to as African, Asian, Australian, Caucasian, and New Guinean. In its original form, it maintains that the mtDNA of today's world population can be traced back to one particular sequence that existed some 200,000 years ago. This sequence would have been found in the body of a woman inhabiting equatorial Africa at that time, among the first modern humans—she was the evolutionary Eve. About 100,000 to 140,000 years ago, populations began to migrate beyond the African continent and eventually populated the rest of the world.

This is where Sykes's research comes in. Also on the basis of mtDNA studies, Sykes introduced the theory that the current population of Europe can be referred back to seven Paleolithic founder tribes or clans that originated in Europe (or began to inhabit Europe, in the case of the one that originated outside Europe) between 45,000 und 8,500 years ago. The assumption is again that, since mtDNA analyses are exclusively about maternal lines, the seven ancestral DNA-sequences of the seven current European clusters were once in the bodies of seven actual women. To suggest their descent from the mitochondrial or African Eve, Sykes refers to these hypothetical female clan mothers as the seven daughters of Eve.[30]

Sykes's research incited such public interest that he decided to make (more) money from it. In the year 2001, he founded an Oxford University spin-off company that rendered the new technologies accessible to the public. Oxford Ancestors, as the firm is called, offers several genetic services. The MatriLine™ package informs the customers "about their own maternal ancestry and their place in the family tree of all humanity,"[31] while the Y-Clan™ and the Tribes of Britain™ services establish male lineages. Tribes of Britain™—to which I will return—is only available to British men, for whom a Celtic, Anglo-Saxon, or Viking origin should be diagnosed. Customers who, for example, decide on an mtDNA analysis for £180 will receive a readout of 400 base pairs and a certificate that identifies them as members of a particular Paleolithic European clan, pertaining to one of the seven daughters of Eve, as well as another certificate locating that clan in the larger picture of the family of world clans going back to African Eve herself. Obviously, Sykes here not only instrumentalizes a powerful religious origin narrative and mother figure, he also imitates cultural practices of national and other identification. Like a passport that links a citizen to a land and nation through her bloodline, these certificates connect the customers to areas within a political region via genetic ancestry. Significantly, the certificates are more than a Monopoly-like make-believe, they bear the authority of natural science, of a well-known geneticist, and of Oxford University.

However, while it is possible for the customer to take recourse to a rich and very alive cultural memory of what it may mean to be of Celtic or Viking descent, the case is not that simple with regard to an identity based on one of the seven daughters of Eve and her clan. These are Sykes's inventions, and their names and specificities in DNA-sequence therefore would be mute for the customer. This is where Sykes's inter-medial system catches. He combines the information and communication on the company's website and the services of Oxford Ancestors, which themselves are connected to his academic research, with popular books.

In *The Seven Daughters of Eve* (2001), Sykes explains not only his approach and theory, but also invents life stories for the seven daughters. He gives fictive biographies of the Stone Age women, rendered plausible by means of archeological and other sources of knowledge about prehistory. Once upon a time there were Ursula, Helena, Jasmine, Tara, Velda, Xenia, and Katrine . . . [32] The strategy is very successful. So successful indeed that many readers of the book and customers of Oxford Ancestors assume that they are informed about women whose bodily remains have actually been found. With this and the other books that accompany the Oxford Ancestor services, Sykes provides point mutations with faces and inscribes into nucleotide-sequences stories that would otherwise be of little interest to the customer.[33] This has obvious consequences for the claim of the organic objects as more authentic record of the past, and for the methods of their analysis as more objective approaches to the histories they store, than either those of physical anthropology and archeology or those of history—an issue to which I will return.

The ties between products and customers are further tightened through good use of the new media. Oxford Ancestor's website is a platform on which customers can exchange their experiences with the services of the company. Those customers wishing to establish genetic kinship also with the living may search the Oxford Ancestors database for people with similar mutation patterns. Sykes describes this production of biosociality as emotionally highly charged and bonding;[34] clan-parties are even organized. Accordingly, the genetic analyses are accompanied by expectations; not least, because they can create as well as correct an existing cultural identity. The former chief executive of Oxford Ancestors, for example, expressed on a previous version of the website his regrets that "[a]lthough both father and son are blond-haired and blue-eyed they, disappointingly, do not carry a Y-chromosome of probable Viking descent."[35] That the website has been changed could be read as a sign that the company is keen to dissociate itself from a history of human classification in anthropology. Rather than providing space for such stereotypes, the representatives call from the webpage: "We are all human and we can prove it!"[36] However, the universalist discourse, which is so typical of human population genetics in general, cannot belie the fact that also here, it is differences that are of interest. The question why the British, and which section of the British, should want to know about their genetic history and genealogy remains unanswered—presumably not to find out that they are human. The sex appeal of the new technologies is more likely to be due to the aura of old myths.

This entanglement of new media and old myths, of cutting-edge science and fantasy to create meaning and identity can be seen in a particularly illuminating way for Sykes's book *Blood of the Isles: Exploring the Genetic Roots of Our Tribal History* (2006), which is obviously linked to the Oxford Ancestors service Tribes of Britain™.[37] What is actually being sold? And how, in analogy to Laurajane Smith's understanding of the cultural heritage, is the genetic heritage inscribed with origin stories? How are the identities of scientists and customers negotiated in the process? In how far is the genetic history applied in Wells's sense—that is, not only commercialized but also effective in the life-world? And what are its relations to other forms of history writing?

The genetic data that inform the book resulted from ten years of DNA-sampling by Sykes's Oxford University team throughout Great Britain. Besides blood and cheek swabs, which Sykes and co-workers collected in England, Wales, and Scotland through blood donation services, at schools and fairs, and by mail (above 10,000), the data from Oxford Ancestors customers was also fed into the project. The research was part of the Oxford Genetic Atlas project, primarily funded by the Wellcome Trust. Adding to the network out of Oxford Ancestors and its website, Sykes's Oxford University team, laboratory, and publications, Blood of the Isles also has its own website, which informs about the project and contains a form through which the volunteer donors can ask for a code that allows them to identify their own data.[38] The mtDNA and Y-chromosome data of the Genetic Atlas project are added to the website as pdfs and can be used under observation of copyright.

Sykes's begins *Blood of the Isles* with the sentence: "This is the very first book to be written about the genetic history of Britain and Ireland using DNA as its main source of information."[39] He thus positions the kind of history writing he is concerned with and continues: "In *Blood of the Isles*, I approach the DNA evidence in the same way as others who write about the past using their different specialties—material artifacts, written documents, human remains and so on. The most important thing about the genetic evidence is that it is entirely independent of these other sources."[40] Sykes not only stresses the novelty and independence of his approach, he also points to its applicability. The genetic reconstruction of origins and history answers very specific needs: "I have experienced the thirst for roots first hand through the company I set up to help people trace their origins using DNA."[41] Sykes's history is a kind of first-aid for the people of today's societies who hunger for orientation. In this regard, Sykes, like Wells, distances his history from that of historians who might discuss in elaborate language the trauma of cultural uprooting through migration in a globalized world, and tries to understand the search for origins as the desire for a meaningful, morally informed, and authentic narrative of the self vis-à-vis the ambiguities and discontinuities of modernity. Sykes prefers to let "the simple man" speak for himself: "'I want to be able to tell my children where their ancestors came from. It gives them a sense of belonging in a world that sometimes moves too fast.'"[42] Sykes sticks to the simply formulated questions of everyday life and the history from DNA-sequences seems to provide equally straightforward answers.

However, one may object that this desire for origin narratives is already met by the many applications of traditional history, as it has become the object of analyses of *public history* and *memory studies* since the 1970s.[43] But Sykes distances his genetic history from humanistic history writing not only on the basis of its lack of complexity—which he sees as an advantage. He also makes use of the notion of heritage as material objects with inherent meaning, the critique of which from *heritage studies* I have mentioned above. Sykes's history is an organic history. The DNA-sequences and, by inference, the histories they encode are just as palpable as the needs of "the simple man." This also accounts for the special status of DNA as a witness of history that lived in the bodies of our ancestors and now lives in us: "It was there."[44] We are dealing with a history that has been inscribed by nature into every human body, a "history within," as it is called on the website of the

Genographic Project. In tune with this connective energy of DNA, the message of *Blood of the Isles* reads: "Ours is a shared history."[45]

Such a unifying power is a quality of myths, and Sykes makes ample use of such, which he finds often more in accordance with his interpretation of the genetic data than the ambiguous archeological evidence.[46] But the DNA-sequences at times also seem to contradict the myths. Sykes's genetically based history undermines the very topical myth of "the Celtic brand," which he regards as being in the service of creating difference through the claim of an ancient Celtic race. "The Celtic brand," as used by Sykes, designates the belief in and cult of the distinctiveness of the West-Scottish, Irish, and Welsh Celts, and those of Cornwall and the Bretagne, who share the Celtic language. In Sykes's view, these "Celts" in the west of the Isles abuse "the Celtic brand" to split the British population and to counter the supposed English dominance. The DNA, to the contrary, tells a uniting story.[47]

At the same time, Sykes is well aware of the affect-laden, colorful cultural heritage "the Celtic separatism" lays claim to. And it is this kind of emotionally charged origin narrative that Sykes makes money with. Therefore, I argue, Sykes does not side with those archeologists, such as Simon James, who deconstruct this notion of the Celtic as myth.[48] To the question of whether genetics may help to see behind "the Celtic brand," its feelings of originality and authenticity, and behind the marketing machine and politics of it, Sykes comes up with a different answer. "The Irish, Scottish, Welsh, and English DNA" tell of a very old, continuous history of the maternal lines, rooted mainly in the Paleolithic and Mesolithic inhabitants of the British Isles: "We are an ancient people."[49] Neolithic farmers did arrive from the Iberian Peninsula along the shores of the Atlantic, but they did not replace the indigenous Mesolithic Britons in great measures. Since then—that is since approximately the last 6,000 years—the British female gene pool has remained more or less intact. Sykes christens this original British lineage "Celtic/Pictish": "On our maternal side, almost all of us are Celts."[50] Even the male lines are mainly Celtic in this pan-British sense. Saxon, Danish/Viking, and Norman Y-chromosomes are there, but they are minorities: "Overall, the genetic structure of the Isles is stubbornly Celtic."[51]

In other words, Sykes argues that the genetics do not support the theory of a great wave of immigration from central Europe into the west of the British Isles. The genetics contradict the notion that the Scotts, Welsh, and Irish are related to those "Celts" that in the first century before Christ moved from Hallstadt and La Tène toward Italy, Greece, and Turkey. But Sykes does not use this argument to undermine an Irish-Scottish-Welsh identity as Celts. Rather, he appropriates the emotionally and politically powerful "brand," founds it genetically, to unite all parts of the Isles beneath it. The term *Celt* is altered to refer back thousands of years to the Paleolithic and Mesolithic inhabitants of the British Isles. Robbed of its foundational power for the aims of devolution and separatism, *Celt* becomes a synonym for *Britishness*. But Sykes's pan-insular notion of the "Celtic brand" itself relies on exclusivity, because it excludes all later immigrants to the British Isles. In fact, in the context of the racial riots in Oldham, Sykes's genetics have been appropriated by the British National Party to argue for a former genetic purity and whiteness of Great Britain that should be reestablished.[52]

However, rather than with such direct biopolitical application of his research results, Sykes seems concerned with the marketing power of the "Celtic brand" for the Tribes of Britain™ Y-chromosomal analysis sold by Oxford Ancestors. He wants to make sure that the change in meaning is not accompanied by a loss of mythic aura. Nonetheless, it is exactly the mythical character of Sykes's narratives that seems to betray his longing for closure. His retelling performs the relation between the known and his reinterpretation with the aim to get at the truth behind the myth, and thereby set an end to the telling. Genetic myths especially seem to turn history into nature and claim the last word. They reduce historical complexity to that simplicity in which things (DNA-sequences) speak for themselves and abstractions become sensual.[53]

On the other hand, Sykes's history seems very much one for the people and by the people, not only because it is identity-forming and commercialized, but because we all carry fragments of it in our bodies. It is therefore symptomatic of the trend towards the individualization of history that has been diagnosed by historians. The subject continuously positions him- or herself in time through an individualized experience of the past. The level of meaning-production and orientation is the unique life. This personalized history nonetheless relies on collectives, as the distancing from others remains central for Western understandings of self. Identities are achieved through ever newly attained experiences of difference.[54] Katja Patzel speaks of the individual as wanderer between major collective memories in a free market of common identities.[55]

Furthermore, Sykes's language of a "Celtic brand" brings to mind the shift from kind to brand or from type to trademark described by Donna Haraway, and that Celia Lury elucidated in an interesting way for the context of this paper with the Benetton and other examples.[56] Lury suggests that nationality and race no longer appear as naturally given. Rather, for the global citizen, choice has become the only necessity. Lury argues that the United Colors of Benetton advertising campaign launched in 1985, which couples the spectacle of human racial diversity with a statement for global unity, conveys race as a matter of style. In the endless play of colors, the distinction between clothes and skin is undermined. With female legs wrapped in colored stockings, skin color becomes an act of choice. Not only race, but also nationality, is turned into a matter of playful choices about style. Lury concludes that "the brand is contributing to the violent erasure of historical links between people, products, places, and practices that is part of a shift from natural and historical understandings of the nation-state to the expansionist, mediated and market-led notions of global nature, global culture."[57]

It is tempting to interpret Sykes's re-creation of the "Celtic brand" as appropriating this very power of brand, associated as it is with "expansionist, mediated

and market-led notions," but thereby retying it to "natural and historical understandings of the nation state," and, in this sense, making it work for the reconstruction of "links between people, products, places, and practices." Sykes deals in
brands, but their flexibility and playfulness, the possibility to change them like
clothes, is under threat when they sell genetically defined origins and histories.
It may prove difficult to wander between biologically founded identities and histories as one pleases. The characteristics typical of applied history, such as the
commercialization, multimediaization, personalization, and interactivity of history, which are associated with openness and choice, are thus accompanied by the
claim for exact science and the naturalization and fixation of mythical and historical knowledge through biological foundation. That this constellation demands a
balancing act, not only between academic and popular, but also between techni-
cal-numerical and narrative-symbolic forms, becomes evident from the genealogy
Sykes offers for his genetic history.

A Genealogy for Genetically Based Applied History

The novelty Sykes claims for his genetic reconstruction of British history may work
to launch an old brand in new garb. At the same time, it may pose difficulties,
since, as analyses of the commemorative practices in science have shown, new
approaches in particular depend on "founding fathers" and traditions.[58] Sykes
establishes a tradition for his science from the physical anthropology of the nineteenth century and the early blood group studies. John Beddoe's research on eye
color, hair color, and skull shapes to reconstruct the British national history is
given as the starting point of this genealogy.[59] Beddoe's measuring forays into the
Isles are rendered as romantic-heroic adventures, with which the geneticist Sykes,
rarely traveling without his DNA-sampling kit, easily identifies: "It is as if John
Beddoe, criss-crossing the country with card and pencil in hand, calipers and tape
in his knapsack, had already anticipated the arrival of the geneticist. How he
would have loved to be alive now!"[60] Possibly, Sykes's identification with Beddoe is
further facilitated by the conclusions that could be drawn from the latter's anthropometric surveys: The Irish were not too different a race to be integrated into
British society. In other words, Irish Home Rule was no anthropological necessity.[61]

    According to Sykes, Beddoe's empirical studies nonetheless suffered from a
certain subjectivity, due to the bias inherent in the anthropological approach,
which he sees resolved in the serology of the early twentieth century.[62] The
attempts to classify human races and to reconstruct their migrations by means of
an analysis of the distribution of blood groups are, in Sykes's logic, one step closer
to being the final arbiter of inheritance than Beddoe's external characteristics.
The empowerment of the DNA-sequence as the most authentic and authoritative
historical document goes hand in hand with a history of anthropology that
appears as journey into the body.[63] The closer to the DNA the analysis, the less is
the environmental contamination. What seems presaged in the article by

Zurckerkandl and Pauling of 1965, has become common knowledge. It is the majority of mutations that have no effect on the phenotype that renders the DNA-sequence the most objective and direct repository of history: "But it is these, the silent passengers of evolution," so Sykes, "that are its most articulate chroniclers."[64]

This is what I identify as the paradox of genetic history writing. The nucleotide sequences are indeed mute, and even the latest technologies may well wrench patterns from them, but no stories. To the contrary, the stochastic nature of the mutation process and the mathematics of the statistical analysis seem opposed to the emotionality and symbolism of narratives. Sykes seems to wrestle with the discrepancy: "Once a number is produced, something, perhaps everything, of value has been lost. Like so many tabulations, the numbers disguise individual stories of heroism and betrayal, triumph and defeat, and force them into bleak summaries. This is no way to treat our ancestors, and you will be glad that I shall not insult them, or you, in this way again."[65] This is a rhetorical attempt to bridge the abyss between the numerical, technology-mediated, and digitalized world of the laboratory science, on which Sykes draws for his claim of objectivity, and the literalized metaphor of the DNA-sequence as embodiment of a narrative kind of history. Sykes spares the reader the hard facts. Understandably so, because it is only in a semi-mythical approach to his object that the DNA-sequences begin to "tell stories," "carry inscriptions," and "witness migrations." Like the biologist Wells, the geneticist Sykes has to reinvent himself in this endeavor, for "[geneticists] are not natural storytellers."[66]

Thus, Sykes finally succeeds at packaging the security, authority, and objectivity of natural science along with myths and history. However, the fathers with whom he adorns his natural scientific history writing are themselves of questionable pedigree. Therefore, both observers and critics of human population genetics have drawn attention to the continuities with the history of physical anthropology and with the serology of the later nineteenth and early decades of the twentieth century. The collection of biological data by anthropologists from royal/national societies was part of unequal power relations and domination also outside the colonial context. The regional and national anthropometric surveys for the study of racial traits, racial composition, and history could become part of government decisions. Concerning the continuities in the history of studies of exterior bodily characters, bones, and molecules of the Irish, mostly by English and American anthropologists, the geographer Catherine Nash observes: "Though recent studies have dropped the language of racial types, the subjects of the research (genetic evidence of the 'political-religious' boundary in Northern Ireland, for example) and the methods (studying phenotypical variation as well as blood type and gene frequencies) suggest the legacy of earlier models of 'national' as well as 'biological' difference."[67]

In today's human population genetics, national and ethnic identities may be established by ways of reference to biology and geography, and it shares certain concepts, practices, and interests with the physical anthropology (of the past), such as that of indigenous populations as historical relics, the collection of bodily material, and the biological reconstruction of kinship and history. As in the example of Sykes, the link to the anthropological projects to reconstruct racial/ethnic composition, migration patterns, and (national) history, may even be explicitly made. However, molecular and physical anthropology are different scientific traditions, which leads to the essential paradox between the technological-quantitative and narrative-holistic approaches discussed for Sykes above. The anthropologist Jonathan Marks can therefore turn on its head the argument that the molecular techniques have introduced objectivity into a historically burdened and methodologically fuzzy anthropology, by denying molecular anthropology its status as a field of anthropology based on its reductionist approach. He also hands back the allegation of bias. Current anthropology implies sensitivity for the role of power and difference in shaping human relations and a critical stance toward "natural facts" that Marks misses in human population genetic projects.[68] Sykes's treatment of the history of anthropology is at best naive.

The suggestion that applied genetic history promising its customers to find their genetic peers, and by inference information about who the genetically others are, would do well to engage more critically with its legacies, may be reinforced with a provocative hint at the historical entanglements between applied and racial history. Instead of starting out from Wells's rupture with the tradition of racial anthropology, I could have begun with its simultaneous apotheosis elsewhere. In fact, the term *applied history* appears on the cover of one of the folkish books by the German high school teacher Heinrich Wolf in 1911. "The education to political thought and will," as it is subtitled, reached a circulation of 35,000 copies in 1926, and in 1940 entered the list of books recommended for schools and libraries of the Reichsministry for science, upbringing, and education. As early as 1930, the *Applied History* had grown to a series that encompassed six individual books, among them the *Applied Race Science: World History on a Biological Basis* of 1927. This explicitly applied biological history combined biology and myth into an instruction in identity politics. For the folkish worldview that was based on race ideology, a historical and prehistorical foundation of Germanic values was central.[69]

The demand that human population genetics engage the past of racial and colonial anthropology in a more self-reflexive way certainly seems justified. But now this past rather belongs to that which the new mnemo-technologies would have us forget. Despite the very common assertion that population genetics brings to light the underlying unity of mankind and the close kinship of all populations, which is to counteract the suspicion of a racial anthropological interest, this happens without critical discussion of the issue. As a consequence, in its commercialized, mediaized, and participatory form that I call applied genetic history, it is innocently enough referred to as *recreational genetics*—a mere pastime. However, I suggest a different understanding of the expression *recreational genetics* as designating a genetics that creates anew. Indeed, genetic ancestry tracing companies work with types and myths genetically recreated as brands. Even in German-speaking Europe, the provider of genetically based genealogy and history, iGENEA, feels safe enough to lure to the gene test through its website by asking the questions: "Would you like to learn about your original ancestry? Do you possibly have Celtic, Germanic, or Jewish roots?"[70]

To Conclude: Genetically Imagined Communities

There is no research following on the suspicion that catchwords such as *Germanic* and *Jewish* are part of the reason why the supposed revolution in identity brought about by applied genetic history has not (yet) taken place in German-speaking Europe. There is also no careful historicization of the genetic-ancestry-tracing phenomenon. Both are part of my larger project. Last but not least, it seems essential to know more about the ways in which different segments of customers deal with the information about genetic identity and history. It may be particularly relevant to further discuss the differences between humanistic and biological applied history, and to integrate the genetic services regarding kinship and history more satisfactorily into the discourses about a possible new eugenics, and about a new biopolitics in general, as they are associated with scholarship on (ethnicized) medical genetics.[71]

When thinking about biopolitics in the age of genomics, it seems appropriate to take population genetic projects and commercial services regarding the reconstruction of ethnic/racial, national and human history into account. The biosocialities they produce between natural science and market differ from those involved in ethnic medical genetics in that group-identity is not built primarily around genetic disposition for certain diseases, but more exclusively on the basis of common descent and history. Through skilled combinations of academic research, the genetic ancestry tracing market, and popular science media, Sykes, for example, fosters the establishment of kinship around DNA-databases. For these genetically imagined communities, traditions are invented and the tools provided for customers to contribute to their further development.[72] Despite the rhetoric of unity, in the genetic reconstruction of the British and Irish national history, Sykes defines clear boundaries: While the current population of Great Britain and Ireland are seen as the product also of migrations, it is the long and unbroken line of descent from the Paleolithic and Mesolithic inhabitants of the regions that is stressed against the historical and present tendencies of decentralization. A pan-insular unity of genetic citizens is thereby invoked.[73] But excluded from this unity are British citizens and inhabitants of the Isles whose immigrations are part of much later diasporic processes, such as those from India, Pakistan, and the Caribbean.

In closing, the possibility that such genetically old and, in a certain sense, purely imagined communities may increasingly have a counterpart in societies at large, is suggested as a possibility by means of an anecdote. As in other regions,

Great Britain has experienced a shortage in sperm donors to meet the demand for artificial insemination. In the eyes of one Glasgow clinician, the problem could be solved by importing sperm from a rich sperm bank in Denmark. The media distribution of the news incited many Scottish men to offer to donate their own sperm to alleviate the shortage—and possibly to prevent a renewed invasion of the Scottish gene pool by Danish genes. This at least was the interpretation visualized in a cartoon published in *The Guardian*. The caricature combined the present situation with the historical event of Viking invasion and settlement in Scotland. Whether through bodily contact or artificial insemination, the outcome presumably remains the same: The Scottish gene pool is reconfigured and the genetically imagined community may have to reinvent its traditions—in this case, its history as a football nation seems to have been a central concern.[74]

NOTES

1. For a discussion of the notion of *applied history* see Wolgang Hardtwig and Alexander Schug, eds., *Angewandte Geschichte* (Stuttgart: Steiner, or Frankfurt a/M: Campus 2008); for an encompassing treatment see Simone Rauhe, *Public History in den USA und der Bundesrepublik Deutschland* (Essen: Klartext 2001); for a definition of public history, see, for example, Charles Cole Jr., "Public History: What Difference Has It Made?" *The Public Historian* 16, no. 4 (Fall 1994):S. 9–35, here 11.

2. See, for example, Astrid Erll, *Kollektives Gedächtnis und Erinnerungskulturen: Eine Einführung* (Stuttgart: Metzler 2005), 2–4; David Lowenthal, *The Heritage Crusade and the Spoils of History* (Cambridge: Cambridge University Press), chap. 1; Rauhe, *Public History*, especially 167.

3. See Christoph Kühbergerand Christian Lübke, *Wahre Geschichte—Geschichte als Ware: Die Verantwortung der historischen Forschung für Wissenschaft und Gesellschaft* (Rahden: Marie Leidorf, 2007).

4. www.ibdna.com/regions/UK/EN/?page=recreationalgenetics.

5. H. G. Wells, *The New and Revised Outline of History: Being a Plain History of Life and Mankind* (1920; rpt. Garden City, NY: Buchaufl, 1931), 1–13.

6. James Harvey Robinson, *The New History: Essays Illustrating the Modern Historical Outlook* (New York: Macmillan, 1912); see also Peter Burke, "Overture. The New History: Its Past and Its Future," in *New Perspectives on Historical Writing*, 2nd ed. (University Park: Pennsylvania State University Press, 2001), 1–24.

7. Carl L. Becker, "Mr. Wells and the New History," in *Everyman His Own Historian: Essays on History and Politics* (New York: Appleton-Century-Crofts, 1935), 189–190. New historians also welcomed *The Outline of History* because Wells aimed at transcending a purely Western perspective and because he was interested in a number of sources and modi of history writing.

8. Carl Becker, "Everyman His Own Historian," *American Historical Review* 37, no. 2 (1932):221–236, quote on 231; all longer citations have been translated by the author.

9. Wells, *The New and Revised Outline of History*, 6.

10. Ibid.

11. Julian Huxley, H. G. Wells, and G. P. Wells, *The Science of Life* (London: Cassell, 1931), 863–864; see also William T. Ross, *H. G. Wells's World Reborn: "The Outline of History" and Its Companions* (Selinsgrove: Susquehanna University Press, 2002), 40–41, here 22–26.

12. Wells, *The New and Revised Outline of History*, 6.

13. Luca Luca Cavalli-Sforza, "Call for a World-Wide Survey of Human Genetic Diversity: A Vanishing Opportunity for the Human Genome Project," *Genomics* 11 (1991):490–491. On anthropology as big science, see Jonathan Marks, "'We're Going to Tell These People Who They Really Are'—Science and Relatedness," in *Relative Values—Reconfiguring Kinship Studies*, ed. Sarah Franklin and Susan McKinnon (Durham, NC: Duke University Press, 2001), 355–383, here 355.

14. See for example Luca Luca Cavalli-Sforza and A.W.F. Edwards, "Phylogenetic Analysis: Models and Estimation Procedures," *American Journal of Human Genetics* 23 (1967): 235–252; for autobiographical rendering of his early blood group studies see Luigi Luca Cavalli-Sforza and Francesco Cavalli-Sforza, *The Great Human Diasporas: The History of Diversity and Evolution* (Reading, MA: Addison-Wesley, 1995), chap. 5.

15. See Laurajane Smith, "General Introduction," in *Cultural Heritage: Critical Concepts in Media and Cultural Studies,* 4 vols., Vol. 1: *History and Concepts,* ed. Laurajane Smith (London: Routledge, 2007), 1–21.

16. See Lowenthal, *The Heritage Crusade*, chap. 1.

17. Cavalli-Sforza, "Call for a World-Wide Survey of Human Genetic Diversity," 490.

18. Ibid., 491.

19. David C. Harvey, "Heritage Pasts and Heritage Presents: Temporality, Meaning, and the Scope of Heritage Studies," in *Cultural Heritage. Critical Concepts in Media and Cultural Studies,* 4 vols., Vol. 1: *History and Concepts,* ed. Laurajane Smith (London: Routledge, 2007), 25–44, quote on 26.

20. See Smith, "General Introduction," 4.

21. Emile Zuckerkandl and Linus Pauling, "Molecules as Documents of Evolutionary History," *Journal of Theoretical Biology* 8 (1965):357–366, quote on 360; see also Marianne Sommer, "History in the Gene: Negotiations between Molecular and Organismal Anthropology," *Journal of the History of Biology* (2008).

22. John H. Relethford, *Reflections of Our Past: How Human History Is Revealed in Our Genes* (Boulder, CO: Westview, 2003), 9.

23. See Jenny Reardon, *Race to the Finish: Identity and Governance in an Age of Genomics* (Princeton, NJ: Princeton University Press, 2005); on the HGDP see, for example, Jonathan Marks, "Your Body, My Property: The Problem of Colonial Genetics in a Postcolonial World," in *Embedding Ethics,* ed. Lynn Meskell and Peter Pels (Oxford: Berg, 2005), 29–45.

24. Relethford, *Reflections of Our Past*, 8.

25. On the Irish Origins Project, see Catharine Nash, "Irish Origins, Celtic Origins: Population Genetics, Cultural Politics," *Irish Studies Review* 14, no. 1 (2006):11–37.

26. On the Genographic Project, see Catharine Nash, "Mapping Origins: Race and Relatedness in Population Genetics and Genetic Genealogy," in *New Genetics, New Identities,* ed. Paul Atkinson, Peter Glasner, and Helen Greenslade (London: Routledge, 2007), 77–100.

27. On genetic services tailored to Native Americans see Kimberly TallBear, "Native-American-DNA.coms. In Search of Native American Race and Tribe," in *Revisiting Race in a Genomic Age,* ed. Barbara Koenig, Sandra Soo-Jin Lee, and Sarah Richardson (New Brunswick, NJ: Rutgers University Press, 2007).

28. Rick A Kittles and Cynthia Winston, "Psychological and Ethical Issues Related to Identity and Inferring Ancestry of African Americans," in *Biological Anthropology and Ethics: From Repatriation to Genetic Identity,* ed. Trudy R. Turner (Albany: State University of New York Press, 2005), 209–229, quote on 222.

29. See Rebecca L. Cann, Mark Stoneking, and Allan C. Wilson, "Mitochondrial DNA and Human Evolution," *Nature* 325 (1987):32–36.

30. The method is explained in Bryan Sykes, *The Human Inheritance: Genes, Language, and Evolution* (Oxford: Oxford University Press 1999).

31. www.oxfordancestors.com.

32. Bryan Sykes, *The Seven Daughters of Eve* (New York: W. W. Norton, 2001).

33. See also Bryan Sykes, *Adam's Curse: A Future Without Men* (London: Bantam, 2003).

34. For the concept of biosociality, see Paul Rabinow, "Artificiality and Enlightenment: From Sociobiology to Biosociality," in *Essays on the Anthropology of Reason*, ed. Paul Rabinow (Princeton, NJ: Princeton University Press, 1996), 91–111.

35. www.oxfordancestors.com, [accessed May 17, 2004].

36. Ibid.

37. Bryan Sykes, *Blood of the Isles: Exploring the Genetic Roots of Our Tribal History* (London: Bantam, 2006).

38. www.bloodoftheisles.net.

39. Sykes, *Blood of the Isles*, 1.

40. Ibid., 2.

41. Sykes quotes an anonymous Australian from New South Wales, in ibid., 54.

42. Ibid.

43. For systematic and historical overviews of memory studies, see Aleida Assmann, "Gedächtnis als Leitbegriff der Kulturwissenschaften," in *Kulturwissenschaften. Forschung—Praxis—Positionen*, ed. Lutz Musner and Gotthart Wundberg (Wien: WUV, 2002); Aleida Assmann, *Der lange Schatten der Vergangenheit: Erinnerungskultur und Geschichtspolitik* (München: C. H. Beck, 2006); Astrid Erll, *Kollektives Gedächtnis und Erinnerungskulturen: Eine Einführung* (Stuttgart: Metzler, 2005); Jeffrey R. Olick and Joyce Robbins, "Social Memory Studies: From 'Collective Memory' to the Historical Sociology of Mnemonic Practices," *Annual Review of Sociology* 24 (1998); on the connection between memory studies and public history, see Rauhe, *Public History*.

44. Sykes, *Blood of the Isles*, 54. On myths as remembered history and their formative power, see, for example, Jan Assmann, *Das kulturelle Gedächtnis: Schrift, Erinnerung und politische Identität in frühen Hochkulturen* (München: C. H. Beck, 1992).

45. Sykes, *Blood of the Isles*, 3.

46. Ibid., 21.

47. Ibid., chap. 3.

48. See Simon James, *The Atlantic Celts: Ancient People or Modern Invention?* (Madison: University of Wisconsin Press, 1999).

49. Sykes, *Blood of the Isles*, 281.

50. Ibid.

51. Ibid., 287.

52. See Catherine Nash, "Genetic Kinship," *Cultural Studies* 18 no. 1 (2004):1–33, here 21–22; for another example of the genetic construction of a specifically white "Britishness," see Kath Cross, "Framing Whiteness: The Human Genome Diversity Project (As Seen on TV)," *Science as Culture* 10, no. 3 (2001):411–438, here 419–427.

53. On these ideas of Hans Blumenberg and Roland Barthes, see Stephanie Wodianka, "Mythos und Erinnerung; Mythentheoretische Modelle und ihre gedächtnistheoretischen

Implikationen," in *Erinnerung, Gedächtnis, Wissen: Studien zur kulturwissenschaftlichen Gedächtnisforschung*, ed. Günter Oesterle (Göttingen: Vandenhoeck & Ruprecht, 2005), 211–230, here 218–223.

54. See Clemens Wischermann,"Geschichte als Wissen, Gedächtnis oder Erinnerung? Bedeutsamkeit und Sinnlosigkeit in Vergangenheitskonzeptionen der Wissenschaften vom Menschen," in *Die Legitimität der Erinnerung und die Geschichtswissenschaft*, ed. Clemens Wischermann (Stuttgart: Franz Steiner, 1996), 55–85.

55. Katja Patzel,"'Alle Erinnerung ist Gegenwart': Zur Selbstverortung des Individuums im Prozeß der Modernisierung," in *Die Legitimität der Erinnerung und die Geschichtswissenschaft*, ed. Clemens Wischermann (Stuttgart: Franz Steiner, 1996), 189–213, here 193–194.

56. See Donna Haraway, Modest_Witness@Second_Millennium.FemaleMan©_Meets_OncoMouse™ (New York: Routledge, 1997), 66–67, 74. In what Haraway calls the New World Order Inc. (postmodern, globalized, technoscientific world), natural kind becomes brand or trademark, such as OncoMouse™, a sign protecting intellectual property claims in business transactions. Another example is GeneBank© at Los Alamos, containing the human genome sequence information: Man the taxonomic type become Man the brand. The transformation from type to brand is associated with the commercialization of life itself, when genomes are patented as a form of intellectual property. It goes along with new kinds of kinship, such that as between a company and its products or consumers.

57. Celia Lury, "The United Colors of Benetton: Essential and Inessential Culture," in *Global Nature, Global Culture*, ed. S. Franklin, C. Lury, and J. Stacey (London: Sage, 2000), chap. 5, quote from 183.

58. See Pnina Abir-Am, "The First American and French Commemorations in Molecular Biology: From Collective Memory to Comparative History," *Osiris*, 2nd Series, 14 (1999): 324–372; Janet Browne, "Commemorating Darwin," *British Journal for the History of Science* 38, no. 3 (Sept. 2000):251–74.

59. John Beddoes, *The Races of Britain: A Contribution to the Anthropology of Western Europe* (Bristol: Arrowsmith, London: Trübner, 1885).

60. Sykes, *Blood of the Isles*, 77.

61. See Henrika Kuklick, "The British Tradition," in *A New History of Anthropology*, ed. Henrika Kuklick (Malden: Blackwell, 2008), 52–78, here 58. Besides surveying the racial constitution of the British people, the committees that were installed by the BAAS were to investigate whether the British, and if so which part of them, were degenerating.

62. Sykes, *Blood of the Isles*, 83. Sykes mentions the Hirschfelds (see L. Hirschfeld and H. Hirschfeld, "Serological Differences between the Blood of Different Races," *Lancet* [18 October 1919]:S. 675–679).

63. Sykes, *Blood of the Isles*, 91.

64. Ibid., 96. The argument is common from the 1960s onward, and can be found in the previously cited Cavalli-Sforza and Edwards, "Phylogenetic Analysis," 233. The version used by Sykes is based on the hypothesis of neutral evolution at the molecular level and the molecular clock (Motoo Kimura, "Evolutionary Rate at the Molecular Level," *Nature* 217 [17 February 1968]:624–626). For the history of the hypothesis see Michael R. Dietrich, "The Origins of the Neutral Theory of Molecular Evolution," *Journal of the History of Biology* 27, no. 1 (1994):21–59; M. Sommer, "History in the Gene: Negotiations between Molecular and Organismal Anthropology," *Journal of the History of Biology* 41 (Fall 2008):473–528.

65. Sykes, *Blood of the Isles*, 112.

66. Ibid., 117.

67. Nash, "Irish Origins, Celtic Origins," 12; see also Marks: "Your Body, My Property, 29–45.

68. Jonathan Marks, "What Is Molecular Anthropology? What Can It Be?" *Evolutionary Anthropology* 11 (2002):131–135.

69. Heinrich Wolf, *Angewandte Geschichte: Eine Erziehung zum politischen Denken und Wollen*, 4th. ed. (Leipzig: Dieterich'sche Verlagsbuchhandlung, 1911); Heinrich Wolf, *Angewandte Rassenkunde: Weltgeschichte auf biologischer Grundlage*, Angewandte Geschichte Vol. 5, 3rd. ed. (1927; rpt. Berlin-Schöneberg: Theodor Weicher, 1943); See also Uwe Puschner, "Völkische Geschichtsschreibung: Themen, Autoren und Wirkungen völkischer Geschichtsideologie," in *Geschichte für Leser. Populäre Geschichtsschreibung in Deutschland im 20.* Jahrhundert, ed. Wolfgang Hardtwig and Erhard Schütz (Stuttgart: Franz Steiner, 2005), 287–307, here 292–293.

70. www.igenea.ch.

71. See, for example, Troy Duster, *Backdoor to Eugenics*, 2nd. ed. (New York: Routledge, 2003); Daniel J. Kevles, "From Eugenics to Genetic Manipulation," in *Science in the Twentieth Century*, ed. John Krige and Dominique Pestre (Amsterdam: Harwood Academic Press, 1997), 301–318. The inclusion of projects and services of human population genetics into the discussion of biological citizenship in advanced liberal democracies, as undertaken by Nikolas Rose on three pages of his latest book, seems unsatisfactory (see Nikolas Rose, *The Politics of Life Itself: Biomedicine, Power, and Subjectivity in the Twenty-first Century* [Princeton, NJ: Princeton University Press, 2007], 176–179).

72. See Benedict Anderson, *Imagined Communities: Reflections on the Origin and Spread of Nationalism*, 3rd. ed. (London: Verso, 2006); Eric Hobsbawm and Terence Ranger, *The Invention of Tradition* (Cambridge: Cambridge University Press, 1983).

73. On the notion of genetic citizenship, see Deborah Heath, Rayna Rapp, and Karen-Sue Taussing, "Genetic Citizenship," in *Companion to the Anthropology of Politics*, ed. D. Nugent and J. Vincent (Oxford: Blackwell, 2004), 152–167.

74. See Bob Simpson, "Imagined Genetic Communities: Ethnicity and Essentialism in the Twenty-first Century," *Anthropology Today* 16, no. 3 (June 2000):3–6.

14

Cells, Genes, and Stories

HeLa's Journey from Labs to Literature

PRISCILLA WALD

In early 1951, an African American woman named Henrietta Lacks consulted a doctor at the Johns Hopkins Medical Center. She had no idea that the vaginal bleeding that had led her there was the result of a remarkably aggressive cervical cancer, which would ultimately prove fatal. Nor could she have guessed that the proliferating cells that were killing her would allow researchers at Johns Hopkins to develop the first "immortal" cell line later that same year. Medical researchers George and Margaret Gey had been trying to keep cells alive and reproducing in Petri dishes, but had been unsuccessful until they received a sample of the aggressive cells that were killing Henrietta Lacks. The trait that made them so difficult to treat in Lacks's body made them thrive where other cells had not, and the Geys had found their elusive immortal line. The HeLa cell line (named for Henrietta Lacks) revolutionized cell biology, leading to new opportunities for research, as well as important medical advances, including the development of the polio vaccine within the decade. It also created a new life form for which there was no precedent.

Henrietta Lacks died in a segregated ward of the hospital without knowing the contribution that her cells would make to science. Although medical researchers would collect blood and tissue samples from Lacks's family, the Lackses also knew nothing about the HeLa cell line until 1975, when Barbara Lacks, the wife of Henrietta's oldest son, happened to be at a dinner party with a medical researcher who was working with HeLa cells and commented on the coincidence of her surname.

Although many have profited from the HeLa cell line, Lacks's family has not shared in that profit. Many familiar with the case, including medical ethicists and Lacks's family, have a perception of wrongdoing on the part of the medical establishment. Discussions about the case have centered on the racism evident in the treatment of Lacks and her family and in the narratives that circulated when the identity of the donor of the HeLa cells became public knowledge. It is, however, difficult to pinpoint the exact nature of the violation. Neither Lacks nor her family gave consent for the use of her cells, but the case preceded such protocols. It seems unjust that Lacks died in poverty and that her family struggled while medical researchers, and especially pharmaceutical companies, profited from the HeLa cell line, but the line was not patented, and the profits were indirect, stemming from products and discoveries it enabled. Unlike subsequent researchers who patented cell lines, the Geys did not get rich from the HeLa cell line. It is certainly wrong that Henrietta Lacks died in a segregated ward and unjust that her cells have been used to develop drugs and other treatments to which many of her descendents might not have access, but it does not make sense to argue that Lacks should not have been on a segregated ward *because* her cells were unique or that her family should have access to better health care *because* of the properties of Lacks's cells. Rather, the Lacks case underscores the institutional racism that has plagued the nation since its inception.[1] Lacks should not have been on that ward because it should not have existed, and her descendents should have access to better health care because such access ought to be a fundamental human right and not a privilege.

Many bioethicists and cultural critics have noted the racism that is evident in the treatment of Lacks and her family by researchers and the media, but failure to recognize its multiple manifestations has resulted in confusion surrounding the exact nature of the violations in this case. Lacks's story offers important insight into the deeper issues of institutional racism that are frequently overlooked, not only in the Lacks case, but also in discussions about race and biotechnology generally.

Her story calls attention to social inequities that are at the center of contemporary debates surrounding health care, but it is equally relevant for the insight it can offer into the spirited debates surrounding race and DNA at present. George Gey had worked conscientiously to protect the identity of his unwitting donor until Stanley Gartler, a geneticist, discovered the far-reaching contamination of subsequent cell lines by the remarkably aggressive HeLa cells, which prompted him to ask Gey about the racial identity of the donor. Gartler used genetic markers associated with DNA from African-descended individuals to identify the contamination of other cell lines by HeLa cells. His announcement of the contamination and the source of the cell line at a conference on cell tissue and organ culture in 1966 would eventually lead to public narratives about Lacks that put assumptions about race, sex, and gender conspicuously on display (Gold 1986; Landecker 2007; Skloot 2009; Weasel 2004). The narratives show how those assumptions have structured social and scientific practices and thereby elucidate why unresolved social tensions surface with any challenge to conventional definitions of the human.

In a 2008 essay in *Genome Biology*, "The Ethics of Characterizing Difference: Guiding Principles on Using Racial Categories in Human Genetics," a multidisciplinary faculty group from Stanford University offered ten principles designed to serve as guidelines in the debates that have surfaced with the acceleration of research in human genetic variation following the mapping of the human genome. Their list of principles emerges from their recognition that scientific research has historically reinforced racial hierarchies and social inequities, and their first principle is their declaration "that there is no scientific basis for any claim that the pattern of human genetic variation supports hierarchically organized categories of race and ethnicity" (Lee et al. 2008). The ten principles register the salient points around which debates about racism and research in the genome sciences and scientific medicine have centered in the past decade.[2] The authors reiterate the distinction that population geneticists have been making since the early years of the field, between the genetic category of a population and the sociopolitical contexts of the terms race and ethnicity, and they attempt to explain the biology of human variation. They urge medical researchers to minimize their use of the categories of race and ethnicity and to be especially careful about how they explain those labels. In the final two principles, they call for funding for interdisciplinary study of human variation that includes humanists, scientists, and social scientists, and they suggest that the teaching of genetics should include historical study of how science has been used to construct a biological, reductivist concept of race and, in turn, to justify racism.

The authors of the Stanford report profess their belief that "the equality of rights of all human beings is an unquestionable, moral claim that cannot be challenged by descriptive, scientific findings" (Lee et al. 2008:404.1–2). Such assertions have a long history, but they have not prevented the abuses to which the piece alludes. While all of the principles are important, and the goal of the piece—to examine how research involving human genetic variation can fuel racism—is commendable, the list also manifests an absence that has characterized these discussions: insufficient attention has been paid to the legacy of racism, specifically to how *racist assumptions have historically structured the definitions of human being on which assertions of inviolable human rights rely*. Those assumptions surface with renewed energy—and can therefore be more readily apprehended—when scientific research and geopolitical transformation underscore the fundamental instability of the concept of "human being."

The period following the Second World War offers such a convergence. The exigencies of war yielded rapid technological innovation and dramatic scientific discoveries in many areas, including genetics, and its legacy included widespread geopolitical transformation and accompanying political theories. From the point of view of science and medicine, the HeLa cell line represented a radical breakthrough, but it also created a new organic entity—a Frankenstein's creature—for which there was no context. Exemplifying some of the ways in which scientific research was challenging conventional biological definitions of the term "human being," it dovetailed with the political theories of such figures as Hannah Arendt and Frantz Fanon, who analogously questioned conventional social definitions of that term. The creation of new and unfamiliar organic entities, such as cell lines, commingled with the haunting images of human beings stripped of their humanity to challenge, in their uncanniness, conventional definitions of human being and humanity.

Both Arendt and Fanon accordingly called for new and expanded definitions of human being and new narratives of human history to accompany them. Many involved in the HeLa research noted its resemblance to science fiction. Indeed that genre crystallized around these questions in the post-war moment and offers theoretical insight into the instability of the concept of human being. In what follows, I will chronicle these questions as they circulate through narratives of scientific innovation and geopolitical transformation and will conclude by following Henrietta Lacks's cells into science fiction writer Octavia Butler's *Xenogenesis* trilogy of the late 1980s. In this context, the dilemma raised by the HeLa cells shows both how the bioethical debate has continued to obscure the unresolved conceptual issues that inform it and how the history of racism has shaped anxious responses about the impact of biotechnological innovations into the present.

Cellular Conundrum

The uniqueness of the first immortal cell line raised questions about the relationship of the entity to the donor who provided the cells. Noting that "the distribution to and presence in laboratories all over the world of what had been a single specimen from one person was an utterly new mode of existence for human matter," Hannah Landecker chronicles the anthropomorphism that emerged from the attempt to make sense of the HeLa cells (Landecker 2007). Landecker is intrigued by the efforts of "scientists and their publics alike . . . to fathom the new conditions of possibility for humans and human bodies in biomedical science" (Landecker 2007:18). Implicit in these attempts is the recognition of the profound instability of the concept of "human being." It is in the anxious responses to that recognition that institutional racism becomes apparent.

Racial identification of the donor of the HeLa cells became important when Gartler sought to identify the extent of the contamination of other cell lines. The very properties that had allowed the cells to survive in the Petri dish in 1951 also posed a serious problem for medical researchers. The remarkable aggressiveness of the HeLa cells made them very difficult to contain, and they contaminated other cell lines, in some cases invalidating years of research. The donor's racial identification was relevant to Gartler for tracking the cells; it had no bearing on their aggressiveness. The anthropomorphism of the cells shows both how the race and gender of the donor permeated the public narrative and how cultural biases surface when scientific research yields new entities.

"In the 1960s, the cells became the enemy within," as one pundit puts it, "contaminating every other cell [line] in America and effectively wasting four years and billions of dollars in research. In the 1970s, Hela [*sic*] got into espionage, infiltrating the Soviet Union and destroying its cancer research too" (Taylor 1997).[3] In the words of another, "Scientists call them HeLa cells. Non-scientists call them She. . . . She was an invaluable lab animal. And she escaped. Extraordinarily virulent, invasive, and vigorous, the HeLa cells reached and ruined scientific experiments from America to Russia. (You would swear she had a sense of humour. Leonard Hayflick, testing his own baby's tissue, found a black enzyme. Mrs. Hayflick protested her innocence. It was Henrietta.)" (Banks-Smith 1997). A third commentator recounts how a researcher discovered the contamination of cell lines he had purchased from the Soviet Union and notes that "Henrietta had got through the Iron Curtain by infecting other lines" (Cooper 1997). These accounts register the confusion of Lacks with her cells, and the image that emerges from these quotations is of a bestialized, invasive, contaminating, sexually promiscuous African American woman.

The racism and sexism evident in these remarks has been widely noted in the ethical debates concerning the original creation and subsequent use of the cell line for several decades. An alternative narrative emerged, originally in the black press, sanctifying Lacks and describing her "sacrifice" for science. She has subsequently been honored in a congressional resolution, as well as by the Smithsonian Institution, Morehouse College, the National Foundation for Cancer Research, and in an annual commemoration ceremony in Turners Station, Maryland, where she lived prior to her untimely death.

Yet, both the demeaning and the sanctifying rhetoric beg the unanswered question at the heart of these discussions: What is the relationship of Henrietta Lacks to her cells? A question such as that one emerges whenever technological developments lead to the creation or identification of new entities. The story is so complicated because the cell line is relevant, not only for its scientific importance, but also because its creation and use are embedded in a capitalist economy—that is, because it is profitable.

The thorny implications of that embeddedness would become the subject of a series of legal cases, beginning in the late 1980s, concerning the cells of John Moore, a white man whose cancer cells similarly were the source of a cell line that was believed at the time to have potentially important medical properties (and financial implications) (Boyle 1996; Landecker 1999; Mitchell 2001; Mitchell 2004; Mitchell 2007; Skloot 2009; Wald 2005; Waldby and Mitchell 2006). The legal and journalistic discussions that followed the case of John Moore and the Mo cell line showed the uncertainties that emerged around the question of the ownership of the cells and that crystallized around the commodification of organic material and personhood.

Moore sued the researchers and the research hospital that he claimed had taken cells from his cancerous spleen for research without his consent and without sharing the profit. Significantly, attorneys for both Moore and the defendants, as well as legal theorists and journalists who wrote about the suit, all evoked the specter of enslavement (bioslavery) to make sense of either the violation that Moore had ostensibly endured or the implications that would follow any acknowledgement that Moore "owned" his cells.

The Moore case also evinces concerns about racism, which suggests that the racial identification of the donor, while significant, does not tell the whole story. The case demonstrated that the entity of a cell line and its relationship to a human being had not been resolved in the intervening decades since the Lacks case. In its irresolution, the case registered the instability of the definition of human being as it manifested the legacy of the perverse institution that haunted the Lacks case. Both cases demonstrate how a challenge to the idea of human being in one context readily summons the (racialized) history of dehumanization.

Human Contingency

The unsettling nature of the HeLa cell line makes sense in the context of the dramatic transformations in the biological sciences of the mid-twentieth century—in particular the rise of evolutionary biology and its spatio-temporal displacement of individual human beings in favor of cells and, ultimately, genes. The most dramatic change in postwar thinking about the biological nature of human beings, and therefore a crucial context for understanding the destabilization evident in the Lacks case, emerged from what was called "the evolutionary synthesis" and marked the crystallization of genetics and natural science into a new articulation of evolutionary theory. Darwin had written the Great Origin Story of the nineteenth century; the evolutionary synthesis updated and revised that tale. The biologist Theodosius Dobzhansky is widely credited with popularizing the idea of the evolutionary synthesis in his 1937 *Genetics and the Origin of Species*, although the actual term did not appear until Julian Huxley's 1942 *Evolution: The Modern Synthesis.*

The synthesis, which resulted from increasing collaboration between geneticists and natural historians, explained how micro-changes at the level of the gene produced macro-changes at the level of the population. A simple copying error on a single allele in the earliest stages of reproduction could ultimately produce a new species. Of course, that process depended upon a multitude of other factors, but the role of chance at that microscopic level was breathtaking. Human being had never before appeared so unstable, so contingent on a single unpredictable mistake.

The evolutionary synthesis, which shifted the primary scale of evolutionary focus from individual human beings to alleles and populations, demonstrated the extent to which contingency and instability characterized every aspect of the human condition. Over time, change was the only constant. Dobzhansky was aware of how population genetics might affect "the race problem" and stressed the contingency of race, noting that "races and species as discrete arrays of individuals may exist only as long as the genetic structures of their populations are preserved distinct by some mechanisms which prevent their interbreeding. Unlimited interbreeding of two or more initially different populations results unavoidably in an exchange of genes between them and a consequent fusion of the once distinct groups into a single variable array" (Dobzhansky 1937:13). Clearly, both biological and social classifications and the hierarchies they named were temporary, as in fact was the species itself. There is an intrinsically apocalyptic element to human evolution that is not often remarked on except in science fiction. Extinction is as much a given in the field as evolution is, and the changes marked by evolution can be sufficiently dramatic over time as to blur the distinction. Natural selection notwithstanding, Mother Nature evidently has no preordained plan for human survival.

The specter of human finitude haunted the evolutionary narrative, and biological contingency had a social analogue in "stateless" or "displaced persons." As Hannah Arendt argues in *The Origins of Totalitarianism*, the category of "displaced persons" demonstrated the contingency of human beings' rights and dignity—of an acknowledgment, in effect, of their social being—on the nation-state: "the conception of human rights, based upon the assumed existence of a human being as such, broke down at the very moment when those who professed to believe in it were for the first time confronted with people who had indeed lost all other qualities and specific relationships—except that they were still human. The world found nothing sacred in the abstract nakedness of being human" (Arendt [1951], 1979). These displaced persons were not the first groups to register this contingency. Those who were enslaved and colonized before them had given the lie to any concept of fundamental rights, displaying how rights depended on persons' relationships to the state, which, as the years leading up to the war had shown, could be severed by the state.

The analogue between the evolutionary synthesis and Arendt's formulation turns on ideas of biological and social nonbeing, and both help to explain an intrinsic ontological anxiety that pervaded the years following the war. Arendt traces that anxiety back to an alienation from nature that grows out of the human capacity to destroy "all organic life on earth with man-made instruments" (Arendt [1951] 1979:298). That anxiety takes on an ontologically apocalyptic quality because of the particular human relationship to nature that she sees as rooted in the concept of the rights of man. For her, that political doctrine constituted human beings' declaration of independence from history and of allegiance instead to nature. It included the tacit assumption "that nature was less alien than history to the essence of man" and implied "the belief in a kind of human 'nature' which would be subject to the same laws of growth as that of the individual and from which rights and laws could be deduced" (Arendt [1951] 1979:298). She chronicles the growing challenge in the postwar years not only to this idea of human "nature," but also to the idea of natural laws generally, as they applied to both political forms and scientific observations. Scientific probing has led, she argues, to a view of the universe as random and chaotic, because of which "nature itself has assumed a sinister aspect" (Arendt [1951] 1979:298). Human beings and their institutions have been denaturalized in every conceivable sense of the word, and the displaced persons embodied the implications of that dehumanization.

The Martinican psychiatrist and political theorist Frantz Fanon notes a similar denaturalization that, for him, was a function of colonialism. In the colonial discourse, the "native" is diseased and disruptive, but the colonial worldview dehumanizes the native through a broader conceptual construction of "hostile

nature, obstinate and fundamentally rebellious," which encompasses indigeneity
in its broadest sense, including "the bush, . . . mosquitoes, natives, and fever," and
which must be "tamed" by the colonizer (Fanon [1961], 1963). Fanon identifies a
vocabulary of colonialism in which the settler "speaks of the yellow man's reptil-
ian motions, of the stink of the native quarter, of breeding swarms, of foulness, of
spawn, of gesticulations" (Fanon [1961] 1963:42). The bestialized native slips readily into the past of the "race of man" and, in the process, into something that no
longer belongs in this world: "those hordes of vital statistics, those hysterical
masses, those faces bereft of all humanity, those distended bodies which are like
nothing on earth, that mob without beginning or end, those children who seem to
belong to nobody, . . . that vegetative rhythm of life. . . . Every effort is made to
bring the colonized person to admit the inferiority of his culture, which has been
transformed into instinctive patterns of behavior, to recognize the unreality of his
'nation,' and, in the last extreme, the confused and imperfect character of his own
biological structure" (Fanon [1961] 1963:42–43, 236). The native is excluded from
full presence and participation in the contemporary moment by this temporaliz-
ing of space, which produces the narrative of "the ascent of man."

The dehumanization entailed in that exclusion enables murder not to seem
like murder to the colonizers, which explains why mass murders—"the 45,000
dead at Sétif," an Algerian town, in 1945, "the 90,000 dead in Madagascar" in 1947,
and "in 1952, the 200,000 victims of the repression in Kenya"—can pass virtually
unnoticed (Fanon [1961] 1963:78). Arendt similarly observes that "natives"
appeared to Europeans as "'natural' human beings who lacked the specifically
human character, the specifically human reality, so that when European men
massacred them they somehow were not aware that they had committed murder"
(Arendt [1951] 1979:192).

Fanon issues a call to arms in *The Wretched of the Earth*, in which he urges citizens of the newly decolonized and decolonizing nations not to emulate Europe,
not to imagine that they have to "catch up" to anyone, but rather to understand
that a new humanity will follow from the new stories of humankind. He believes it
falls to "the Third World [to start] a new history of Man, a history which will have
regard to the sometimes prodigious theses which Europe has put forward, but
which will also not forget Europe's crimes. . . . the differentiations, the stratification, and the bloodthirsty tensions fed by classes; . . . racial hatreds, slavery,
exploitation, and above all, the bloodless genocide which consisted in the setting
aside of fifteen thousand millions of men" (Fanon [1961] 1963:315). With "bloodless
genocide," Fanon depicts colonization as the systematic destruction of native
cultures and the attendant dehumanization as a form of mass murder. Colonialism registers the genocidal underside of the European past and the need for both
new world leadership and a new origin story that justifies it.

Decolonization therefore mandated a radical challenge to conceptions of
both nature and humanity. At the beginning of his 1961 *The Wretched of the Earth*,
Fanon calls, in classic revolutionary language, for "quite simply the replacing

of a certain 'species' of men by another 'species' of men" (Fanon [1961] 1963:35). Revolution is the mutation that starts humanity on its road to evolution. "Species" is set off in quotation marks, but the term is not entirely metaphorical. The author of the 1952 *Black Skin, White Masks* had already explored the role of racism in the constitution of subjectivity—had insisted, in fact, on the need for revision of psychoanalytic theory to account for that role—and had spent nearly a decade studying the impact of colonialism on the psychology of the colonized while practicing as a psychiatrist in Algeria before and during the Algerian revolution. The call for a new "species" of men conveyed the magnitude of the mental, physical, cultural and political changes that revolution would usher in. As a psychiatrist and a theorist of decolonization, Fanon understood the need for a new and more comprehensive conception of human being that would address that ostensibly biological justification for social exclusions.

The three decades following the Second World War witnessed the massive acceleration of decolonization and a rapid geopolitical reorganization of what would become known, during this period, as "the Third World," a term that expressed the relationship of emerging nations to the politics of the Cold War. As one of the foremost theorists of decolonization, Fanon, like his teacher Aimé Césaire, insisted on the importance of culture as well as politics to the process. The native and settler had brought each other (as types) into existence through the colonial encounter, and the humanity of each was at issue. Decolonization was more than an undoing; it was a "historical process" that "influences individuals and modifies them fundamentally. It transforms spectators crushed with their inessentiality into privileged actors, with the grandiose glare of history's floodlights upon them. It brings a natural rhythm into existence, introduced by new men, and with it a new language and a new humanity. Decolonization is the veritable creation of new men" (Fanon [1961] 1963:36). That process had to be accompanied by new accounts not only of a specific history, but also of human history generally, and it entailed a radical revision of an entire worldview.

The future depended on those narratives of the past for Fanon and Arendt, both of whom called for the rewriting of new and more inclusive narratives of humanity. Like Fanon, Arendt accompanies her call with the haunting figure of an image of humanity utterly divested of its earthly qualities—not, in her case, the colonized native, but the concentration camp survivor who cannot "believe fully in his own past experiences. It is as though he had a story to tell of another planet," she writes, "for the status of the inmates in the world of the living, where nobody is supposed to know if they are alive or dead, is such that it is as though they had never been born" (Arendt [1951] 1979:44). There is no place—no category—within the current story of human history for such figures, who thereby haunt the story and its conception of nature in their utter alienness. Alien they were, yet visible and all too present in the post-war years. They embodied the paradox of human (or natural) rights: that the immateriality of those rights became apparent at precisely the moment they were most necessary.

Both political theorists saw the failed narrative—the story that subsequent events had shown to be inadequate—as the story of the rights of man. In their effort to imagine inviolable, or non-contingent, rights, human beings had in fact abnegated their responsibility for their actions. Nature, godlike, endowed them with rights they did not need to work to define, refine, or maintain. For both Fanon and Arendt, humanity could not move forward without new accounts of human nature that would be so thoroughly haunted by the unearthly images of human beings stripped of their humanity that they would have to begin with a more inclusive and inviolable conception of humanity—in effect, a new species of human being. The new articulation of humanity for Fanon and Arendt had to be rooted neither in a deified Nature, nor in biology. Arendt invokes Aristotle's distinction between *zoe* and *bios*, biological and cultural existence, to mark the difference between being alive and meaningfully existing. Bare life showed nothing but the paradox of natural/human rights, as the stateless refugees or the camp survivors embodied their contingency. In that context, species-thinking (as in the emphasis on survival of the species, rather than of humanity) marked the road to annihilation.[4]

No one better captured the conceptual implications of the radical geopolitical changes for the ideas of human being and humanity that were precipitated, or at least accelerated, by the war. Their work exemplifies the pervasive shift across fields and disciplines, as cultural observers, from social scientists to political activists, from religious leaders to novelists and filmmakers, explored new conceptions of human being and, consciously or otherwise, produced new narratives of the history and nature of humanity. The otherworldly figures through which they explored the limits of contemporary conceptions of humanity resonated with the burgeoning genre of science fiction, in which such figures proliferated. The theoretical insights of that genre have not yet been sufficiently explored.

Humanity's Borders

The rise of biotechnology as a multi-billion-dollar industry in the 1970s offered new potential for understanding, manipulating, and managing human life, and it dovetailed with political theorists' interest in the strategies and consequences of dehumanization. The public narrative of Henrietta Lacks and the HeLa cells emerged in this context, and the anxieties raised by the uncertainties of the nature of a cell line and its relationship to its donor—explicitly expressed a decade later in the Moore case—are evident in efforts to make sense of HeLa through its personification. Lacks as a Cold War Mata Hari, infiltrating the Iron Curtain; as a sacrificial heroine, paving the way for human immortality; as a vengeful fury, contaminating the research of the scientists who spurned her—Lacks as angelic, demonic, supernatural—obscures the lack of resolution about the relationship of Lacks to the HeLa cells as it evinces the uncanniness that accompanies any blatant destabilization of the concept of the human.

The political philosopher Michel Foucault fashioned his theory of biopolitics—how the state exercises control through "the administration of bodies and the calculated management of life"—in this context as well (Foucault 1977:140).[5] In a series of lectures delivered at the Collège de France in the 1970s, he developed this theory through an account of the co-emergence of a liberal conception of government and the (bio)power that it articulates in the language of human welfare: specifically, the responsibility of liberal government for the welfare of bodies and populations. Biopolitics is rooted in a justification of liberal governance that appears to emanate not from the state, but from society, which, like the U.S. Constitution's "We the People," paradoxically constitutes the state that brings that body into existence. The state constitutes the people that it has ostensibly arisen to govern as a population, which it marks through forms of measurement, such statistics collected to assess the well-being of the population, including rates of birth, death, and disease. Foucault calls this turn "the entry of life into history" (Foucault 1977:141). The health and welfare of the population becomes the responsibility of, and justification for, the state as the population subtly becomes the means of its representation.

Like Arendt and Fanon, Foucault returns to the eighteenth-century rise of a liberal conception of governance (premised on the doctrine of the rights of man) to understand the dangerous confluence of human survival and the conception of human life and to chronicle the strategies of control that it enabled. He sees genocide as the logical outcome of the incorporation of the life sciences into the governance of the state, calling it "the dream of modern powers . . . not because of a recent return of the ancient right to kill; [but] because power is situated and exercised at the level of life, the species, the race, and the large-scale phenomena of population" (Foucault 1977:137). This logic was exemplified in Nazi Germany, in which concern for the welfare of the German people as a population led to eugenics: the effort to cleanse the gene pool of polluting characteristics. It is in that sense the "dream of modern powers," the fulfillment of a wish: the ultimate expression of the subjugation of bodies and the management of populations that at once engenders and emerges from biopower.

The rapid growth of biotechnology, especially genetics, despite the Nazi taint, offered new information that shaped everything from new accounts of human history to dangerous excuses for "the administration of bodies and the calculated management of life." It is, then, not surprising that the biologizing of life represented such a dramatic danger in Foucault's historical narrative, which resembles the dystopian narratives about the dangerous governmental misuses of biotechnology offered in science fiction works in this decade, such as *THX 1138* (dir. George Lucas, 1971) and Ira Levin's 1971 *This Perfect Day*. While Foucault's analysis offers insight into the uncanniness that accompanies the manipulation of living organisms, it does not explain why the uncertainties generated by the production of cell lines and other biotechnological developments should be so readily racialized in the United States.

The racialization that surfaces with the destabilization of the human is the result of historical specificities, and it bears witness to the institutional racism that has troubled biotechnology—and clouded ethical discussions of its developments—from the outset. Those specificities are evident in cultural productions that reflect on the possibilities of changing notions of the human, which was a central topic, particularly of science fiction, in the decades following the war. With her interest in science and race, the science fiction writer Octavia Butler was almost certainly familiar with the famous unwitting donor, whose cells had made news in the 1970s following Gartler's announcement that many researchers were unknowingly working with HeLa cells that had contaminated other cell lines. But whether or not it was intentional, the striking resemblance between Henrietta Lacks and the protagonist of Butler's *Xenogenesis* trilogy (now known as *Lilith's Brood)* situates the Lacks case in the broader context of the imbrication of biotechnology in a history of racism and colonialism.

Butler wrote the trilogy—*Dawn* (1987), *Adulthood Rites* (1988), and *Imago* (1989)—at the end of a decade that had witnessed significant advances in the genome sciences, culminating in the initiation of the Human Genome Project in 1990. Her treatment of the themes surfacing around biotechnology is suffused with her analysis of the history of racial slavery and colonization. Notably, the trilogy engages themes of genetic hybridity and malleability and illuminates nuances of genetic identity that are often oversimplified in contemporary genomics.

In *Dawn*, Butler's aliens, the Oankali, rescue the dying population of Earth following a full-scale nuclear war, and they rejuvenate the dying planet. After several centuries of suspended animation, they awaken the first human being, an African American woman from L.A. named Lilith, and begin the process of repopulating the planet. With a genetic predisposition to cancer, Lilith provides her rescuers with an example of cells whose rapid growth teaches them invaluable lessons about cellular reproduction. They consider cancer the great gift of the human species—a "talent" for cell growth—and they find themselves ineluctably drawn to these compelling beings.

The trilogy turns on the fundamental incompatibility between the Oankali and the human beings whom they have rescued. The Oankali understand themselves as saviors. They offer health, longevity, and harmony, but they are gene traders who believe that interbreeding is the key to the health of a population, and they want to accelerate human evolution through an exchange of genes. Over the course of the three novels, no human being willingly accepts the Oankali. Some agree to the Oankali terms, but none is ever fully satisfied with the choice.

While the Oankali speak for the collective good, the human beings feel that their dignity is violated. The question of consent is especially controversial. The Oankali refrain from interacting with human beings without consent, but their definition of consent does not imply conscious acquiescence; rather, they read bodily impulses and ignore the conscious will, which to them represents interference with the desires and needs of human bodies. It is a matter of perspective whether the Oankali are "reading" human beings or coercing them when they perform genetic alterations that enable human survival and reproduction. For the human characters, that survival comes at the expense of their humanity, which they define as conscious, reasoned choice and believe to be synonymous with freedom.

The trilogy raises questions about the assumptions that underlie that definition of humanity. The Oankali are committed ecologists in every sense of the word. They are drawn to strangers because they understand that strangers promote growth: the social and biological health of a group (conceived as a population). They take seriously that biodiversity is necessary to that health. Evolution, for them, enables survival and improvement, while for the human beings, evolution implies extinction. If a succeeding generation differs too much from its progenitors (literally, xenogenesis), then the progenitors have ceased to exist in a meaningful way. "Humanity" and "population," in other words, represent different ways of thinking about survival and meaningful existence in the trilogy, as they do for Fanon, Arendt, and Foucault. For the human beings, "humanity" names a collection of individuals and focuses on the present, while "population" suggests only their species being—*zoe*. For the Oankali, however, "population" implies interdependence and looks to the future—the vocabulary of population genetics. The trilogy does not finally endorse either point of view.

Where the Oankali embrace difference, Butler's human beings are stubborn in their resistance to the unfamiliar and insist on the Oankali's utter and irreconcilable strangeness. They are violent and intolerant and do not even unite in opposition to the Oankali; their communities of resistance tend to be racially and linguistically homogeneous. The Oankali discover in the genes of human beings what they label "the central contradiction": intelligence and hierarchy that, in combination, lead inevitably to self-destruction. Yet, if Butler's human characters as a whole conform to the image that the Oankali have of them, the Oankali in turn justify the human complaint that they treat human beings like children, as well as the suspicion shared by human beings who choose to live among the Oankali that their attachment to their Oankali mates and kin is coerced: that they are captives. Lilith understands her need for her Oankali mates as a "literal, physical addiction to another person," and she explains the Oankalis' desire for human beings as a kind of cannibalism (Butler 1989). "If you [ate meat]," she tells Nikanj, one of her mates, "the way you talk about us, our flavors and your hunger and your need to taste us, I think you would eat us instead of fiddling with our genes" (Butler 1989:155). Nikanj indeed admits to Jodahs, one of their progeny, that "We feed on them every day. . . . And in the process, we keep them in good health and mix children for them. But they don't always have to know what we're doing" (Butler 1989:156).

The trilogy demonstrates the ethical consistency of both positions, even while depicting their incompatibility and exploring basic assumptions about human rights and dignity. Most difficult for the novels' human characters (and perhaps for contemporary readers) is the Oankalis' sterilization of human beings who refuse to mate with them. Preventing childbirth within a group falls under the definition of genocide in the U.N. Convention on the Prevention and Punishment of the Crime of Genocide. Yet, even that disturbing position represents a consistent Oankali ethics and stems from what they believe is their deep concern for human beings. The Oankali are travelers, and eventually, as Nikanj explains to its hybrid child, "we [will] break the Earth and go our ways" (Butler 1989:87). The resistors will have lived out their long lives by then. The Oankali are reluctant to sacrifice human lives, so they prevent the continuation of a species that would not survive the Earth's dissolution. The Oankali are indeed keeping terrible secrets, even from their human mates; Nikanj's justification sounds like colonial paternalism. Yet, Butler also never allows her reader to forget that human beings would long before have destroyed the Earth if the Oankali had not restored it after nuclear war and that nothing endures forever, that resources are finite. Populations endure only if they change, and the sterilization, however horrific and resonant with the worst eugenics practices in human history, thus makes sense as Oankali ethics. However unpalatable, the Oankali solution represents a consistent, if dangerous, ethical position in a future that is radically different from the past and cannot reliably use it as a reference.

The Oankali's ecological practices are at once compelling and troubling. The trilogy implicitly summons the history of racism to explain why those practices elicit the human conviction that human beings are more than the expression of biology and that without their humanity, biological survival is meaningless. While "humanity" implies free will, choice, and emotional range, it also relies on a recognizably human lineage that extends both backwards through historical memory and endlessly into the future. The need for this genealogy is alien to the Oankali, for whom memory is genetic. They intrinsically remember all of their incarnations and experience their changes as productively developmental. Without either genetic memory or a recognizable lineage, however, human beings experience themselves as excluded from history and accordingly find life meaningless. Historian Orlando Patterson calls that experience "social death," referring specifically to the dehumanization that is at the heart of enslavement (Patterson 1982). The trilogy shows how the social death—the erasure of and exclusion from history— that was a key feature of both enslavement and colonization continues to inform the experience and definition of humanity. The human beings believe that if they cannot project a mirror image of themselves into the future, they will cease to be.

Lilith and her offspring, *Adulthood Rites*'s Akin and *Imago*'s Jodahs, are all hybrids of some sort, bridge figures who negotiate between the human and Oankali perspectives, showing the difficulty, the anguish, and the cost of that position. Each protagonist convinces the Oankali to modify the policies the human beings find most repugnant, but in so doing, each promotes the eventual assimilation of human beings and Oankali. Throughout the trilogy, Lilith never stops wondering whether she and her offspring are teaching her people to die.

Butler's hybrid protagonists evoke the long history of hybridity, which, beginning in botany and zoology, eventually became synonymous with "mixed-blood" to describe the children of parents from different races. Human hybridity manifests the conflation of social and biological taxonomies that characterizes racism and is disturbing in its threat to undermine the racial logic of social hierarchies. It attests to the permeability of social and cultural boundaries and the impermanence of racial classifications. In representing the ineluctability of social and biological transformation, mixed-race hybrids at once embody the principle of ecology—the health of the population—and represent a threat to the reproduction of a "humanity" that defines itself by stasis: the ability to look into the future and imagine a mirror image of contemporary social and biological configurations.

To understand that fear in terms of social death is to see the traumatic residue of the experience of enslavement and colonization, both of which demonstrated the mechanisms of oppression and power in one group's attempts to erase the history and culture of another. Racism may indeed shape the human response to the Oankali—not because human beings experience the Oankali as another race, but because they cling to a definition of humanity that encompasses the disavowed memory of what it means to be excluded from history. "Humanity" is an unstable term from which the exclusion of persons and groups has enabled the justification of exploitation and genocide. It is unclear whether the Oankali represent the antidote to or most recent application of this racist logic.

The trilogy does not resolve that question, but its analysis of racist history and its relation to the instability of the concept of "humanity" offers insight into how biotechnology gets entangled with that troubled history. The most disorienting and compelling of the Oankali to the human beings are the Ooloi, whose name means "treasured strangers." These third-gender beings are natural scientists: genetic engineers who effect reproduction and healers who can cure everything from harmful genetic mutations to gunshot wounds and cancer. The trilogy offers insight into how the racialized history of social death can turn the creation of a cell line into a potential challenge to humanity and, conversely, how any such unsettling recalls the history of racism. This analysis helps to explain why both the prosecution and the defense invoked the specter of bioslavery in the John Moore case and why HeLa was so readily and so problematically racialized and gendered.

Lilith's sense of being tampered with—of no longer owning herself (which is her first thought on awakening among the Oankali)—anticipates the outraged response, including charges of racism, of indigenous groups to population geneticists' proposals to collect the DNA of indigenous populations allegedly facing "extinction."

Spearheading such research, Stanford population geneticist Luigi Luca Cavalli-Sforza, one of the authors of "The Ethics of Characterizing Difference" (Lee et al. 2008), has been as puzzled by the response to his work as the Oankali are by the human animosity they encounter. While Cavalli-Sforza believes that his research would help to prove that racism is "unscientific," he fails to understand the historical context for the response that launched a group called Indigenous Peoples Council on Biocolonialism (Reardon 2004; Wald 2006). Their critique addresses the inscription of his proposed genomic research in the social and economic inequities that reflect centuries of colonization in which resources, including human labor and human beings, were exploited and populations were oppressed often to the point of annihilation. Cavalli-Sforza and his colleagues do not understand the concern of indigenous peoples about how the researchers will use their genetic information and who will control the interpretive stories that emerge from their research, and the scientists charge their critics with misunderstanding the science. Like the Oankali, these geneticists lack an understanding of the history of institutional racism in which the absence of informed consent of research subjects from oppressed populations was a manifestation of their exclusion from (and of the unstable definition of) human being and "humanity."

Researchers risk reproducing that history not only in their treatment of their research subjects, but also in their slippery use of terms such as "race" and "ancestry," which characteristically slide between biological and social definitions, despite efforts, such as the Stanford group's, to distinguish between them and prevent such slippage. The history of racism explains Lilith's suspicions and the human resistance to the Oankali.

At the same time, the trilogy never entirely confirms the human beings' suspicions, and it complicates the critique. The history of racism includes not only racialized groups' subjection to scientific medical research, but also their exclusion from its benefits (Washington 2006). In its depiction of the human resistance to the Oankali, the trilogy reproduces that paradox, showing, in the process, the problem with "humanity" (and human rights) as a term of ethical resistance. If fear of a racist use of science yields efforts to articulate an inclusive definition of "humanity," the fear and abjection of hybrids is historically an expression of that racism and also underlies efforts to stabilize the definition, and static reproduction, of "humanity." Butler's hybrids show both that the distinction between "humanity" and species-being is murky and that "population" as an evolutionary term can offer an alternative in which hybrids embody the breakdown of exclusionary categories, social as well as biological.

The Xenogenesis trilogy, which is explicitly a creation myth projected into the future, shows how radical biological and social metamorphoses produce new origin stories. From the human perspective, that story takes the shape of a classic heroic struggle for freedom against an apocalyptic threat to "humanity." From the Oankali perspective, it is an ecological story of incorporation and the emergence of a new species. The perspective of the hybrid protagonists, however, presents the creation myth through the lens of the complicated history of racism and the unresolved uncertainties it underscores. From their perspective, the trilogy suggests the need to keep the concepts represented by both terms (humanity and population) in mutually modifying dialogue in the interest of a social justice that begins with recognition of interdependence and the inevitability of change.

What the hybrids manifest, in other words, is that "humanity" is not what remains when species-being is factored out; it will never emerge as a timeless and enduring term, but will, like life itself, evolve.

Engagement with the long-term future implications of human evolution is rare outside of science fiction. Butler's trilogy offers insight into how the definition of humanity rests on a projection of contemporary formations into an unending future; the contemporary obsession with ancestry similarly registers the desire for a continuous and recognizable line from the past to the present. In the aftermath of genocide, it is not surprising that political theorists sought an enduring definition of "humanity" on which to build political institutions, even while they recognized the implausibility of that project. The trilogy, too, demonstrates the importance of definitions, but shows how the inevitably destabilizing and unpredictable factor of change produces different narratives of transformation. Nothing is more fluid than narrative, and nothing is more foundational; each seismic change in the evolution of humanity in geopolitical and biological terms shakes the stories on which even the most apparently stable institutions are founded.

Human being and humanity will always be contingent—biologically as well as socially—and the trilogy suggests both the impossibility of stabilizing their definitions and the urgency of attending to the narratives through which human beings make sense of seismic change and shape political institutions accordingly. "The universe is made of stories, not of atoms," observed the poet Muriel Rukeyser; thus are human beings, as Arendt would say, world makers, constructing stories in many forms, including theories and interpretations, that shift as scientific innovations generate new insights. Butler's novels illustrate the foundational quality—the biopower—of stories in all of their incarnations. Those stories, as the varying accounts in Butler attest, can be inclusive or exclusive and therein lies the project of social justice.

NOTES

1. Stokely Carmichael coined this term in speeches in the 1960s to mark persistent racialized social inequities that are intrinsic to and perpetuated by the institutions and practices that structure social life.

2. Much has been written on this debate. I reviewed and historically contextualized this debate in an essay that I am drawing on for this piece, "Blood and Stories" (Wald 2006).

3. It is important to note that all three of these comments are drawn from pieces that appeared in the London press as reviews of *The Way of All Flesh*, a BBC documentary about Henrietta Lacks and the HeLa cells. They at once describe and reproduce the rhetoric surrounding discussions of the HeLa cells that followed Gartler's announcement and the subsequent identification of Lacks several years later. On that process, see especially Landecker and Skloot.

4. Giorgio Agamben builds and reflects on Arendt's discussion of this distinction in *Homo Sacer: Sovereign Power and Bare Life* (1998).

5. Numerous critics have extended Foucault's concepts of biopower and biopolitics to explore biotechnological developments and governance in late modernity. See

especially Rabinow 1996; Rabinow 1999; Rabinow 2003; Rabinow and Rose 2006; Rajan 2006; Rajan 2010; Rose 2007).

WORKS CITED

Agamben, Giorgio. 1998. *Homo sacer: Sovereign power and bare Life.* Translated by Daniel Heller-Roazen. Palo Alto, CA: Stanford University Press; first edition, *Homo sacer: Il potere soverano e la vita nuda* (1995).

Arendt, Hannah. [1951] 1979. *The origins of totalitarianism.* New York: Harcourt Brace Jovanovich; original edition, 1948.

Banks-Smith, Nancy. 1997. The horrors of long division. *The Guardian* (March 20), T6.

Boyle, James. 1996. *Shamans, software, and spleens: Law and the construction of the information society.* Cambridge, MA: Harvard University Press.

Butler, Octavia. 1989. *Imago.* New York: Warner Books.

Clarke, Adele E., Laura Mamo, Jennifer Ruth Fosket, Jennifer R. Fishman, and Janet K. Shim, eds. 2010. *Biomedicalization: Technoscience, health, and illness in the U.S.* Durham, NC: Duke University Press.

Cooper, Glenda. 1997. *The Independent* (March 14), 2.

Dobzhansky, Theodosius. 1937. *Genetics and the origin of species.* New York: Columbia University Press.

Fanon, Frantz. 1963. *The wretched of the earth.* Translated by Constance Farrington. New York: Grove Press; first edition, *Les damnés de la terre,* 1961.

Foucault, Michael. 1978. *The history of sexuality, Part I: An introduction.* Trans. Robert Hurley. New York: Random House, 1978.

Gold, Michael. 1986. *A Conspiracy of cells: One woman's immortal legacy and the medical scandal it caused.* Albany: SUNY Press.

Huxley, Julian. 1980. *Evolution: The modern synthesis.* London: Allen & Unwin, 1942.

Landecker, Hannah. 1999. Between beneficence and chattel: The human biological in law and science. *Science in Context* 12, 1:203–225.

———. 2007. *Culturing life: How cells became technologies.* Cambridge, MA: Harvard University Press.

Lee, Sandra Soo-Jin, et al. 2008. The ethics of characterizing difference: Guiding principles on using racial categories in human genetics. *Genome Biology* 9:404.2.

Mayr, Ernst, and William B. Provine, eds. 1980. *The Evolutionary Synthesis: Perspectives on the unification of biology.* Cambridge, MA: Harvard University Press.

Mitchell, Robert. 2001. Owning shit: Commodification and body wastes. *Bad Subjects* 55 (March), eserver.org/bs/55; and the expanded version, $ell: Body wastes, information, and commodities. 2004. In *Data made flesh: Embodying information,* edited by Robert Mitchell and Phillip Thurtle, 121–136. New York: Routledge.

———. 2006. The rhetorical ecology of "dignity," "waste," and "information" in U.S. tissue economies. In *Tissue economies: Blood, organs, and cell lines in late capitalism,* edited by Catherine Waldby and Robert Mitchell. Durham, NC: Duke University Press.

———. 2007. Sacrifice, individuation, and the economies of genomics. *Literature and Medicine* 26.1 (Spring):126–158.

Patterson, Orlando. 1982. *Slavery and social death: A comparative study.* Cambridge, MA: Harvard University Press.

Rabinow, Paul. 1996. *Making PCR: A story of biotechnology.* Chicago: University of Chicago Press.

———. 1999. *French DNA: Trouble in purgatory.* Chicago: University of Chicago Press.

———. 2003. *Anthropos today: Reflections on modern equipment.* Princeton, NJ: Princeton University Press.

Rabinow, Paul, and Nikolas Rose. 2006. Biopower today. *Biosocieties* 1:195–217.

Rajan, Kaushik Sunder. 2006. *Biocapital: The constitution of postgenomic life.* Durham, NC: Duke University Press.

———. 2010. *Biomedicalization: Technoscience, health, and illness in the U.S.,* edited by Adele E. Clarke, Laura Mamo, Jennifer Ruth Fosket, Jennifer R. Fishman, and Janet K. Shim. Durham, NC: Duke University Press.

Reardon, Jennifer. 2004. *Race to the finish: Identity and governance in an age of genomics.* Princeton, NJ: Princeton University Press.

Rose, Nikolas. 2007. *The politics of life itself: Biomedicine, power, and subjectivity in the twenty-first century.* Princeton, NJ: Princeton University Press.

Skloot, Rebecca. 2009. *The immortal life of Henrietta Lacks.* New York: Crown Publishers.

Taylor, Sam. 1997. *The Observer* (March 16), 81.

Wald, Priscilla. 2005. What's in a cell?: John Moore's spleen and the language of bioslavery. *New Literary History: Essays Probing the Boundaries of the Human in Science and Science Fiction* (special issue) 36.2 (Spring):205–225.

———. 2006. Blood and stories: How genomics is rewriting race, medicine, and human history. *Patterns of Prejudice* 40.4–5 (September/December):303–333.

Washington, Harriet A. 2006. *Medical apartheid: The dark history of medical experimentation on black Americans from colonial times to the present.* New York: Doubleday.

Weasel, Lisa H. Feminist intersections in science: Race, gender, and sexuality through the microscope. *Hypatia* 19.1 (Winter 2004):183–193.

15

The Case of the Genetic Ancestor

JENNIFER A. HAMILTON

DNA is a very powerful and reasonably priced tool, and is the only true answer to positively proving our roots.–DNA Heritage customer, www .dnaheritage.com, accessed May 25, 2006.

As usual, Nancy was intrigued at any hint of a mystery. She studied the row of odd figures. Suddenly it dawned on her that they might be a message in code!–*The Secret of Red Gate Farm* (A Nancy Drew Mystery)

I begin this chapter with reference to the now iconic figure of Nancy Drew, fictional American girl sleuth extraordinaire. In her blue convertible and cashmere twin sets, she follows clues, relies on her power of deductive reasoning, pieces together evidence, and solves the mystery. Against the backdrop of moss-covered mansions and dusty attics, Nancy looks for secrets in old clocks, hidden staircases, missing maps, ciphers, and secret diaries. As each story progresses, readers experience a little thrill as connections emerge and pieces begin to fall into place, a sense of satisfaction as the narrative of a crime or the details of a deeply hidden family secret begin to emerge. Following clues and interpreting their meanings, Nancy brings to light things hidden, haunted, unknown, and forgotten, usually to the great joy of those she chooses to help (and much to the chagrin of local miscreants). Though her methods are decidedly low-tech by modern standards,[1] Nancy's sleuthing restores a kind of social order, effectively making sense of the past and the wrongs committed then, and creating a clear and just path forward for the future.

But let us now imagine that Nancy is at the center of a new twenty-first century mystery, a mystery in which contentious questions about relatedness, injury, citizenship, and justice are reframed within a logic of genetics. In this new mystery, that we might call *The Case of the Genetic Ancestor*, the key parts of the story revolve around an emergent technology, genetic ancestry tracing (GAT). Also called genetic genealogy, GAT is an increasingly popular commercial venture that markets DNA tests as "powerful tools for inferring human population history, exploring genealogy and estimating individual ancestry" (Shriver and Kittles

2004:611). Encompassing a series of technologies originally developed in the context of population genetics, GAT purports to link individual genotypes to genetic—more recently called *biogeographical*—ancestries, roughly defined as African, European, Asian, and Amerindian (Johnston and Thomas 2003; Shriver and Kittles 2004). With slogans such as "History unearthed daily" (Family Tree DNA), "Trace your DNA. Find your roots" (African Ancestry), and "Your ancestry discovered" (Roots for Real), genetic ancestry companies appeal to both the already well-established hobby of genealogical research (family trees) and the increasing interest in "genetic origins" (Nash 2002; Nash 2004).

During the past several years, GAT has been featured prominently in the media and has captured the public imagination, especially in the United States. Since 2005, the *New York Times* alone has run dozens of stories discussing genetic ancestry. PBS recently aired its second installment of *African American Lives*, a documentary in part featuring high-profile African Americans discussing the role and meaning of DNA-tracing technologies in constructing their family genealogies. Yet questions of genetic ancestry have not been limited to the realm of "recreational genomics," but have taken on important social, political, and legal dimensions. For instance, in April 2006, the *Times* published an article—later widely circulated—about genetic ancestry tracing technologies and some of their emergent uses in the United States. The article provocatively suggested that genetic ancestry could be used as proof in identity-based claims such as affirmative action benefits or membership in an American Indian tribe. This triggered further discussion about the relationship between race and genetics (Harmon 2006). In response to this growing interest among consumers as well as a growing awareness of the potential political implications of these technologies, experts have written a series of cautionary pieces about GAT (Bandelt et al. 2008; Bolnick et al. 2007; Greely 2008; Lee et al. 2009). And in late 2008, the American Society of Human Genetics issued a set of recommendations, warning consumers about the problematic scientific bases of these technologies and citing concerns about the validity and utility of the information (ashg.org/pdf/ASHGAncestry TestingStatement_FINAL.pdf, accessed February 16, 2011). Host of *African American Lives*, Harvard professor Henry Louis Gates Jr. tried different tests from several companies and was surprised to find that different companies yielded different results, spurring him to create a new company (Winstein 2007). Yet despite these controversies and concerns, consumers are using GAT technologies with increasing frequency, and these technologies have become a standard part of the already popular hobby of personal genealogical research.[2] The increasingly widespread use of GAT, especially in the United States, demonstrates the appeal of these tools, and work exploring how people use and understand them is moving forward (Nash 2006; Nash 2007; Nelson 2008a; Nelson 2008b).

GAT technologies promise to shed light on, while perhaps not definitively to solve, questions of ancestry, belonging, and kinship. Who am I? Where do I come

from? Who are my people? Where do I belong? Given the centrality of these questions to an American cultural imagination, it is perhaps not surprising that
genetic genealogy has spread beyond the confines of recreational genomics and
into the realm of law. GAT technologies have emerged as potential evidentiary
tools in a series of legal cases, cases broadly involving issues of race and identity
in U.S. courts. This chapter examines two of these cases, what I call "cases of the
genetic ancestor." In particular, I explore two examples in which GAT has been
tentatively used in legal disputes, disputes in which plaintiffs invoke the figure of
a genetic ancestor to make marginal histories relevant in the legal realm.

In the first case, a group of African American plaintiffs attempted to use
genetic ancestry tracing technologies to bolster their legal right to litigate a slavery reparations case in federal court.[3] By providing results from GAT tests to the
court, the Farmer-Paellmann plaintiffs challenged an earlier ruling that denied
them "standing," a legal principle that determines whether or not someone has
the right to initiate a lawsuit.[4] Through an appeal to genetic ancestry, the plaintiffs tried to constitute a particular kind of legal subjectivity that would be cognizable to the court.

In the second case, the Freedmen of Oklahoma, also known as "Black Indians,"
appealed to GAT in their battle with both the federal Bureau of Indian Affairs (BIA)
and various tribal governments to be recognized as tribal citizens. The Freedmen
are the descendents of enslaved Africans and members of the "Five Civilized
Tribes" (Cherokee, Chickasaw, Choctaw, Creek, and Seminole) who were forcibly
relocated to Oklahoma during the Trail of Tears in the early part of the nineteenth
century (Ehle 1997). While since the late nineteenth century, the federal government has considered certain Freedmen to be members of these tribes, based on
post-Civil War treaties, contemporary tribes have a legal right to determine their
membership requirements, a right recognized by the United States Supreme
Court.[5] Recently, some of these tribes, most famously the Cherokee Nation of
Oklahoma, have reconfigured their membership requirements in ways that
remove some Freedmen from tribal rolls. In particular, the tribal government
now requires that members be able to trace their direct lineage to an ancestor
included in an early twentieth century census, the Dawes Rolls. In response, some
of the Freedmen are challenging the legality of these reconfigurations in a variety
of legal spheres and have appealed to genetic ancestry tracing technologies to
demonstrate the presence of "Indian blood" (Koerner 2005).

Thus, I examine two cases wherein the "genetic ancestor" is constituted in
law as a way to configure, in the present, legitimate, legally cognizable subjects,
who can make claims to rights and benefits under the law. I look at GAT technologies as a way to explore the use of genetic knowledge to bolster legal claims by
considering the processes of subject formation in both genetics and law. I begin
with the premise that such legal claims embody the epistemic commitments of
agents as well as the complex interplay among norms, practices, and subjectivities. More specifically, I focus on how existing legal subjectivities and emergent

genetic ones overlap and coalesce in ways that reveal connections among broader fields of inquiry and domains of knowledge, including bioscience, biomedicine, kinship, ethics, and, of course, the law. Moreover, as we shall see, the genetic ancestor looms large in ways that are deeply connected to both historical and the contemporary understandings of race in the United States.

The Genetic Ancestor

But what or who is the genetic ancestor? Or, to reinvoke the figure of Nancy Drew, what is the "message in the code," and how do we decipher it? The genetic ancestor, in these cases, is not a specific historical person, but rather a figure forged out of genomic science and animated in the realm of law. It leaves clues to its identity in DNA, which, when uncovered, seem to supplant older notions, like phenotype and blood quantum, with a new and ostensibly legitimate, objective, and quantifiable science. The genetic ancestor promises to right the wrongs of the past and allow for a more just future. Yet, an analysis of these cases suggests that the genetic ancestor is a more complex and problematic figure than might first appear.

In 2004, the legal scholar Alain Pottage provocatively argued that law is the original biotechnology. This contention makes apparent the close relationship between Western cultural notions of biology and relatedness on the one hand and the codification of these categories in both law and science on the other. As Pottage asserts, "The question which at once associates and distinguishes law and biotechnology is the question of how law and life, or the social and the biological, are bound together" (Pottage 2004:255). In this scheme, the legal and scientific figure of the genetic ancestor is more than simply a reflection of a natural order, more than a discovery of that which already exists. It is, instead, a figure that is created, by both law and science, in such a way that they mutually reinforce and naturalize each other.

As a result, the science is designed in such a way that it cannot help but naturalize the legal, creating a continually naturalized legal/scientific notion of ancestry. The genetic ancestor, then, is not simply a figure discovered by genomic science and integrated into law, but is, rather, an assemblage materialized at the intersection of legal and scientific practice.

When we seek to uncover the genetic ancestor, we are already engaged with Western notions of biology and kinship that have been encoded not only in law but also in science. To put it another way, the genetic ancestor is not the mere result of consumer genetics, shaped by available scientific knowledge and creatively engaged by plaintiffs to strengthen their legal claims. It is, in fact, a much more complicated entity, created and constantly renegotiated by the longstanding interplay of science and law.

The Case of the Genetic Ancestor: Farmer-Paellmann

In early 2004, a U.S. District Court judge in Illinois dismissed an African American slavery reparations lawsuit asserting, in part, that the plaintiffs lacked sufficient legal standing to bring the suit.[6] The plaintiffs, "on behalf of themselves and their enslaved ancestors, and all other persons similarly situated,"[7] sought reparations from "blue chip U.S. corporations [that] benefited and continued to benefit from acts including piracy, slavery, torture, rape, murder, theft of property and services, and other human rights violations."[8] According to the plaintiffs, these corporate defendants and their predecessor companies—representing the financial, insurance, transportation, and raw materials industries—were for generations "unjustly enriched" by their participation in the Trans-Atlantic slave trade. The plaintiffs further alleged that by owning slaves, using slave labor, and financing and insuring various aspects of the slave trade, these companies and their predecessors not only violated international law and amassed enormous wealth, but also contributed to the creation of a fundamentally unequal America, based on race, a nation whose racial inequalities continue to differently shape experiences and opportunities for its African American citizens.

While Judge Charles Norgle argued that "[i]t is beyond debate that slavery has caused tremendous suffering and ineliminable scars throughout our Nation's history," he nevertheless maintained that the "Plaintiffs' claims . . . fail based on numerous well-settled legal principles."[9] In concert with many of the arguments submitted by the defendants, Norgle dismissed the lawsuit, asserting that the Plaintiffs' "Complaint is *devoid of any allegations that connect the specifically named Defendants or their predecessors and any of the Plaintiffs or their ancestors.*"[10] Essentially, because the plaintiffs could not make a legally cognizable claim that they had personally suffered at the hands of the defendants (nor could they demonstrate appropriate relatedness to an ancestor who had), Norgle asserted that their claim was insufficient to invoke federal judicial action. He similarly argued that the statute of limitations on such a suit was long past and that the courts were an inappropriate venue for what were, at heart, "political questions."

According to Norgle, the plaintiffs' claims were "conjectural and hypothetical" because they had not "personally suffered a concrete and particularized injury as a result of the Defendants' putatively illegal conduct."[11] Norgle asserted that the plaintiffs could not satisfy the basic requirements of standing because they could not "establish a personal injury sufficient to confer standing by merely alleging some genealogical relationship to African-Americans held in slavery over one-hundred, two-hundred, or three-hundred years ago."[12]

It is at this point in the litigation process that genetic ancestry tracing makes its appearance. Shortly after the judge's dismissal in 2004, lead plaintiff Deadria Farmer-Paellmann filed a new slavery reparations suit, this time in the state of New York, against three companies named in the original complaint—FleetBoston, Lloyd's of London, and R. J. Reynolds Tobacco.[13] In an attempt to address some of the legal shortcomings identified by Norgle in his dismissal of their initial lawsuit, Farmer-Paellmann and the other plaintiffs reformulated their claim not in terms of "unjust enrichment," but in terms of *genocide.* The plaintiffs employed the technology of genetic ancestry tracing in support of their legal claims, arguing that they are direct, *genetic* descendants of former slaves imported from Africa and exploited by early U.S. companies, who are the corporate progenitors of the defendants. Plaintiffs sought to firmly establish (rather than "merely alleging") a *gene*-alogical relationship to their enslaved ancestors by introducing genetic ancestry tracing in a court of law.[14]

The plaintiffs had compellingly argued that their case was hindered, not only because of the sheer lack of archival evidence concerning their enslaved ancestors, but also because the defendants had purposefully withheld, and in some cases destroyed, records and other key documents that might have been used to establish some kind of genealogical relationship. In *Farmer-Paellmann,* the plaintiffs attempted to address these concerns by demonstrating their "specific connection," using genetic ancestry tracing. They argued that "scientific testing in the form of DNA testing has proven beyond a doubt the direct relationship between the instant plaintiffs and the instant defendants."[15]

Deadria Farmer-Paellmann and the other plaintiffs in the 2004 reparations suit availed themselves of the services of *African Ancestry*, a genetic ancestry tracing company, and proposed to use the results as a way of addressing the issues of legal standing articulated by Judge Norgle. Plaintiff Farmer-Paellmann argues that, through her mtDNA, she is a "direct descendant of persons from the Mende tribe in Sierra Leone."[16] In so doing, she articulates a *genetic* kinship to a contemporary group as an attempt to make a legally cognizable connection. What is especially novel about this claim is that, while it relies on genetic technology, it is outside of the usual purview of court-sanctioned DNA applications that link one individual to a particular sample or to another *individual*—think, for example, of paternity tests and DNA fingerprinting. I suggest that what the genetic ancestry claim does in part is attempt to forge a certain kind of collective identity—an identity that U.S. courts have been traditionally unable or unwilling to accommodate within the framework of civil law—in the more familiar idiom of kinship, genetics, and, indeed, *race.*

The Case of the Genetic Ancestor: Freedmen of Oklahoma

The legal history of Indian identity in the United States is both complex and often contradictory. "Who is an Indian?" has been a key question in the United States throughout its history, but especially since the mid-nineteenth century (Brownell 2001; Hamilton 2008; Meyer 1999:234). While the question "Who is an Indian?" and, by extension, who is not, is not an exclusively legal one, it has nevertheless dominated questions of federal Indian law. At various times throughout U.S. legal history, establishing who is and is not Indian has been central to determining collective and individual identities. These identities are, in turn, tied to questions of land and resource distribution, property, inheritance, treaty payments, state and federal benefits, civil and criminal jurisdiction, tribal membership, and certain political rights (Biolsi 2001; Ray 2006; Turner Strong and Van Winkle 1996).

Arguably one of the most salient aspects of Indian legal identity in the United States has been, and continues to be, "blood quantum." Determination of Indian identity both politically and culturally is often based on blood quantum, usually a measurement of "how much" of an individual's "blood" (as a unit of heredity) has been inherited from Indian ancestors. While concepts of blood quantum have evolved over time, and they vary throughout the United States, they have nevertheless been consistently associated with extant and emergent ideas of race in American society (Garroutte 2003; Kauanui 2008; Spruhan 2006).[17]

In the first part of the twenty-first century, a range of disputes around tribal membership practices have emerged, and questions about who is an Indian continue to be important in Indian country. One of the most famous involves running disputes between the Freedmen of Oklahoma and the tribal governments of the Five Civilized Tribes. Recently, some of these tribes, including the Cherokee Nation of Oklahoma, which will be focus of this section, have reconfigured their membership requirements in ways that remove some Freedmen from tribal rolls. In response, some of the Freedmen are challenging the legality of these reconfigurations in a variety of legal spheres and have appealed to genetic ancestry tracing technologies to demonstrate the presence of "Indian blood" (Johnston 2003; Kaplan 2005; Koerner 2005).

Much of the mainstream media discussion has linked "disenrollment" practices among Indian tribes to the development of legal gaming on reservations in the latter part of the twentieth century. While it is certainly true that tribal gaming has substantially shifted political and economic relations both on and off the reservation (Cattelino 2008), anthropologist Circe Sturm suggests that contemporary attempts at disenrollment reference a more complex and contentious racial and judicial history, implicating issues around treaty rights, land ownership, and the reach of tribal governance (Sturm 2002).

To determine membership, tribes in Oklahoma currently rely on early twentieth century documents produced by the U.S. government: the Dawes Rolls. These rolls were a bureaucratic technology that emerged from the passage of the Dawes Act, also known as the General Allotment Act, in 1887. This policy emerged as part of the federal government's attempt to extinguish Indian to title the land and to implement a "civilizing" system through which any collective systems of land ownership were dismantled and Indians (and by extension the Freedmen) were given individual plots of land in order to practice agriculture. Historians typically understand the Dawes Act as a major and overwhelmingly negative moment for American Indians in the United States, for, in addition to its often devastating effects on the traditional lifeways of American Indians, the Dawes Act also served as a key technology for the widespread dispossession of them from their lands (Carter 1999; McLaughlin 1996).

The purpose of the Dawes Rolls was in part to determine who counted as "Indian" (and who did not) in order to distribute individual land holdings. Bureaucrats determined the composition of the Dawes Rolls based on their interpretation of "phenotypic" features and whether or not individuals appeared to as "African" or "Indian," regardless of an individual's family history (that is the presence of "full-blooded" Indian relatives) or cultural affiliation (Sturm 2002). Thus, bureaucrats relied on counting and racial categorization; these "technologies" were deeply implicated in the distribution of resources and had implications for those categorized and their descendants beyond what anyone could have imagined.

In their contemporary incarnations, tribal citizen requirements in Oklahoma generally rest on whether or not an individual can trace a direct descent from an "Indian by Blood" listed on the Dawes Rolls. Clearly, such cases intersect with older legal discourses and practices. Despite their longstanding membership in the various Oklahoma tribes, the Freedmen are now often denied tribal citizenship because they were not classified as "Indian by blood" on the nineteenth-century rolls.

In addition to a variety of lawsuits and other legal measures in both federal and tribal courts, some of the Freedmen plaintiffs also employed genetic ancestry tracing as a potential way to bolster their claims to tribal citizenship (Kaplan 2005; Koerner 2005; Johnston 2003; Robinson 2010). In 2004, geneticist and co-founder of *African Ancestry*, Rick Kittles, approached some of the Freedmen with an offer to perform genetic ancestry tests at no cost to them, in order to determine the percentage of "Indian blood." As Freedmen plaintiff Marilyn Vann expressed: "It's important that we be able to establish that we are Indian people, not just African people who were adopted into the tribe. . . . If you're the average tribal member, you don't want to be discriminated against because you look Indian. So how can you discriminate against other people just because they have some African features?" (cited in Koerner 2005). Yet, in widely reported findings, Kittles expressed both surprise and disappointment that genetic markers characterized as "Native American" were not especially prevalent among the tested Freedmen and that the percentage of Native American "genes" were substantially lower than the 20 percent he anticipated (Kaplan 2005; Koerner 2005). Instead, the percentages ranged from 3 percent to 6 percent, a result that Kittles implies is less compelling. Nevertheless, some of the Freedmen have understood these results as bolstering their claims, especially because this evidence supports rather than contradicts their family histories, both written and oral (Kaplan 2005).

Thus far, genetic ancestry claims have not been particularly successful, both because the results of the tests themselves have been equivocal and because tribal leaders have continued to rely on the Dawes Rolls as the defining criterion of citizenship:

> Our citizenship laws require you to have a Cherokee ancestor who was on the Dawes Roll. Can a DNA sample prove that? . . . If I did a DNA test, it might show that I have some German DNA. That doesn't mean I could go back to Germany and say, I have German ancestry and I would like to be a German citizen.—Cherokee spokesperson Mike Miller. (cited in Koerner 2005)

Whether or not the Freedmen's claim to citizenship in the Cherokee Nation is analogous to Miller's German example is debatable. Nevertheless, his analogy is a powerful reminder of the political and legal status of American Indian tribes in the United States and the exclusive right of tribal governments to determine membership criteria.

Mainstream media reports have generally been sympathetic to the cause of the Freedmen. Brendan Koerner's 2005 piece in *Wired Magazine* has been especially influential, and the photographs of individuals who are and are not legitimate members of the Cherokee Nation have become iconic of the racial politics of the issue. Vann's earlier reference to discrimination based on "some African features," suggests that a key dimension of the genetic ancestry tests is to challenge assumptions about phenotype through appeal to genotype. The tribal government of the Cherokee Nation vehemently denies that blackness is any kind of factor in determining membership: "The Cherokee Nation is a great Indian nation that embraces our mixed-race heritage. . . . Our sole purpose is to weave together a great Indian nation, made up of many ethnic groups which are knit together through one common cultural thread—a shared bond to an Indian ancestor on the base roll" (freedmen.cherokee.org/; accessed November 24, 2009). A key insight about race in Indian country is that the shape of American Indian national identities cannot be understood outside of the emergence of dominant national identities and the racial logics that shape this process (Sturm 2002). In other words, the contemporary logics of indigeneity cannot be understood outside of the twin poles of whiteness and blackness that influence the contours of race in the United States. The genetic ancestor is, of course, also a part of such logics. As we will see in the following section, genetic ancestry has become somewhat of a proving ground for legal identity, although what it means to "prove" is not at all clear.

GAT: The Proving Ground for Legal Identity?

What would Nancy Drew make of *The Case of the Genetic Ancestor*? In what ways is DNA analogous to old clocks, hidden staircases, missing maps, ciphers, and secret diaries? What assumptions and aspirations are embedded, or perhaps embodied, in these appeals to genetic ancestry? The way these technologies have been tentatively used in the cases presented here simultaneously suggests something about the power of these technologies and about the role of DNA in reworking and rewriting marginal histories (and the present) of race in America. Unlike some of the other prominent uses of DNA technologies (for example, forensic investigations or paternity), in both of these cases, we are asking GAT technologies in some ways to tell us things we already know. In other words, the kinds of "facts" that GAT can determine, shed light on, prove or disprove, are often facts that either are not in dispute or are not verifiable in conventional ways. These are what Agamben calls the "aporia of historical knowledge": "a non-coincidence between facts and truth, between verification and comprehension" (2000:12).

Thus, we must ask what kinds of work GAT technologies are performing in these legal contexts. Or, another, slightly different formulation is to ask what do we already know that we are asking GAT to do?

In the *Farmer-Paellmann* case, that the plaintiffs are the descendants of enslaved Africans is not in dispute. Rather, the legal dispute hinges on whether or not the plaintiffs can demonstrate a legally cognizable relationship with their ancestors sufficient to establish standing in order to bring a civil suit against a series of corporate defendants. In the case of the Oklahoma Freedmen, the status of the plaintiffs/complainants as Freedmen is also not in dispute. That some people self-identify as Cherokee and can demonstrate kin relationships to shared tribal ancestors in a variety of ways (for example, official documents, family genealogies, oral and written histories) is also not in dispute. Thus, GAT technologies are not used to establish certain kinds of "facts," but are rather used to create a kind of legal subjectivity that is legitimate to make the claim in legal spaces.

These cases leave us, then, with more questions than answers about the role of GAT in law. Why does genetics resonate so profoundly with people seeking to establish legal identities? And, more generally, what can further investigation into the genetic ancestor tell us about the operation of kinship, history, belonging, and law?

One of the most compelling aspects of GAT technologies for users is that they seem to have the potential to fill deep lacunae in the written historical record. For many African Americans in particular, the absence of genealogical records, due to the legacy of slavery, make GAT an almost indispensable tool for tracing personal histories. DNA in these scenarios takes on the role of archive in a language of kinship. Additionally, both of these (archive and kinship) are extraordinarily important dimensions of evidentiary support in Anglo-American law. One of the key processes here is the transformative attempt to make GAT speak to the courts in a legally cognizable way. Genes have long been understood in terms of blueprints, as an underlying code and plan that structure living things and life itself. Yet, if we think about genes as "relics as well as blueprints" (Wasserman 2003:45), potential relationships among DNA, race, and history come into focus.

What can we make of the figure of the genetic ancestor in scenarios like those I have described, scenarios that could be described as a "genetico-legal" politics of recognition? Additionally, what are we to make of what are arguably socially and legally progressive claims and the "meaningfulness" of biology in an age of social constructivism? Anthropologist Marilyn Strathern contends that "[c]hanges in the ethical terrain with which science operates have been going on all the time, until we suddenly find ourselves on a 'new' social map that needs interpretation" (2002:985). The cases of the genetic ancestor begin to reveal the contours of such a map and open up space for further investigation.

Scholars in the fields of legal studies as well in science and technology studies have independently argued that the social is not merely refracted through legal or scientific technologies, but is rather already embedded within them. How might we extend these insights by showing the ways in which "the case of the genetic ancestor" brings these fields and these insights into conversation with one another? As issues of race, ethnicity, and indeed indigeneity are becoming newly entangled with contemporary ideas of the genetic (TallBear 2003; 2007), how are long-circulating idioms of racial science marshaled and reinvigorated in discourses of law and genetics?

That the tests themselves are deeply problematic and that their accuracy is at best debatable and contested, although important, is not the key issue explored in this chapter. Instead, I point to these cases of the genetic ancestor as indicators of how kinship, collectivities, and a politics of recognition are being tentatively reconfigured in the twenty-first century.

Earlier, I posed the question about what genes represent and embody in these cases of the genetic ancestor. How can we read the case of the genetic ancestor as a palimpsest that reveals historical assumptions and motivates contemporary readings of race, genetics, and law? In closing, I want to suggest that genetic ancestry tracing, with its attendant conceptions of biogenetic kinship, is being used to produce new configurations of politically and legally cognizable (af)filiation within a broader political economy of recognition (Faubion and Hamilton 2007). The specific contours of these configurations remain to be seen.

ACKNOWLEDGMENTS

I would like to thank the editors of this volume for their invitation to participate in such a rich conversation and for their support in bringing this chapter to print. David Delaney and Sally Merry offered thoughtful comments on the manuscript at the Northeast Law & Society Association Meeting in 2010. Special thanks to Alondra Nelson and Jacob Speaks for their careful reading and editorial advice.

NOTES

1. And despite jokes about the admissibility of Drew's evidence in twenty-first-century legal frameworks: "New DNA Evidence Forces Investigators to Reopen Nancy Drew Mystery," *The Onion,* www.theonion.com/content/radio_news/new_dna_evidence_forces [Accessed November 13, 2009].

2. See, for instance, the incredible success of Gates' own television series and more recently, actor Isaiah Washington's acceptance of citizenship in Sierra Leone, based in part on his results from a GAT test: www.gondobaymangafoundation.org/#/home/; edition.cnn.com/2009/WORLD/africa/05/03/av.isaiahwashington/index.html [Accessed November 29, 2009].

3. *Farmer-Paellmann v. FleetBoston,* Complaint with Jury Demand, 04 CV 2430.

4. "A party seeking to demonstrate standing must be able to show the court sufficient connection to and harm from the law or action challenged." definitions.uslegal .com/s/standing/ [Accessed September 9, 2010].

5. *Santa Clara Pueblo v. Martinez,* 436 U.S. 49 (1978).

6. *In Re African-American Slave Descendants Litigation,* 272 F. Supp. 2d 755, 2003 U.S. Dist. 12634.7. *In Re African-American Slave Descendants Litigation,* First Amended and Consolidated Complaint (FACC), p. 5.

8. FACC, p. 8.

9. *In Re African-American Slave Descendants Litigation*, Judge's Opinion and Order, p. 73.

10. Judge's Opinion and Order, p. 16; my emphasis.

11. Judge's Opinion and Order, p. 27.

12. Judge's Opinion and Order, p. 34.

13. *Farmer-Paellmann* v. *FleetBoston*, Complaint with Jury Demand, 04 CV 2430.

14. To my knowledge, the *Farmer-Paellmann* case was the first to introduce genetic ancestry tracing as evidence in a U.S. court.

15. *African American Genocide & DNA Case*, pp. 15–16.

16. *African American Genocide & DNA Case*, p. 7.

17. Such practices include, for instance, the similarity of measurements like "blood quantum" (an older method largely imposed on tribes to determine membership and to regulate the distribution of land and resources) and "genetic ancestry."

WORKS CITED

Agamben, Giorgio. 2000. *Remnants of Auschwitz: The witness and the archive.* New York: Zone Books.

Alsever, Jennifer. 2006. DNA kits aim to link you to the here and then. *New York Times,* February 5.

Bandelt, Hans-Jürgen, Yong-Gang Yao, et al. 2008. The brave new era of human genetic testing. *Bioessays* 30 (11–12):1246–1251.

Biolsi, Thomas. 2001. *Deadliest enemies: Law and the making of race relations on and off Rosebud Reservation.* Berkeley: University of California Press.

Bolnick, Deborah A., Duana Fullwiley, et al. 2007. The science and business of genetic ancestry testing. *Science* 318 (5849):399–400.

Brownell, Margo. 2001. Who is an Indian?: Searching for an answer to the question at the core of federal Indian law. *University of Michigan Journal of Law Reform* 34:275.

Carter, Kent. 1999. *The Dawes Commission and the allotment of the Five Civilized Tribes, 1893–1914.* Orem, Utah: Ancestry.com.

Cattelino, Jessica. 2008. *High stakes: Florida Seminole gaming and sovereignty.* Durham, NC: Duke University Press.

Faubion, James D., and Jennifer A. Hamilton. 2007. Sumptuary kinship. *Anthropological Quarterly* 80 (3):553–559.

Garroutte, Eva Marie. 2003. *Real Indians: Identity and the survival of Native America.* Berkeley: University of California Press.

Greely, Henry T. 2008. Genetic genealogy: Genetics meets the marketplace. In *Revisiting Race in a Genomic Age,* edited by B. A. Koenig, S. S.-J. Lee, and S. S. Richardson, 215–234. New Brunswick, NJ: Rutgers University Press.

Hamilton, Jennifer A. 2008. Of Caucasoids and kin: Kennewick Man, race, and genetic indigeneity in *Bonnichsen v. United States.* In *Indigeneity in the courtroom: Law, culture, and the production of difference in North American courts,* 71–88. New York: Routledge.

Harmon, Amy. 2006. Seeking ancestry in DNA ties uncovered by tests. *New York Times,* April 12.

Heffernan, Virginia. 2006. Taking black family trees out of slavery's shadow. *New York Times,* February 1.

Johnston, J., and M. Thomas. 2003. Summary: The science of genealogy by genetics. *Developing World Bioethics* 3(2):103–108.

Johnston, Josephine. 2003. Resisting a genetic identity: The Black Seminoles and genetic tests of ancestry. *Journal of Law, Medicine and Ethics* 31 (2):262–271.

Kauanui, J. Kehaulani. 2008. *Hawaiian blood: Colonialism and the politics of sovereignty and indigeneity.* Durham, NC: Duke University Press.

Koerner, Brendan I. 2005. Blood feud. www.wired.com/wired/archive/13.09/seminoles.html [Accessed Aug 27, 2009].

Lee, S. S., D. A. Bolnick, et al. 2009 Genetics: The illusive gold standard in genetic ancestry testing. *Science* 325 (5936):38–39.

McLaughlin, Michael R. 1996. The Dawes Act, or Indian General Allotment Act of 1887: The continuing burden of allotment. *American Indian Culture & Research Journal* 20:59.

Meyer, Melissa L. 1999. American Indian blood quantum requirements: Blood is thicker than family. In *Over the edge: Remapping the American West*, edited by V. J. Matsumoto and B. Allmendinger, 231–252. Berkeley: University of California Press.

Nash, Catherine. 2002. Genealogical identities. *Environment and Planning D: Society & Space* 20 (1):27–52

———.2004. Genetic kinship. *Cultural Studies* 18 (1):1–33.

———.2006. Irish origins, Celtic origins. *Irish Studies Review* 14 (1):11—37.

———.2007. Mapping origins: Race and relatedness in population genetics and genetic genealogy. In *New genetics, new identities*, edited by P. Atkinson, P. E. Glasner, and H. Greenslade, 77–100. New York: Routledge.

Nelson, Alondra. 2008a. Bio science: Genetic genealogy testing and the pursuit of African ancestry. *Social Studies of Science* 38 (5):759–783.

———. 2008b. The factness of diaspora: The social sources of genetic genealogy. In *Revisiting race in a genomic age, edited by* B. A. Koenig, S. S.-J. Lee, and S. S. Richardson, 253–268. New Brunswick, NJ: Rutgers University Press.

Pálsson, Gísli. 2002. The life of family trees and the book of Icelanders. *Medical Anthropology* 21 (3–4):337–367.

Ray, Alan S. 2006. Native American identity and the challenge of Kennewick Man. *Temple Law Review* 79:89–154.

Robinson, Judy Gibbs, Freedmen's descendants discover past. *The Oklahoman,* cacreview .blogspot.com/2005/06/freedmen-descendants-use-dna-to-show.html   [Accessed January 13, 2010].

Shriver, M. D., and R. A. Kittles. 2004. Opinion: Genetic ancestry and the search for personalized Genetic histories. *Nature Reviews Genetics* 5 (8):611–618.

Spruhan, Paul. 2006. A legal history of blood quantum in federal Indian law to 1935. *South Dakota Law Review* 51:1–50.

Strathern, Marilyn. 2002. Still giving nature a helping hand? Surrogacy: A debate about technology and society. *Journal of Molecular Biology* 319 (4):985–993.

Sturm, Circe. 2002. *Blood politics: Race, culture, and identity in the Cherokee Nation of Oklahoma.* Berkeley: University of California Press.

TallBear, Kimberly. 2003. DNA, blood, and racializing the tribe. *Wicazo Sa Review* 18 (1):81–107.

———. 2007. Narratives of race and indigeneity in the Genographic Project. *Journal of Law, Medicine & Ethics* 35 (3):412–424.

Turner Strong, Pauline, and Barrik Van Winkle. 1996. "Indian blood": Reflections on the reckoning and refiguring of Native North American identity. *Cultural Anthropology* 11 (4):30.

Wade, Nicholas. 2006a. If Irish claim nobility, science may approve. *New York Times,* January 18.

———. 2006b. New light on origins of Ashkenazi in Europe. *New York Times,* January 14.

Winstein, Keith J. 2007. Harvard's Gates refines genetic-ancestry searches for blacks. *Wall Street Journal* Online, November 15.

16

‧‧

Making Sense of Genetics, Culture, and History

A Case Study of a Native Youth Education Program

MICHELLE M. JACOB

To be an Indian in modern American society is in a very real sense to be unreal and ahistorical.–Vine Deloria, Jr., *Custer Died for Your Sins*

In recent years Native peoples, who have land-based identities, find that their homelands and legal status are under assault by a genetics-based science that dismisses Native cultural beliefs as irrelevant to knowing about the past. In qualitatively studying the discourse surrounding the controversial Kennewick Man case (skeletal remains of an ancient man found in Kennewick, Washington), as taught during a contemporary Native youth education program, complexities of the relationships among indigenous culture, legal status, genetics, and history are revealed.

This chapter examines the stakes of genetic analysis from the perspective of Native peoples, and concludes with a discussion of how Native peoples and non-Native teachers, including youth, interpret genetic information to make claims relating to their homeland. The chapter concludes that an "intercultural framework" is needed in order to simultaneously advance a genetic scientific enterprise and protect indigenous cultures.

Culture and Identity

Native peoples have land-based identities. In diverse religious and cultural ceremonies a special recognition is given to the indigenous homeland that has sustained Native peoples for countless generations. In tribal communities, knowing one's roots in the land is an important aspect of identity formation. "Where are you from?" is a question that is commonly asked (Smith 2001). To know where one is from, to know the land, the mountains, rivers, foods, is to know the people. Land is the backbone of Native identity. Native peoples, as the first peoples in what is now the United States, believe that they were placed on their homeland by the Creator. Surviving the multiple onslaughts of discovery, missionization, colonization, genocide, and assimilation policies, Native peoples persist in their efforts to exist as indigenous peoples, with cultures that continue to teach of their land-based identity, passed down from generation to generation through the traditional mechanisms of oral tribal histories, songs, and ceremonies (Connolly Miskwish 2007; Hunn 1990).

In contrast, the rising influence of genetic information tells another, sometimes starkly contrary, story about identity: one that is rooted in scientific testing of genes and explanations derived from large databases of evidence from scattered populations. In this framework, DNA test results tell who you are and where you come from. In the realm of genetics, scientists are the experts of explaining identity and history. Tribal elders' traditional knowledge systems become irrelevant or even obstructionist in this genetics enterprise. It is with this dramatic cultural conflict, of competing definitions and explanations of identity and history, that this chapter is concerned.

This chapter uses a case study of a Native education program to understand how Native peoples persist in maintaining land-based identities, and also uses the growing genetic information and its claim to explain identity and history.

My case study examines tensions surrounding the meaning of Kennewick Man in the context of the American Indian Recruitment Programs (AIR), and what that tension contributes to our understanding of identity, history, and social construction processes at work in tribal communities today. The case study of this teaching program bringing Native peoples together with non-Native teachers allows us to witness, on the ground, the collision of genetics, identity, and history, and to examine the stakes of that collision.

Constructing Identity: Culture, Race, and Power

Cultural teachings serve as the backbone of indigenous identity. However, because of a distinct political status, American Indians are not only members of a cultural group, but they are also members of sovereign Indian nations. Official enrollment practices stem from a colonial policy of the U.S. government, and continue to be administered by the Bureau of Indian Affairs (BIA). The BIA policy for enrollment criteria consists mainly of a person proving at least one-quarter blood quantum of a single Indian tribe, which is a continuance of American policies of assimilation, ideals of racial purity, and a desire to control Native peoples and lands. The ideas of blood and descent continue to influence identity politics within Indian communities. However, some tribes are resisting this government standard of racialized and bureaucratized identity. While some tribes are turning to DNA testing to "prove" who should be officially enrolled in a tribe (or disenrolled, as is sometimes the case), other tribal peoples continue to follow the more traditional cultural teachings, which dictate that identity is based on cultural knowledge and practice. This indigenous conception of identity stands in seemingly stark contrast with a genetics-based identity. The indigenous conception of identity is rooted in cultural knowledge and participation, which necessitates a group-based identity and a sense of belonging to one's homeland.

In contrast, a genetics-based explanation simply necessitates a DNA test and scientific interpretation to "prove" individual identity; there is no social or cultural relevance in such a definition of identity. As the Deloria quote that opened this chapter foreshadows, in the realm of genetics it is quite possible that Native culture and peoples themselves do not have a real or historic value in explaining history and identity.

As an ethnic studies scholar who is concerned about the well-being of indigenous peoples, I ask: What influence does genetic information have in tribal identity and history? The politics surrounding the Kennewick Man case provides some insight on this question. The racialized discourses and the warring views of history surrounding the case have sent shock waves throughout Indian Country, as DNA testing of an ancient skeleton served to undermine the legitimacy of tribal histories. This chapter also examines some of the aftermath of the Kennewick Man case.

In fall 2007, I observed a Native education program in which tribal peoples taught Native high school students about the Kennewick Man case. As part of the curriculum, the education program explicitly addressed the "threats" that genetic information may pose to tribal cultures, histories, and claims to land. In examining the education program this chapter addresses an important gap, as little is known about the ways in which Native youth participate in the social construction processes that assign meaning to identity, genetics, and history.

Truth and Science: Critical Social Theory in Marginalized Communities

The starting point of any analysis of indigenous identity, genetics, and history must begin with an analysis of the rich and diverse body of social critique that is rooted in marginalized peoples' struggles for freedom. Indigenous Studies scholars demand that theorists engage with contemporary, real-life issues that matter to indigenous peoples (Deloria 1988; Duran 2006; Smith 2001). Such arguments overlap with feminist and womanist concerns, as marginalized groups point to the "everyday world as problematic" (Smith 1987), and demand that critical social theory "speak the truth to people about the reality of their lives" (Collins 1998:198).

Patricia Hill Collins writes, in a discussion about the importance of critical social theory, "All groups need to see how their views of truth remain limited by the workings of unjust power relations" (Collins 1998:xv). This "critical perspective" is valuable in discussions about Native identities and tribal histories. Since first contact with explorers and settlers, Native peoples have seen their views of truth undermined, delegitimized, and ignored by more powerful social actors. This pattern continues into the present, with some white anthropologists still claiming greater expertise in indigenous cultural and archeological matters. For example, in Jeff Benedict's (2003) book *No Bone Unturned,* a top Smithsonian archeologist is portrayed as an American hero fighting for truth and justice in the quest to study and understand America's past. The heroic white, male anthropologist, Dr. Owsley, is introduced to readers as having his office jammed full with boxes holding human remains. Readers are expected to assume this is a good thing. Benedict tries to persuade readers of this, writing, "To Owsley the skeleton was a human being, an intimate friend whom he knew almost as well as a family member. 'You can learn more about a person from his bones than from anything else,' he said. . . . Each box represented a treasure more valuable than gold or silver. The bones, he explained, were caches of knowledge" (Benedict 2003:x). Through the course of Benedict's book we discover that Owsley is one of the main actors seeking to undermine tribal sovereignty and the Native American Graves Protection and Repatriation Act legal protections in the famed Kennewick Man case.

That Owsley feels he knows and understands Native peoples' ancestors better than Native people themselves speaks volumes about the foundation of the putatively "value neutral" and "apolitical" science of archaeology. Owsley ultimately accuses the federal government and tribes of "playing politics" when arguments are made to return Kennewick Man's remains back to the tribes who seek to protect him. He feels that repatriating the remains would be an example of tribal religious beliefs being forced on him as a scientist (Benedict 2003:238). Speaking from a privileged position, Owsley fails to understand how his training as a scientist has taught him that it is acceptable to force his beliefs onto indigenous peoples as he unearths, scrapes, ships, radiates, and studies their ancestors' bones. Thus, the idea that Native peoples do not know much about the world, history, or themselves persists when the top Smithsonian scientist works within an institution that holds over 30,000 American Indian human remains and the scientist himself "has handled more skeletons" than anyone in the world (Benedict 2003:xi), and studied as a graduate student under a professor who "had personally recovered more American Indian remains than any other anthropologist in the United States" (Benedict 2003:11). The idea that science is value-neutral, while appealing to some, is clearly part of the social and institutional "Curriculum" which Collins (1998) critiques as managing and suppressing historically oppressed groups.

Eduardo Duran argues that those who believe "science based on data is truly objective" are believing in a "misrepresentation at best," because of the historic relationship between science and racist ideologies, lack of representation of marginalized peoples in positions of power within scientific inquiry processes, and an ignorance of indigenous cultures and traditions generally among scientists (Duran 2006:8). Duran draws from Gayatri Chakravorty Spivak's (1988) notion of epistemic violence in order to understand the context and process by which white, colonial views and norms have come to dominate systems that are meant to serve Native peoples. In his work with scientists and practitioners in the health fields, Duran finds that both Natives and non-Natives are so conditioned to hegemonic power relations that oftentimes the destruction of Native families and communities is taken as an expected outcome of social and cultural behavior.

Frantz Fanon also writes about the devastating effects that colonialism has on Native peoples, "[e]very effort is made to bring the colonized person to admit the inferiority of his [sic] culture which has been transformed into instinctive patterns of behaviour, to recognize the unreality of his [sic] 'nation,' and, in the last extreme, the confused and imperfect character of his [sic] own biological structure" (Fanon 1968:45). All of these critical scholars point to the unequal power relations that continue to exist in the scientific enterprise.

Power, Resistance, and "Truth": Producing Critical Social Theory

As Collins argues, critical thinking holds tremendous potential for liberation because, "[a]lthough far too many classrooms present the Curriculum as universal truth, they simultaneously provide potential spaces of participatory democracy" (Collins 1998:xi). This critical approach guided the work with Native youth in the American Indian Recruitment Program (AIR), the afterschool program I observed in the fall of 2007. The students had never heard of NAGPRA. Thus, their combined decades of education had failed to teach them about the importance of respecting tribal traditions, customs, and ultimately repatriation. In working with the students, project staff had in-depth discussions about the objectivity of science, basic definitional information about NAGPRA legislation, and court case examples. All of the curricular work was done with the two guiding principles that (1) students needed to be exposed to indigenous perspectives on these issues, and (2) students needed the time, space, and encouragement to develop their critical thinking skills regarding these issues. Project staff felt it was of central importance to create a "vocation of space" to help the AIR students understand their identities and cultural traditions as they relate to questions about science, genetics, and history (Pulido 2006).

As part of a larger community service learning project with the American Indian Recruitment Program's non-profit program (AIR), students from my ethnic studies college courses serve as tutors and mentors to local American Indian high school students on a weekly basis. Nearly all of my university students (mentors) are non-Indian, while all of the AIR (high school) students are Indian, with most attending the program from Kumeyaay Indian Reservations throughout San Diego County. The AIR Program has been in existence for over fifteen years. It was founded by a small group of American Indian college students who, in the early 1990s, noticed that there were few Indians attending college. They decided to address the problem by starting their own after-school tutoring and mentoring program, targeting American Indian high school youth. In a effort to literally indigenize the academy, the AIR founders decided that sessions should be hosted at college campuses. At AIR, Indian youth are tutored and mentored by college students and alumni. The sessions are peppered with discussions that demystify higher education and promote Indian educational and professional success. This organization is a good case study of a tribal community producing critical social theory.

AIR Program requirements include a collaborative research project (and a final presentation given at the end of the semester) on a topic determined by AIR staff. The fall 2007 semester project focused on the Native American Graves Protection and Repatriation Act (NAGPRA), a federal law passed in 1990, and this led to a focus on the case of Kennewick Man, an ancient human being whose remains were found on the shore of the Columbia River in Washington State in 1996.

The Kennewick Man case is important because of the way in which DNA testing undermined the strength of NAGPRA, since DNA testing of bone shavings revealed "inconclusive" results and the scientists and national media interpreted these findings to mean that he was not an American Indian. The debate over the meaning of Kennewick Man, then, is a flashpoint in a broader controversy in genetics evidence, historical claims, and indigenous identity. An indigenous perspective would interpret the "results" as reinforcing the idea that Western science does not necessarily equal "truth" or "fact." Indeed, as Umatilla religious leader Arnold Minthorn has publicly stated, scientific tests can be unnecessary and unwarranted. From an indigenous perspective, Native religious traditions, teachings, and oral histories trump scientific tests. Culturally sensitive anthropologists also support indigenous perspectives (Jones and Stapp 2003); however, such views did not triumph during the court proceedings surrounding Kennewick Man. His remains continue to be locked up in a university museum, an offensive example of what Rebecca Tsosie defines as "cultural harm."[1] In a critique of the culturally biased proceedings of the case, Tsosie acknowledges, "The court disregarded NAGPRA's statutory requirement that accords oral history and tribal narrative the same evidentiary weight as scientific data in the assessment of cultural affiliation" (Tsosie 2007:407). That Native people's narratives were not given equal evidentiary weight as scientific claims is a testament of the need for ongoing work to decolonize the institutions that rule over Native peoples' lives, cultures, and histories.

Plateau tribal peoples respectfully refer to Kennewick Man as the Ancient One, and tribes continue to work collaboratively to recover the Ancient One's bones in order to give him a proper reburial and thus restore balance and peace, according to tribal beliefs. The Ancient One has come to be a strong symbol of indigenous struggle and claims. His bones are, literally, what brought the AIR participants together to debate the relevance of DNA testing and the sources of historical knowledge.

Over the course of the semester, the AIR group debated the importance of Kennewick Man's case. Project research revealed that there has been great contention over the "truth" of Kennewick Man's "race." While Kennewick Man's "race" has proven important for determining what would happen to his bones, there are much larger stakes involved with this case than simply a respectful reburial of his remains. Kennewick Man's case has helped to solidify the privileging of DNA testing as the "gold standard" in producing historical "fact." For example, although DNA testing was not conclusive, the public perception (largely due to biased media reports) was that Kennewick Man's DNA tests did not show he was Native. While this is true, it is also true that the Ancient One's DNA tests did not show he was anything else, either—because the DNA testing did not show any conclusive results. Because of the bias that privileges DNA testing as the "gold standard," it was enough for media reports to simply say that the tests did not support tribal claims. Thus, the "magician's sleight of hand" convinced the public to largely side with scientists' ideas that the Ancient One was not Indian. Coleman and Dysart discuss this powerful "magical" communication strategy as one that directs "attention to one particular point while obscuring another" (Coleman and Dysart 2005:7).

The logic, although flawed, was that, if tribes are wrong, then scientists who argued that Kennewick Man was white must be right, even though the DNA testing did not prove this. This flawed logic matched well with a media frenzy that was most excited about the possible Caucasoid roots of Kennewick Man (Crawford 2000). The ideological power of DNA testing as the gold standard that upholds truthful science was enough to undermine tribal legitimacy in the public's view. Such views of scientific standards ignore indigenous traditions, including oral histories, and render our elders' historical knowledge useless in court cases that decide the fate of indigenous people and indigenous homelands. As indigenous scholar Kimberly TallBear writes, a "contemporary and perhaps more sophisticated form of eugenics equates genetic markers with cultural continuity and seeks to use DNA to support or deny an individual or group claim to cultural and political rights" (TallBear 2003:82). Indigenous critiques of science are important because they challenge the hegemonic power of scientific inquiry that is rooted in society's racialized systems of oppression and domination.

The Need for Indigenous Consciousness

Frantz Fanon, in his discussion of the damages of colonialism, writes, "[c]olonialism is not satisfied merely with hiding a people in its grip and emptying the native's brain of all form and content. By a kind of perverted logic, it turns to the past of the oppressed people, and distorts, disfigures and destroys it. This work of devaluing pre-colonial history takes on a dialectical significance today" (Fanon 1968:37). The AIR Program activities provides an opportunity to understand how damaging the colonial project can be. My analysis reveals that indigenous students immersed in an educational system that operates with colonialist assumptions (for example, that Western science is value-neutral and bias-free or that indigenous histories do not matter or are untrue) have difficulty articulating a counter-narrative.

The AIR project, in many ways, highlighted how disputes over evidence in the Kennewick man case reflected deeper disagreements over the nature of evidence and cultural values. During the weekly AIR Program activities, students engaged in library research and listened to guest speakers from the Kumeyaay Culture and Repatriation Committee (KCRC), who discussed repatriation battles generally and the details of past cases that had been resolved. Additionally, participants discussed examples of on-the-ground work surrounding the Ancient One's case as represented in Northwest Tribal newspaper articles.

Students began demonstrating an interest and concern for the Ancient One fairly early on in the program. By week two, students were asking about the Ancient One's well-being, with questions such as: "Where is the Ancient One now?" and "Who is taking care of his bones?" The students, with their curious questions, were demonstrating their traditional cultural values, which mandate that the dead be cared for so that their spirits may be at rest.

Throughout the semester, the AIR students and mentors expressed disbelief at the way in which the Ancient One was treated. A review of Web site resources resulted in online photos of scientists touching and analyzing the Ancient One's bones, a tremendous violation of tribal cultural norms. However, when AIR staff would play "devil's advocate" and discuss how the DNA testing was "inconclusive" in determining tribal lineage, AIR students seemed confused on the matter. They demonstrated their confusion by being silent or asking questions such as: "Doesn't DNA testing prove who you are?" Or they made statements such as "Well, if the DNA tests don't prove he's Native, then I guess he isn't." Additionally, when a member of the KCRC asked the students if cases like Kennewick Man proved tribal histories were wrong, students responded with confusion and apathy. The need to indigenize students' consciousness was evident. Staff clearly saw how students needed to understand "racialized ideas of 'Indianness' and how such ideas actually undermine political and cultural authority" (TallBear 2003:82). Most important, staff saw how the students needed to understand that tribal identity is "based in particular histories, cultures, and landscapes" (TallBear 2007:416).

In times of confusion, AIR staff would ask the students basic questions that were rooted in the students' traditional culture. For example, the students were asked, "According to your tribal history, how long has your tribe been here?" Students responded that they were the first people to live in the area, that they had been here for thousands of years. Then, when the discussion was broadened to have a more pan-Indian focus, students were asked, "Who were the first people here in America?" Students were quick to respond that they knew American Indians were the first people.

However, when staff discussed aspects of the Kennewick Man case that challenged the students' understandings of history, students grew quiet or confused. The cultural assumptions of mentors and students, views that shaped the meaning of Kennewick Man from both sides, came into view. In week three, students were asked, "What does it mean if Kennewick Man was white? What does it mean if scientists are saying that the first people here were not American Indians?" Students were also shown images from Web sources, such as the "Friends of America's Past" and the "New Nation News" Web sites. Included on the sites were the artistic renditions of what some white scientists and artists believed the Ancient One looked like. The popular *Star Trek* rendition (also appearing on the cover of *Time* magazine) was the image, ingrained in American imagination. Even the *Christian Science Monitor* weighed in on the story. In the story "An ancient man's bones of contention," the *Christian Science Monitor* shares the mainstream perspective, "He was a sturdy man of middle years who may have looked a bit like British actor Patrick Stewart of *Star Trek* fame, about 5-feet, 9-inches tall, and living in a dangerous world" (Knickerbocker 1999).

When students were presented with such images and verbiage they giggled and made fun (especially of the images). However, when pressed to articulate the reasons why the images and articles were perhaps flawed, students struggled to speak with confidence from an indigenous perspective. They had not yet learned how to critique the idea that "[s]cience cannot prove an individual's identity as a member of a cultural entity such as a tribe" (TallBear 2003:84). It was interesting to imagine how the students had been so exposed to white, Western perspectives, that they were unable to effectively articulate what might be wrong with such perspectives. That is, they failed to have a strong indigenous consciousness. Some students, uncomfortable with the challenge posed to them (critiquing the images), slumped their shoulders in a sign of resignation. Others wanted to "give up" on the discussion and sought comfort in distracting side-conversations. While students did, through their giggling and making fun, signal that they knew something was wrong with the images and arguments, they were not confident expressing an argument against a major national news publication or a Web page on the Internet. For many of the students, if something was "in print" or "on the Web" then it "must be true." The students seemed to hold the view that many journalists do. In a critique of the media's coverage of the Kennewick Man's case, Colman and Dysart argue, "scientific perspectives may enjoy preferential treatment because they are inherently attractive to journalists, reflecting values that resonate with journalistic credos of subjectivity and objectivity" (2005:8). It is this assumption that the staff wanted to challenge. Within tribal communities, elders' testimonies are at least as valuable as "scientific" perspectives.

During moments of contention, when students were unable to answer challenging questions posed to them, they looked to staff for guidance on how to respond to such challenging statements as "the scientists and other groups say whites were here first." Fortunately, a KCRC member took the lead in these discussions, reminding the students of the importance of tribal histories. These discussions were some of the richest teaching and learning moments of the entire project, as would later be revealed when the students conducted their final presentations at the end of the semester.

Ideas, Discourse, and Argumentation

As American Indian staff members developing and presenting the curriculum to the students, AIR staff members were able to choose to put indigenous perspectives at the center of the program. Students learned about the importance of tribal histories, the oral tradition (including songs), and the shortcomings of a scientific approach that claims to be bias-free. Staff walked the students through a critique of the famous *Time* magazine image, asking them what impact they think it had that the Ancient One was being assumed to look like a white *Star Trek* actor. Students began to understand that the Ancient One's case was an example of warring ideas and discourses. They started to understand that it was a matter of how powerful one's argument was in the public's perception. Once students grasped this, it was easier to talk about how tribal perspectives are undermined by Western science, Western education systems, and Western media. Staff offered students alternatives through discussions of KCRC's work, discussing examples of the Plateau tribes working together to recover the Ancient One's remains, and sharing indigenous media coverage of the case. Bringing alternative discourses to the discussion provided students with multiple perspectives from which they could choose in constructing their own ideas about DNA, race, and history.

Staff members were pleased that the AIR program provided the space in which to do this decolonizing work, but were also keenly aware that the students were immersed in an educational system that would not build up their indigenous consciousness. Thus, although the students were able to understand and articulate an indigenous perspective of the issues, staff worried that students would lose confidence in their ability to do so if their perspectives were not honored and encouraged in spaces outside of the two-hour weekly program.

My analysis of the program activities confirms the importance of tribal peoples educating their youth on the value and relevance of tribal histories. If youth, such as the AIR students, do not have a solid grasp of the reasons why their tribal stories matter, they will not be able to respond to opposing viewpoints, nor will they be able to feel confident articulating who they are. Clearly, the identities of the future generations are at stake.

Students Find Their Voices: Evidence from the Final Presentations

Evidence from the Program's final presentations demonstrates the importance of role-modeling for the youth. I argue that, largely due to the involvement and dedication from KCRC members, students focused on the importance of culture in determining tribal identity, and resisted the DNA "gold standard." To help demonstrate this point, I will draw from my ethnographic notes as well as an analysis of video footage of the four group presentations, which the students decided to perform as "skits." Each student was assigned to one of four groups. Each group was instructed to do a presentation that would demonstrate what they had learned over the semester. Staff members were not involved with the planning of any skits, in an effort to honor the group's academic freedom and to encourage the articulation of a presentation that was rooted in the students' understanding of the semester's material.

An analysis of the final presentations reveals that the idea of scientists "digging up" human remains left a very powerful impression on the students. All of the skits discussed or represented such acts. Some groups did comical impersonations of over-eager anthropologists digging for gold (or rather Indian bones). Others staged protests at dig sites set on the auditorium stage on which the skits were performed. For example, Group I acted out what they imagined to be a digging site. The skit began with a digging scene and then a phone call was made from the site, with one of the diggers exclaiming, "Professor, come right away, I've found something!" The professor, once on scene, concludes, "Oh yes! This needs MORE study!" Immediately after uttering these words, other students enter the scene and begin chanting "NAGPRA! NAGPRA! NAGPRA!" in protest of the dig. Students explain the basics of the acronym and the meaning of the federal law. One of the students tells what she thinks of the dig site and the scientists' work, keying into basic points of contention from the Kennewick Man case and applying it to her own tribal people, "You say the bones don't match our DNA. But do you know that the world is always changing? We are changing, but we are still Kumeyaay. That is why the DNA doesn't match. We are Kumeyaay and we know from our tribal history that we have been on this land for thousands of years. We are the only people who can claim this ancient being as our ancestor. We want this ancestor to be respected."

The skits revealed that dig sites are popular imagery with the students. They liked imagining the setting and the excitement, perhaps lust, which diggers (ironically a derogatory name given to California Indians by white settlers) felt in seeking out Indian artifacts and bodies. The students, through their skits, demonstrated that they understood how science could turn Indian bodies into commodities that scientists own, control, and study for the supposed "public good."

Skit two also included a dig site. The opening scene had two mentors digging away, with one of the mentors eventually exclaiming, "Wow! I hit the jackpot! (pausing as if to reflect) Pottery last week . . . and now remains!" The other digger looks a little envious that his digging partner had found the bones. The skit is obviously trying to portray the sense of excitement that goes with the "discovery" of remains.

Skit two then changed scenes to a courtroom.

A scientist tells the court that "Much research is needed." Thus, the students are able to present their understanding of why remains are sought. After the scientist spoke, I was surprised to see one of the shyest students perform a monologue. She states, "The Ancient One is not at peace. You've upset the balance. The Ancient One needs to be put back in the Earth. The Earth has shifted and changed over time and so have we, that is why there is a gap in the DNA. This is our ancestor and people. The Ancient One needs to rest."

It was striking to see the student speaking confidently from an indigenous perspective. It was a dramatic shift from the silence and confusion the students displayed early on in the semester. Additionally, the students were able to consider the problem from a pan-Indian perspective, with clear transnational implications. While the "Ancient One" title came from the Plateau peoples and specifically the Kennewick Man case, Kumeyaay students decided to use that name as an important part of their skit. This stood in contrast to the earlier, apathetic response students had in comments such as "if the DNA doesn't prove he's Native, he must not be Native." It is also interesting that the student contests conflicting DNA results. She offers an explanation of a "gap" in DNA test results. Thus, the rigid authority of DNA testing is undermined. The students can now articulate that tribal identity is cultural, not scientific. This shift is especially important within the Southern California context. In the San Diego area, there are a handful of wealthy gaming tribes. Some of the AIR students attend school with or are related to families that are caught up in the enrollment politics linked to the wealth of Indian gaming. The question of "Who is Indian" is very complex in this context, wrought with identity politics and questions of legitimacy. As Joane Nagel (1996) argues, when resources are at stake, identity categories become narrower. Some tribes have turned to government rolls, missionary records, and DNA testing to resolve questions of members' identities. Students who are of mixed racial/ethnic backgrounds, multiple tribes, or lacking a traditional cultural upbringing can find identity questions to be especially troubling within this context of high-profile disenrollment cases. That students were able (in their skits) to articulate a firm sense of "who they are" is an important accomplishment. That they chose to use an indigenous and transnational approach for doing so was further evidence of their rejection of colonial systems that so often divide indigenous peoples and communities.

Perhaps the most powerful skit was performed by Group 4. This group decided to perform a court scene about a fictitious case based on the Kennewick Man case. The court was deciding what to do with the remains of "Mission Gorge Woman" (a fictitious case named after a local site in San Diego). The audience is told that Mission Gorge Woman was dug up at a construction site where new condos were being built (a savvy and realistic observation about development on Kumeyaay homeland).

In the court scene, a museum curator testifies first. She has a brief statement, saying, "We want to study remains to learn about early humans." This demonstrates, as with earlier skits, that the students understand scientists' points of view on the matter.

The student who speaks next identifies herself as a member of the Kumeyaay Culture and Repatriation Committee. Commenting on the Mission Gorge Woman's case, the student states, "Her remains should be returned to be buried in the traditional way. I am here to ask the court to do this."

Another student speaks next, as chair of the Kumeyaay Culture and Repatriation Committee, "Kennewick Man set a bad precedence by giving him to the museum (referring to the fact that the Ancient One is being held at the Burke Museum at the University of Washington). It [Kennewick Man case] establishes that remains that are thousands of years old are not Native. We have shown that the Kumeyaay have been here at least 12,000 years."

The students, choosing roles as members of KCRC, demonstrated the power of role-modeling for youth. As part of the AIR curriculum, members of the KCRC spoke about the importance of traditional culture and tribal histories. The students were moved by these teachers' lessons. That the students chose to privilege an indigenous perspective in their skits was evidence of what they had learned.

In their work with the youth, the staff clearly sought to teach the youth to think about scientific projects, such as genetic research, from an indigenous perspective. In doing so, tribal histories and cultural teachings were privileged. This work in critiquing some uses of science is rooted in a nation-building project that seeks to simultaneously promote cultural survival and resist colonialism. Science and colonialism are deeply intertwined in indigenous communities. The colonial mentality of "taking" whatever one wants from indigenous communities persists. As Trope and Echo-Hawk point out, science has a long history of taking from Indians. Trope and Echo-Hawk use a quote from Franz Boas to help demonstrate their point. In the quote, Boas, speaking as a scientist in the late-1800s, laments, "it is most unpleasant work to steal bones from graves, but what is the use, someone has to do it" (Trope and Echo-Hawk 2000:126–127). We hope that scientists, in their desire to produce knowledge, will pause long enough to consider the many rich forms of knowledge that may be possible when they partner with, and learn from, indigenous communities who engage in cultural survival.

Native peoples do not object to science, genetic testing, and research. However, my analysis reveals that Native peoples do object to all of these when they are conceptualized, planned, carried out, and used to inform future science, law, and policy agendas without indigenous histories and cultures being respected on the same level as scientific perspectives.

Conclusion

What, in the end, does the story of the meaning of Kennewick Man tell us about the collision of DNA, identity, and history? In our quest for knowledge is there room for "both" perspectives—the "indigenous" perspective and the "scientific" perspective? Based on my analysis of the AIR program case study, I conclude that the answer is yes, but only when there are relationships built on mutual respect and equality that make meaningful dialogue and collaboration possible. The case study of the AIR program highlights the promise and the pitfalls in this ongoing search for mutual respect and equality.

From an indigenous perspective it is clear that the burden lies on the scientific community to "undo" the vast damage that has been done in the name of science and DNA testing. As Rebecca Tsosie argues, "interests of Native groups cannot be accurately understood or addressed within our legal system unless we attempt to understand the different normative conceptions of property, ownership, and privacy that exists for these groups" (Tsosie 2007:396). The scientific community must take a critical look at itself and its relationship with upholding the colonial project. The "discovery" mode of genetics, described elsewhere in this volume, is highly suspect within indigenous communities. Possible solutions could stem from proposed legal paradigm shifts, such as what Tsosie (2007) suggests; this includes a scientific enterprise that is guided by an "intercultural framework" that honors "group-oriented" and "collective ownership" principles. Such an approach would prevent a totalizing science that dominates Native peoples' lives and cultures. Perhaps then a greater, more respectful, quest for knowledge is possible. Efforts toward collective human subject agreements have proven to be useful in tribal communities (Foster, Bernsten, and Carter 1998; Sharp and Foster 2002). Perhaps scientists can draw inspiration from the words of the AIR Group 1's concluding scene, where a scientist has the "final say" about what should happen next, "It is important for scientists like me to study, but it's MORE important to respect tribes' beliefs." Using such advice as project guidance, scientists could then perhaps resolve problems of individual consent versus group rights (Mitchell and Happe 2001).

Throughout the project, the AIR staff sought to empower the youth, so that they would be encouraged to seek knowledge, to attain a higher education, to participate fully in society, but above all else, to privilege tribal traditions and an indigenous perspective over a scientific one. Cultural survival is a top concern among American Indian communities. Tsosie describes the urgency of this matter, "When indigenous people across the globe argue for a right to 'cultural survival,' they are arguing for a collective right as groups, to protect and preserve their cultural practices, which have been attacked both directly and indirectly by dominant politics focused on cultural assimilation and appropriation of Native lands and resources" (2007:402). In the era of genetic and genomic research "Native resources" includes tissue samples and the right to define scientific projects that speak about the past, present, and future of Native peoples, cultures, and lands. At the heart of the work with the AIR youth was a commitment to cultural survival. AIR staff members are optimistic that future generations of Native youth will resist colonialism, and hope that the scientific community will follow suit.

APPENDIX: ACRONYMS

AIR   American Indian Recruitment Programs. Nonprofit organization that partners with colleges to provide after-school programs serving Native youth in the San Diego area.

KCRC   Kumeyaay Culture and Repatriation Committee. Local, reservation community members' group that is responsible for repatriation issues. Some community members are involved with both AIR and KCRC.

NAGPRA   Native American Graves Protection and Repatriation Act. Federal law passed in 1990 to "protect burials, sacred objects, and funerary objects on federal and tribal lands" (Mihesuah 2000).

NOTE

1. Tsosie calls for a legal system that not only seeks to bring justice to those who have suffered from "economic harm" but also "cultural harm." She defines two conditions of cultural harm: (1) access to one's own group's cultural systems being blocked; (2) cultural appropriation, meaning one group asserting the right to control aspects of another group's culture (Tsosie 2007:403).

WORKS CITED

Benedict, Jeff. 2003. *No bone unturned: The adventures of a top Smithsonian forensic scientist and the legal battle for America's oldest skeletons.* New York: HarperCollins.

Coleman, C. L., and E. Dysart, 2005. Framing of Kennewick Man against the backdrop of a scientific and cultural controversy. *Science Communication* 27:3–26.

Collins, Patricia Hill. 1998. *Fighting words: Black women and the search for justice.* Minneapolis: University of Minnesota Press.

Connolly Miskwish, M. 2007. *Kumeyaay: A history textbook.* El Cajon, CA: Sycuan Press.

Crawford, S. J. 2000. (Re)constructing bodies: Semiotic sovereignty and the debate over Kennewick Man. In *Repatriation reader: Who owns American Indian remains?*, edited by D. A. Mihesuah, 211–236. Lincoln: University of Nebraska Press.

Deloria, Vine. 1988. *Custer died for your sins.* Norman: University of Oklahoma Press.

Duran, Eduardo. 2006. *Healing the soul wound: Counseling with American Indians and other native peoples.* New York: Teachers College Press.

Fanon, Frantz. 1968. *The wretched of the Earth.* New York: Grove Press.

Foster, M. W., D. Bernsten, and T. H. Carter. 1998. A model agreement for genetic research in socially identifiable populations. *American Journal of Human Genetics* 63:696–702.

Friends of America's Past. 2008. www.friendsofpast.org/kennewick-man/ [Accessed February 20, 2008]

Hunn, E. S. 1990. *Nch'I-Wana "The Big River" Mid-Columbia Indians and their land.* Seattle: University of Washington Press.

Jones, P., and D. Stapp. 2003. An anthropological perspective on Magistrate Jelderks' Kennewick Man decision. *High Plains Applied Anthropology* 1:1–16.

Knickerbocker, B. 1999. An ancient man's bones of contention. *Christian Science Monitor* (October 21), 1.

Mihesuah, D. A. 2000. Introduction. In *Repatriation reader: Who owns American Indian remains?*, edited by D. A. Mihesuah, 3. Lincoln: University of Nebraska Press.

Mitchell, G. R., and K. Happe. 2001. Informed consent after the Human Genome Project. *Rhetoric and Public Affairs* 4 (3):375–406.

Nagel, Joane. 1996. *American Indian ethnic renewal: Red power and the resurgence of identity and culture*. New York: Oxford University Press.

New Nation News. 2008. newnation.org/NNN-kennewick-man.html [Accessed February 20, 2008].

Pulido, A. L. 2006. A vocation of space: Race and ethnicity as a responsible and necessary challenge to U.S. Catholic education in the 21st century. *Journal of Catholic Social Thought* 3 (1):179–194.

Sharp, R. R., and M. W. Foster. 2002. Community involvement in the ethical review of genetic research: Lessons from American Indian and Alaska Native populations. *Environmental Health Perspectives* 110 (Supplement 2):145–148.

Smith, D. E. 1987. *The everyday world as problematic: A feminist sociology*. Boston: Northeastern University Press.

Smith, L. T. 2001. *Decolonizing methodologies: Research and indigenous peoples*. New York: Zed Books.

Spivak, Gayatri Chakravorty. 1988. Can the subaltern speak? In *Marxism and the Interpretation of Culture*, edited by C. Nelson and L. Grossberg, 271–313. Urbana: University of Illinois Press.

TallBear, Kimberly. 2003. DNA, blood, and racializing the tribe. *Wicazo Sa Review* 18:81–107.

———. 2007. Narratives of race and indigeneity in the genographic project. *Journal of Law, Medicine, and Ethics* 35 (3):412–424.

Trope, J. F., and W. R. Echo-Hawk. 2000. The Native American Graves Protection and Repatriation Act background and legislative history. In *Repatriation reader: Who owns American Indian remains?*, edited by D. A. Mihesuah, 123–168. Lincoln: University of Nebraska Press.

Tsosie, Rebecca. 2007. Cultural challenges to biotechnology: Native American genetic resources and the concept of cultural harm. *Journal of Law, Medicine, and Ethics* 35 (3): 396–411.

17

∞∞

Humanitarian DNA Identification in Post-Apartheid South Africa

JAY D. ARONSON

This chapter focuses on the convergence of DNA and history in the context of post-apartheid South Africa. It examines the relationship between the recent use of forensic DNA profiling to identify missing and disappeared (primarily black) political activists from the apartheid era, and continuing debates over the history of the anti-apartheid struggle from elite and non-elite perspectives. It also puts in the foreground issues of identity in a country struggling to come to terms with its past. I begin with a general overview of the issues associated with the identification process in the post-apartheid era. I then focus in detail on two specific cases, those of the "Mamelodi 4" and the "Mamelodi 10," in order to illustrate the complexity and ambiguity in the use of DNA identification to clarify history and perform political work in the new South Africa. In this story, DNA is not being used to define the boundaries of race, or to trace the origins of a particular group of people, but rather to ameliorate past injustices to a historically marginalized group defined entirely by race.

The families of the missing in South Africa, and especially those whose loved ones were affiliated with the armed struggle against apartheid, are seeking to recover more than just mortal remains in their quest to locate and rebury their missing loved ones. They are also seeking to restore the social, political, and historical identity of their loved ones. In other words, the process of post-conflict DNA identification involves multiple forms of *recognition*.[1] First, there is the kind of biological recognition that comes when the mortal remains of the individual are located and then identified by DNA or other forensic methods. Second, families want to recover the social identity of the people identified by scientists and investigators—they want to reclaim them as *their* flesh and blood and provide them with the proper burial they had lacked for so long. Finally, they seek collective social recognition of the heroic sacrifice that their loved ones made for what they believe to be the freedom of all South Africans. Providing this third kind of social recognition means going far beyond the DNA identification process to

295

ensuring appropriate commemoration of the life of the formerly missing person. Thus, any effort to identify the missing must simultaneously integrate biological, social, and historical aspects of personhood.

Background

There are as many as 2,000 people *known* to have gone missing during the apartheid era in South Africa. Of these, 477 were officially recognized by the Truth and Reconciliation Commission (TRC) during its investigations, based on corroboration from details of cases submitted to the Human Rights Violations Committee or information provided by perpetrators during amnesty hearings. It should be noted that this figure does not count all disappearances uncovered during amnesty hearings and was assumed to be an undercount by the TRC. The majority of missing South Africans disappeared during the intensification of the government's repression of blacks in the 1980s (Commission 1998–2003:vol. 6). During this period, military units and police organizations were willing to kill individuals if they were deemed to threaten national security or the authority of the National Party, which were for all intents and purposes one and the same.[2] At the same time, many politically active individuals went into exile and did not return to South Africa once democracy was restored in 1994 (either because they died or started new lives elsewhere).

The exact number of deaths attributable to death squads is disputed, but estimates put the number as high as 1,000 (Gottschalk 2002:231). According to one scholar of South African death squads, in the aftermath of the 1976 Soweto Revolt, the apartheid government had adopted murder as a "conscious element of internal security policy" (Gottschalk 2002:234).[3] This cold-blooded killing was first conducted by state operatives, and then in the twilight years of apartheid (1985–1993) by hired vigilantes of all colors and creeds (Gottschalk 2002). In the early 1990s, the government also fomented fighting amongst rival political parties, leading to significant bloodshed during that period (Commission 1998–2003:vol. 6). Although families were often able to retrieve the remains of their loved ones after death, in many cases bodies were either buried in unmarked graves or mutilated beyond recognition (Commission 1998–2003:vol. 2; Gottschalk 2002). Many members of the armed wings of the major liberation groups, as well as politically unaffiliated individuals, met this fate.

Almost all Southern African ethnic groups—even those that have been Christianized—believe that there is a strong and continuous relationship between the living and the dead (Dennie 1996; Eppel 2006). Appropriate burial rituals must be performed in order to ensure that the recently deceased individual is able to take a place as an ancestor (Dennie 1996; Eppel 2006). When these rituals are not performed, all but the most devoutly Christian Africans believe that the deceased will be forced to wander the nether world between the land of the living and the ancestral homeland. This liminal state both robs the deceased of rest and comfort, and denies the living the protection and counsel that they normally receive from their ancestors. In this situation, the living are thought to be more susceptible to death, disease, economic misfortunate, and bad luck. Because the worlds of the living and the dead intertwine, serious problems emerge when the appropriate rituals are not performed. Further, although it is not universal among all Southern African cultures, in most it is desirable for the body of the deceased to be buried near where he or she was born, in order to ensure easy communication between the living and their ancestors. At a more socio-political level, the presence of the graves of relatives reinforces the claims of the living relatives to belong to, and in, a particular place (Dennie 1996; Eppel 2006).

Efforts to locate the missing began during the investigatory phase of the Truth and Reconciliation Commission (TRC), which lasted from 1996 to 1998. The majority of the 477 people declared missing by the TRC were African National Congress members, especially of its military wing, Umkhonto we Sizwe (MK). This situation arose for several reasons, including: the fact that the TRC was mandated to deal only with human rights violations that were explicitly political in nature; because the ANC suffered very heavy losses during the struggle compared to most other political groups; and also because ANC members were mobilized to give testimony at a higher rate than many other subgroups within South African society (Hamber et al. 2000).

Since the initial effort to collect the names of the missing at the TRC, civil organizations such as the Centre for the Study of Violence and Reconciliation (CSVR) and the Khulumani Support Group have documented more than 1500 additional (but as yet not officially verified) cases, many of whom had no direct ties to the ANC. Although it is beyond the scope of this chapter, disputes have emerged among various parties over which categories of disappearances ought to be investigated by the government (Aronson 2011).

Although only a few graves were exhumed by the TRC, the commission recommended that a team be formed within the NPA to continue the work. Because of her own interest in the subject, and interactions with victims and survivors of the apartheid era, former TRC historian Madeleine Fullard began lobbying government officials to create a team to resolve cases involving missing people (Dewhirst 2008; Fullard 2008). President Thabo Mbeki backed this move in 2003, and the NPA's Missing Persons Task Team (MPTT) has been working to resolve this situation ever since. To date, the MPTT has exhumed more than sixty-six individuals, approximately fifty of whom have been positively identified at the individual level, using DNA and/or other forensic techniques, and returned to their families (Fullard 2011).

The Mamelodi 4

One of the MPTT's most compelling successes is that of the identification of the "Mamelodi 4." The Mamelodi 4 represent two separate cases. In the first incident, which took place in July 1987, South African Police Service's Security Branch (based at the infamous Vlakplaas farm outside Pretoria) abducted Jackson Maake, who was at the time working as an informant for the security police, after they came to believe that he was a double agent who used his state-provided car to bring weapons into the country for use by the MK (van Vuuren 1996:343). Maake initially denied the accusation, but under heavy torture he admitted to being a spy and also confessed that he was involved in a plot to bomb the police's offices in the area (van Vuuren 1996:344). He then gave his interrogators Andrew Makupe's name as his contact with the highly secretive MK (van Vuuren 1996:356). Makupe was then brought to the same location, and after being subjected to torture, he revealed that his job was to bring arms into the country and gave Harold Sefolo's name as his leader within the MK (van Vuuren 1996:350). Sefolo was then brought to the scene (after Makupe, also Sefolo's friend and business partner, was forced to telephone him to tell him to trust the people who were coming to pick him up) so that the police could obtain more information about the ANC cells in the region. In order to compel Sefolo to provide more information, the police shoved a knife up his nose and ultimately electrocuted Maake and Makupe to death in front of him. According to his interrogators, he would not divulge any important information, and eventually asked them to kill him. First, though, he was granted the opportunity to sing "N'Kosi Sikelea Afrika" (the song of resistance that is now South Africa's national anthem) at his request (van Vuuren 1996:351). Once dead, the security officers piled their bodies on top of a land mine. They were then blown to bits in an attempt to make them unrecognizable (van Vuuren 1996:353). The stated justification for the killing was that the identity of the interrogators, and the information gained during the interrogation, had to be protected (van Vuuren 1996:356).

In a separate incident, Justice Mbizana, also from Mamelodi and a known member of an MK unit based out of Swaziland, was arrested by security police soon after returning to the country after a period of exile. He was then taken to an isolated farm where he was interrogated and tortured for more than a week (Prinsloo 1999). During the course of this process, he was prodded with a burning log in the head and (possibly) the anus, shot at close range, drugged with an overdose of sleeping medication, and then finally bludgeoned to death with a gardening spade. He too was blown up using land mines to destroy the evidence of wrong-doing and to prevent his comrades from knowing what happened to him. The remains of the four men were buried together in a pauper's cemetery at Winterveld, all in a single casket because they happened to show up in the morgue in the same month (Fullard 2011).

The TRC amnesty hearings, and simultaneous criminal prosecutions of perpetrators who did not qualify for amnesty, provided relatives of the Mamelodi 4 with their first opportunity to find out what happened to their loved ones. Subsequently, Elizabeth Maake (Jackson's mother), Lizzie Thandi Sefolo (Harold's wife) and Mabel Matlakala Makope (Andrew's wife) testified before the TRC's Human Rights Violations committee (HRVC). In addition to recounting their stories and their suffering, the women made several demands, including: information about their missing loved ones and the opportunity to visit the sites that were relevant to the their deaths; help for the families to locate the bodies of the Mamelodi 4 so they could be properly buried; and that the TRC hold the perpetrators accountable for their actions as far as possible. (Maake 1996; Makope 1996; Sefolo 1996). As Elizabeth Maake testified:

> I would . . . like to rebury him so that we can also be able to go to the cemetery, to the grave of our loved one like other people. We don't know if it's really true that they killed him. We don't know if he's alive or dead. We just heard that he's dead. We would really like to know the truth and we would also like to see where he died. [The police officials involved] must show us where he is. We would also like to request his remains so that we can bury him in our graveyard. That's the thing we would really like to request from you, from the Truth Commission. (Maake 1996:2)

All three women spoke in some detail about the fruitless efforts they undertook to find out what happened to the three men, and the extent to which the lack of information was as painful for them as the absence of their loved ones. Not knowing prevented them from moving on with their lives and fulfilling their duties toward their remaining family members and their community. This testimony resonates with the experiences of families of the missing in other parts of the world. In her book on DNA identification in the aftermath of the Srebrenica massacre, for instance, Sarah Wagner describes in detail the insufficiency of the notion of a "missing person," and the idea that someone is *probably* dead. She writes that such knowledge is incomplete and hollow for families of individuals who have disappeared: "the term *missing* signals the absence of a story, a personal history yet untold, for each victim." Further, the term itself intensifies the anguish associated with loss—it reminds of them of the heinous physical violation of their relatives' remains (Wagner 2008:7).

After testifying at the TRC in 1996, the families of the Mamelodi 4 heard nothing more about the fates of their loved ones for nearly a decade. Thanks to the amnesty hearings, in which the security police who were responsible for the deaths of the Mamelodi 4 told the TRC how and why they were killed in exchange for amnesty from punishment, the families at least knew generally what happened to their loved ones, but they did not know how much of it was true, and they still had no way of retrieving the bodies for proper reburial.

Then, in 2005, the Mamelodi 4 families were contacted by Madeleine Fullard to let them know that the MPTT was going to investigate the case. Through a combination of archival research and archaeological investigations, the grave that contained the remains of the Mamelodi 4 was located in the pauper's section of Winterveld Cemetery, in the outskirts of the Pretoria townships (Fullard 2007). The likelihood of individual identification looked slim when the MPTT opened up the graves and found a mass of comingled bones in a decaying coffin.

Once the remains were sorted out, MPTT investigators realized they had only a few hip and leg bones to work with. Fullard sent the materials to the Human Identity Laboratory at the University of Western Cape, which had personnel who had been trained to extract DNA from ancient bone fragments and had an ongoing collaboration with a leader in this field from Sweden (Laet 2008). Ultimately, the laboratory was able to extract DNA from the bones and individually identified the four men by comparing their DNA profiles to living relatives (Davison et al. 2008). After the identifications were made, the Mamelodi 4 received the remains of their loved ones at a ceremony at Freedom Park in Pretoria (a monument to all freedom fighters in South Africa, including those Afrikaners who fought against British imperial rule) and reburied them at the local cemetery near their homes in Mamelodi.

Early in my research, I assumed that this case was an exciting example of how science could be used could resolve historical questions in a racially and politically charged atmosphere, and also bring peace and closure to family members of the disappeared. When I arrived in Mamelodi to meet with relatives of the Mamelodi 4 in May 2007, I expected to be greeted by relieved mothers and wives who had finally achieved some measure of justice and comfort after nearly twenty years of uncertainty. Instead, I was confronted by angry women who had been freshly wounded by the identification and reburial process. I was quite frankly shocked, but over the course of the time that I spent with them, the source of their anger became understandable to me. To appreciate their claims fully, however, requires a brief detour into the complex dynamics of the anti-apartheid movement, with its competing philosophies of liberation, parallel tactical and intelligence operations, personal and organizational rivalries, unresolved class conflicts, and debate about who deserves credit for the emergence of democracy in the country.

The Liberation Struggle

The ANC is a curious institution, having gone through many forms during the course of its history: a small organization of black elites who demanded citizenship (1912 to early 1940s); a structured, explicitly multiracial organization that focused on change through mass political action (mid-1940s to 1960); an officially banned liberation organization whose leaders were either in exile, imprisoned, or operating underground (1960–1989); an unbanned organization with multiple organizational nodes and intense jockeying for power (1990–1994); the chief agent of the negotiated political transition (1991–1994); and finally, with the election of Nelson Mandela in 1994, the dominant political party in South Africa (Barrell 1993; Butler 2007; Dubow 2000; Meli 1988; Suttner 2007).

The history of the organization is long and complex, but for the purposes of this chapter, it is important to understand that after being banned in 1960, the central leadership of the ANC was dispersed to prisons, exile military bases in bordering countries, and major cities around the world. By the early 1970s, there were two main centers of the ANC in Africa—Lusaka, Zambia and the Robben Island prison, where Mandela, Walter Sisulu, Goven Mbeki (father of former South African President Thabo Mbeki) and others were being held. Each had its own character, style of work, and even understandings about what the struggle against apartheid ought to look like (Suttner 2002). Among the first priorities of the wing of ANC exiles in Lusaka was the creation of a military wing, called Umkhonto we Sizwe (MK, translated as "Spear of the Nation") that would eventually lead black South Africans in armed overthrow of the apartheid state. Beginning in the late 1970s, the ANC also sought to establish a network of underground cells within South Africa that could be mobilized as necessary to carry out covert action, and ultimately armed insurrection under the leadership of MK forces.

Paralleling this development, the Pan-African Congress, a group that had broken away from the ANC in 1959 because it believed that Africans should not collaborate with Whites, Coloreds, or Indians in the liberation struggle, formed the Azanian People's Liberation Army (APLA) to foment armed insurrection against the apartheid state. Making no effort to hide its intentions, APLA adopted the slogan "one settler, one bullet" (Heribert and Moodley 1993:177).

This militarization produced a general feeling among the ANC rank and file that non-violent activities, political negotiations, and mass action would have little role in the return of the country to majority rule. But while ANC combatants were methodically preparing in exile for their moment of military glory, and also carrying out targeted, if largely symbolic, attacks against the apartheid state, the activist community within South Africa was not standing idly by waiting for MK forces to liberate them. Protests flared across the country, most famously in the 1976 Soweto uprising, which began as a peaceful demonstration against Afrikaans-medium schooling for black students before it turned confrontational and bloody when the police moved in to quell the march. In numerous other townships, including Mamelodi, students protested for better education and people of all ages marched for higher quality, more affordable housing (Butler 2008). The 1980s saw heightened mass action within organized labor and civil society as well, the goal of which was to "make apartheid unworkable and South Africa ungovernable" (Suttner 2007:2). These actions were carried out under the auspices of various labor unions and a domestic umbrella organization called the United Democratic Front (Seekings 2000).

By the late 1980s, ANC leaders concluded that the military strategy was not going to be sufficient to end apartheid (Sheehan 2002; Thompson 2000), while the ruling white National Party simultaneously came to the conclusion that, given disturbances in the realms of labor and civil society, it could not systematically separate and dominate the black community forever (Sparks 1995; Thompson 2000). Further, the global recession of the late 1980s and the fall of the Soviet Union (a major financial and ideological supporter of liberation movements around the world) called into question the long-term viability of the ANC in exile (Sparks 1995; Thompson 2000). And finally, through secret discussions between leaders of the state and anti-apartheid forces (most notably involving Nelson Mandela and other ANC members, but also members of the liberal white business community, union leaders, and intellectuals of all ethnic and racial backgrounds) it slowly became clear to most parties that a non-violent solution to the situation in South Africa was not only desirable, but possible (Butler 2008; Sparks 1995; Thompson 2000). Although even the most liberal whites certainly did not imagine handing power over to non-whites at any point in the near future, they did recognize that something would have to be done in order to prevent economic devastation and untold violence (Butler 2008). Thus, when the apartheid state unbanned the ANC in 1990, it did so with the understanding that the organization would become its major partner in reforming the political and social situation in the country in a way that would satisfy the majority non-white population (deKlerk 1998; Mandela 1995; Sparks 1995; Waldmeir 1997).

The decision to shift the ANC's modus operandi from revolution to negotiation, made by the elite leadership without any real input from the rank and file, ultimately led to a sense of betrayal and anger amongst two groups: the ordinary people who had put up with the indignities of life under apartheid while simultaneously working to undermine it; and those who had dedicated the better part of their adult lives to military training (in often squalid conditions in exile) for the day that they would retake their homeland by force (Mashike 2007; Suttner 2007). This bitterness was heightened by the fact that post-independence, the upper echelons of the ANC took positions in the government, the military, finance, and industry, while the rank and file members were sent back to their homes in the townships and rural areas with little or nothing to show for their efforts. Mashike also notes that the shift in tactics left many former MK combatants with the feeling that the skills they had sacrificed so much to acquire were not only irrelevant in the transition to democracy, but also left them with no means of sustaining themselves in the new South Africa (Mashike 2007; Mashike 2008; Suttner 2007).

Thus, while the ANC has a firm grip on political power, it must also address the demands of important constituencies that feel they have not been appropriately recognized and rewarded for their contributions to the struggle. Thus, efforts to identify the missing can be opportunities for the ANC government to "care for" its citizens and establish some sense of control over them, even if they don't directly articulate the latter aim in their official pronouncements (Wagner 2008). Indeed, the stated goal of the MPTT is to

> offer families some recognition of their plight. This official recognition and devotion of state time and resources to their case is a fundamental step in re-incorporating these 'lost citizens' into the body of post-apartheid South Africa. Listening to their stories, recording the events and recovering documentation forms part of the recognition process and the restoration of dignity to the families and the life of the disappeared person (Missing Persons Task Team 2006:20–21).

It is important to remember that there are three forms of recognition in the context of the identification of missing victims of the apartheid struggle: biological recognition, familial recognition, and communal recognition. The relatives I spoke to said that they were elated when they heard that the MPTT was able to individually identify their remains and that they would finally be able to give their loved ones a culturally appropriate burial. But they told me that the happiness they felt had subsided because of the failure of the local ANC branch to provide what they considered to be an acceptable funeral and commemoration for their loved ones. Their perception of proper funereal rights was in large measure political. It was based on what they had seen in the first reburial to take place in Mamelodi, that of the well-known ANC/MK figure Reginald Kekana, whose reburial was used by the Department of Justice as the national kick-off for the Missing Persons Task Team (Fullard 2008). Indeed, the handover ceremony at Freedom Park was an all-star affair, with full military honors accorded to Kekana, and three other MK operatives whose bodies were recovered at the same time, and a guest list that included prominent politicians, military officials, and famous leaders of the struggle. Kekana was praised as a military hero who died to make his people and his country free from colonial rule (Ntuli 2005). For Mabel Makope, the honors he received "shows everybody that this guy has fought" (Makope 2007).

All three women I interviewed told me that they expected the same of the ceremony for their loved ones. But in the end, there was no significant military presence, no pomp and circumstance, not even the mayor of Mamelodi bothered to show up. Makope told me that "it was like we were burying an old person. We are not happy at all. There were no flags. There were no MKs to march for them to show people that these people have fought for this country. It was like a normal funeral" (Makope 2007). For Lizzie Sefolo, the "sickness was removed [when the bodies were initially recovered], but now it's coming back. Because it's like they were not really people who fought for this country, it was just remains." She continued:

> It was not proper. No matter, they put some stones, the headstones. That doesn't interest us. We wanted these people to be buried as soldiers and respected as people who fought for this country. We are here now, we are free, because of the people like them. Why [are they] not being respected like others? . . . So the truth must be said. And then you keep quiet and say 'you mustn't talk about that' and at the end of the day you—it's you who is getting the pain, and you are suffering alone. So they must know that we are not happy at all (Sefolo 2007).

During the course of the discussion, they explained to me that the desire to have their sons and husbands memorialized as military heroes in the armed struggle against apartheid (or, in other words, to give their deaths historical meaning *and* to make them eligible for state benefits that accrue to family members of people who die in the line of duty), was just as important as identifying their physical remains through DNA profiling. Simply finding the bones was not enough. The women argued that the ANC elite only truly cared about the missing people who fit into their own self-congratulatory narrative about the downfall of apartheid—that is, one that privileges the return from exile and Robben Island, along with the settlement negotiated by F. W. de Klerk and Nelson Mandela, over the street demonstrations, riots, and acts of civil disobedience by ordinary people that made the country ungovernable for the apartheid state. This interpretation of the current situation was strengthened in their minds by the fact that Kakena had spent a significant amount of time in exile, while their loved ones were primarily internal operators (Maake 2007; Makope 2007; Sefolo 2007). Ultimately, the relatives of the Mamelodi 4 that I spoke to were deeply disappointed that the exhumation and identification process did not provide them with an opportunity to clarify history.

The women place the blame squarely on the shoulders of the local ANC branch, which operates largely autonomously from the national ANC organization. Indeed, in his analysis of South African politics after 1994, Lodge states that, when ordinary South Africans profess disdain about the state of governance and service delivery in the country, the target of their anger is generally at the regional or local level (Lodge 2003:33). The women told me that the local ANC branch didn't even bother to inform the community that a reburial of formerly missing MK comrades would be taking place at the cemetery. While they did pay for proper headstones for the cemetery as noted above, they did not give the families money to buy food for family members and friends who were taking part in the ceremony (Maake 2007; Makope 2007; Sefolo 2007).

Delving deeper into the problems with the reburial ceremony, the women told me that there was tension between long-standing members of the ANC and those who had joined more recently for reasons that weren't always grounded in ideology or a shared sense of struggle, which is typical in this organization, which had less than 15,000 people in 1990 when it was unbanned, and more than 500,000 by the end of 1991 (Lodge 2003:33). Further, one of the women had close family members who were part of the MK Military Veterans Association in Mamelodi (MKMVA). She told me that MVA would have liked to take control of the burial but they felt that the local ANC branch had jurisdiction because of their relationship to the national government. They said that there is now deep regret that they let the ANC handle the reburial.

For the three women, resolution had not yet come at the time that I initially spoke to them, in May 2007. They had begun to go to ANC meetings, despite not all of them being members, to demand an explanation for what they perceived as ill-treatment. For them, this process was yet another necessary part of the healing process. As one of the women told me, "closure must be there in a proper way . . . we are still waiting" (Sefolo 2007). When I returned to Mamelodi in 2008 and 2009, it was clear to me that, while their anger had mellowed somewhat, they still felt that the government had not met its obligations to them as relatives of fallen military veterans.

When I asked Madeline Fullard of the Missing Persons Task Team what went wrong with the Mamelodi 4 handover and reburial, she suggested that the women were perhaps reading too much into the differences between the two funerals that they had witnessed. She explained to me that the Kakena ceremony was part of the government's kick-off for the Missing Persons Task Team, and was meant to be a singular event to raise public awareness for the program and the issue of disappearances more generally. She noted that the Department of Justice's TRC unit was responsible for the handover and the local political party for the reburial, so she was not heavily involved in the planning of the events. In retrospect, she laments that the false expectation of such a grand proceeding was created for the Mamelodi families, because it is impossible to provide each and every identified person with such an extravagant ceremony—however appropriate it would be to do so. "A whole series of acknowledgments should take place," she told me, "but it's going to be a faulty process because it's government, and government generally doesn't fulfill peoples' fantasies at any level" (Fullard 2008).

Mamelodi 10

While the case of the Mamelodi 4 illustrates the importance of the commemorative dimension of post-conflict identification, another case from the same community, that of the "Mamelodi 10," provides a window into another, equally crucial part of the process: the provision of information and access to the physical evidence associated with the deaths of the missing that can enable recognition, even in the absence of confirmatory DNA test results.

The case of the "Mamelodi 10" (Rooibaard Geldenhuis, Jeremiah Magagula, Steve Makena, Abram Makolane, Samuel Masilela, Morris Nkabinde, Jeremiah Ntuli, Thomas Phiri, Elliott Sathege, and Sipho Sibanyoni; also known as the "Nietverdiend 10" after the site where they were killed) involved ten politically active teenagers from Mamelodi, who were "recruited" in June 1986 by Joe Mamasela, a black security police officer posing as an MK agent, to go into exile with the MK in Botswana to receive military training. En route, the minibus that they were being transported in was ambushed by security forces at a pre-arranged spot. The young men were then ordered off of the bus by the hit squad, who then injected them with tranquilizers to incapacitate them. They were then loaded back into the bus, along with several liters of gasoline, a limpet mine, and an AK-47. The bus was then run into a tree and set alight to make it appear as if there had been a road accident (Rademeyer 2005).[1] The heavily fragmented remains of the ten young men were discovered by local villagers and then taken by local police to an undertaker, who subsequently buried them in pauper's graves at Winterveld Cemetery. It should be noted that this kind of incident was not uncommon in apartheid South Africa, although the remains of the victims were often returned to the families by authorities, such as in the case of the KwaNdeble 9, who were killed under very similar circumstances by Mamesala and colleagues a few weeks later.

Because several former security police applied for amnesty on the Mamelodi 10 case, it fell under the remit of the MPTT, which in 2005, with the help of members of the Argentine Forensic Anthropology Team, succeeded in locating ten bodies believed to belong to the Mamelodi 10 (Missing Persons Task Team 2006). Fullard and her colleagues were fairly certain that the remains belonged to the Mamelodi 10 because they were able to locate documentation that confirmed chain of custody from the security police all the way through to burial records at Winterveld. The only complicating factors were that the ten bodies were buried along with four paupers who arrived at the undertaker at around the same time, and that there were some serious discrepancies between the cemetery records and actual burial patterns on the ground. Thus, the team opened several graves that clearly belonged to people other than the Mamelodi 10 victims. Ultimately, though, they did succeed in locating ten bodies that bore the kind of trauma that one would expect in the deaths that these young men experienced.

In order to obtain confirmation of the identity of the bodies, Fullard sent bone samples to an American company called Bode Technology for identification. After nearly a year of hearing nothing, Fullard received what she described for the record as "disappointing" results (Fullard 2007), which suggested that the ten bodies were unrelated to the families of the Mamelodi 10 (Missing Persons Task Team 2006:17). The results created emotional chaos for everyone involved in the process, including members of the MPTT (Fullard 2007).

Fullard, however, was not convinced that Bode had done all they could to properly analyze the DNA from the Mamelodi 10 samples, so she turned to Neil Laet, from the University of Western Cape. Unfortunately, Laet could not generate individual identifications for nine of the ten bodies, although he did convincingly demonstrate that they could not be ruled out as being part of the Mamelodi 10. The news on the tenth body surprised everybody—it was positively excluded as being a member of the Mamelodi 10 (MPTT 2008). This meant that the MPTT would have to continue searching graves in Winterveld Cemetery—as of June 2011, the tenth body has not been found.

Because of the inconclusive DNA results, Fullard asked an American expert on bone trauma named Steve Symes to come to South Africa to examine the presumptive Mamelodi 10 remains. In his analysis, Symes concluded that the nine sets of remains belonged to men in the age range of the Mamelodi 10 and that their condition was consistent with their bodies being subjected to explosives and intense heat. Based on that information, along with the chain of custody records and the presence of a particular type of coffin associated with pauper burials, the MPTT declared that the nine bodies did indeed belong to the Mamelodi 10 and began to make preparations to hand them over to the families. As it became clear that there would be no conclusive individual identification of the Mamelodi 10, and that there was no guarantee that the tenth body would be found anytime soon, the families of the victims decided to bury the nine bodies together in a shared grave, leaving space for the tenth if and when he was ever recovered (Ntuli 2008).

In July 2008 interviews, the women uniformly stated that they were deeply disappointed that the remains could not be individually identified. However, they all understood the difficulty of extracting DNA from bones that had been subject to the intense heat of the minibus fire and then buried in the acidic soil of South Africa. Although collective burial was not ideal for the women, it was at least a major improvement over the previous state of affairs for both family members and the deceased. Thus, their overarching goal from the process shifted from hoping for individual identity to ensuring that the located remains were those of the Mamelodi 10 collectively. As Maria Ntuli, mother of Jeremiah stated: "they have been burned and from that they went to their grave, and in the grave there was no more coffin, they were just lying in the ground there. Now, how can the DNA be there? At my side, I am very satisfied with what they have done for us. Really, I am satisfied. Even my children, I told them that the DNA doesn't come out. It doesn't match to any remains, so the only thing we can do is to bury those remains and get over with it" (Ntuli 2008).

For Katherine Magagula, mother of Jeremiah Magagula, what was critical for the mothers in the absence of positive DNA results was the information that was carried through; all along the investigation of finding the remains was what gave them hope that these would be the remains of their loved ones (Magagula 2008). The MPTT made sure that the women had access to the photographs of the crime scene (which were recovered by the team from security police records), the opportunity to examine the mortuary records, and a detailed understanding of the investigation process from start to finish. At the mothers' request, Fullard also arranged for Symes to return to South Africa to give the women a presentation on why he felt confident declaring that the remains were those of their children (Magagula 2008; Ntuli 2008).

One of the most interesting aspects of the bones was the extent to which they were markers of the collective, but not individual, identity of the people who died. This is more in line with the situation in forensic anthropology in the era before widespread use of DNA identification. During one of my meetings with the Mamelodi 10 relatives, there was a long and fascinating discussion about how the women reacted to seeing the bones of their loved ones for the first time—that is, during the exhumation itself. All of the women who spoke reported that they felt conflicting feelings of curiosity, anxiety, and even excitement to see human remains on the one hand, and almost indescribable pain and heartache on the other. It is interesting to note that this emphasis on bones is quite different from the situation in the former Yugoslavia, where ICMP case managers discourage viewing of bones because they "offer no visible link to the image that family members have of the person in the final moments at the fall of the enclave" (Wagner 2008:145). In the Balkan context, much more emphasis is placed on the personal effects recovered with bodies (Wagner 2008).

At yet another level, Lizzie Sefolo, wife of Harold from the Mamelodi 4, said that witnessing the exhumation was a kind of validation of the process of identification, that they were a part of the investigation rather just being recipients of information. She said that the relatives are able to follow the entire process through to see exactly how investigators deal with particular remains when they find them. She noted that there is always the possibility of the remains in question not being the ones you are looking for. For the women, watching the actual exhumation and initial investigation gave them a sense of "how you prove or disprove of the identity" (Sefolo 2008). Sefolo concluded that watching gave them a sense that exhumations are long, involved processes, and "not just digging" (Sefolo 2008). Another woman went further, suggesting that had they not actually gone to the gravesite to witness the exhumation, they would have had serious doubts about the veracity of the MPTT's findings.[4]

Thus, we can see that at least in the case of the women from Mamelodi, being present at the exhumation and gaining access to all relevant information about the events leading to the deaths of their loved ones fulfilled two important purposes. The first was to help them bring the period of uncertainty in their lives to a close by given them the knowledge they lacked for so long. This, of course, is not a new phenomenon. The presence of families at exhumations was a key component of the Argentine Forensic Anthropology Team's protocol and, as a result, has been widely adopted by forensic teams in subsequent investigations throughout Latin America (Sanford 2003).

Second, the exchange of information between the investigators and the relatives of the missing helped them recognize the damaged, degraded remains as their own. They came to understand the process used to confirm identity and to trust the scientists and investigators doing the work. While the outcome was obviously not as satisfying as it would have been if individual identification would have been possible though DNA identification, the fact that the bodies were recovered seems to have gone a long way to ameliorating the pain and uncertainty that they felt. Even the Mamelodi 4 relatives, who were deeply dissatisfied by the memorialization efforts for their loved ones, still fully accepted, and were grateful for, the work done by the MPTT (Maake 2007; Makope 2007; Sefolo 2007).

Once again this brings us back to the issue of commemoration and memorialization—the third form of recognition. The mothers of the Mamelodi 10 were very adamant that they wanted to have a better experience than the relatives of the Mamelodi 4 victims, one that was dignified and in accordance with the sacrifice that they believed their children had made for the country. The Mamelodi 4 relatives felt the same way. Indeed, Lizzie Sefolo declared that the families of the 4 were going to work with the Mamelodi 10 mothers to ensure that they would have a better experience (Sefolo 2008).

Their efforts were, on the surface, quite successful, as the Mamelodi 10 reburial was far more reminiscent of Reginald Kakena's than that of the Mamelodi 4. Indeed, along with speeches from religious figures and MKMVA officials, their ceremony included appearances by the mayor of Tshwane (the administrative district including Pretoria and its former townships) and the premier of Gauteng state, as well as a tribute from Kgalema Motlanthe, the interim President of the country (who took over from the deposed Thabo Mbeki) (MKMVA 2008b).

Thus, the Mamelodi 10 succeeded in using the occasion of the discovery of their of their loved ones' remains to insert their loved ones into the history of the new South Africa in a way that the Mamelodi 4 families had not.

Yet, they were still deeply unhappy with the process by which their loved ones were buried for the same reasons that the Mamelodi 4 were, namely the failure of the local ANC branch to follow through with their obligations to fallen military veterans. Specifically, the ANC did not provide the women with the food that they were required to serve to relatives at a funeral, and they did not provide the coffins that were to be used to bury the remains of the Mamelodi 10. Instead, the MKMVA had to arrange donations of coffins from local undertakers. While such complaints may seem trivial, it is important to remember that the women I spoke to care deeply about the symbolic actions of the government that is supposed to represent them.

Conclusion

In her work on the identification of the missing in Bosnia, Sarah Wagner notes that the "path leading from the unrecognized to the recognized also forces open the term *identity*. Identity not only signifies the relationship between a name and a set of physical remains, but also encompasses the social ties that bind a person to a place, a time, and, most importantly, to other human beings" (Wagner 2008:11). From my analysis of the situation in post-apartheid South Africa, it is clear that DNA identification facilitates the process of biological recognition, but it does little to ensure that family members recognize the loved ones that they lost so long ago as social beings, or that society at large will recognize the recently recovered individuals as military heroes in the struggle against apartheid. But history, of course, does not write itself. To achieve the kind of social recognition that is so crucial to relatives of missing MK operatives, serious political work must be undertaken alongside of DNA identification. Thus, DNA identification provides the *opportunity* to produce some sense of closure for families of the disappeared, rather than closure itself.

ACKNOWLEDGMENTS

This work has been supported by a grant from the U.S. National Institutes of Health's Ethical, Legal, and Social Implications of Human Genomic Research (ELSI) Program, R03 HG004655, "DNA Identification in the Aftermath of Genocide and Mass Violence." The human subjects protection procedures practiced by the author have been reviewed and approved by Carnegie Mellon University's IRB (Project ID: HS09–076 Date: 20 February 2009). The author wishes to thank the South African Missing Persons Task Team and Khulumani Support Group for logistical assistance, and, most important, the relatives of the missing and disappeared, who welcomed me into their community and their homes and shared their harrowing stories with me.

NOTES

1. Although my own understanding of the situation in South Africa was developed before I read the work of Sarah Wagner on the identification of the missing in the aftermath of Srebrenica, I have adopted her use of the term "recognition," because it properly describes identity as something that is actively constructed through a particular social process, rather than something that exists in a static form (Wagner 2008:10).

2. Gottschalk 2002; Pauw 1997; Commision 1998–2003, volume 2. It is important to recognize that the number of people killed by security forces in South Africa was much lower than in similar conflicts around the world. In other words, apartheid was characterized more by "everyday oppression" as opposed to systematic, extreme violence.

3. In numerous personal communications, Madeleine Fullard has downplayed the overall significance of extreme violence in the apartheid system. For her, political oppression, everyday harassment, and economic servitude played an equal, if not greater, role in the injustice of apartheid.

4. This statement was made during a group discussion in Mamelodi in July 2008. Upon listening to the recordings, I could not determine exactly who expressed this view, but it is clear that the other relatives in the room at the time agreed.

WORKS CITED

Aronson, Jay D. 2011. The strengths and limitations of South Africa's search for apartheid-era missing persons. *International Journal of Transitional Justice*:262–281.

Barrell, Howard. 1993. Conscripts to their age: African National Congress operational strategy, 1976–1986. Ph.D. diss., Oxford University.

Bloch, Maurice, and Jonathan Parry. 1982. Introduction: Death and the regeneration of life. In *Death and the regeneration of life*, edited by Maurice Bloch and Jonathan Parry, 1–44. Cambridge: Cambridge University Press.

Butler, Anthony. 2007. The state of the African National Conference. In *State of the Nation: South Africa*, edited by Sakhela Buhlungu, John Daniel, Roger Southall, and Jessica Lutchman, 35–51. Cape Town: HSRC Press.

———. 2008. *Cyril Ramaphosa*. Johannesburg: Jacana Books.

Commission, Truth and Reconciliation. 1998–2003. *Final report*. Cape Town: Juta and Co.

Davison, Sean, Mongi Benjedou, and Maria Eugenia D'Amato. 2008. Molecular genetic identification of skeletal remains of apartheid activists in South Africa. *African Journal of Biotechnology* 7, no. 25:4750–4757.

de Klerk, F. W. 1998. *The last trek—a new beginning: The autobiography*. Basingstoke: Macmillan.

Dennie, Garry Michael. 1996. The cultural politics of burial in South Africa, 1884–1990. Ph.D. diss., Johns Hopkins University.

Department of Justice and Constitutional Development. 2008. Notice 1539 of 2008, Invitation to submit comments on proposed exhumation policy on cases reported to the TRC. *Government Gazette* 3172:3–17.

Dewhirst, Polly. 2008. Transitional justice and disappearances, a briefing paper. International Center for Transitional Justice.

Dubow, Saul. 2000. *The African National Congress*. New York: Sutton Publishing.

Eppel, Shari. 2006. "Healing the dead": Exhumation and reburial as truth-telling and peace-building activities in rural Zimbabwe. In *Telling the truths: Truth telling and peace building in post-conflict societies,* edited by Tristan Anne Borer, 259–288. Notre Dame, IN: University of Notre Dame Press.

Fullard, Madeleine. 2007, May. Personal interview with author. Cape Town, South Africa.

————. 2008, June. Personal interview with author. Pretoria, South Africa.

————. 2011, February 28. E-mail exchange with author.

Gottschalk, Keith. 2002. The rise and fall of apartheid's death squads, 1969–93. In *Death squads in global perspective: Murder with deniability*, edited by Bruce B. Campbell and Arthur D. Brenner, 229–260. London: Macmillan.

Hamber, Brandon, Dineo Nageng, and Gabriel O'Malley. 2000. "Telling it like it is": Understanding the Truth and Reconciliation Commission from the perspective of survivors. *Psychology in Society* 26:18–42.

Hamber, Brandon, and Richard Wilson. 2002. Symbolic closure through memory, reparation, and revenge in post-conflict societies. *Journal of Human Rights* 1, no. 1:35–53.

Heribert, Adam, and Kogila Moodley. 1993. *The opening of the apartheid mind: Options for the new South Africa*. Berkeley: University of California Press.

Laet, Neil. 2008, July. Personal interview with author. Cape Town, South Africa.

Lawyers for Human Rights. 2008. *Proceedings from a conference on the International Convention for the Protection of All Persons from Enforced Disappearances: Implications for South Africa and the region*. Pretoria: Lawyers for Human Rights.

Lodge, Tom. 2003. Politics in South Africa: From Mandela to Mbeki. Bloomington: Indiana University Press.

Maake, Elizabeth. 1996, 30 April. Testimony before the Truth and Reconciliation Commission Human Rights Violations Committee, Johannesburg.

————. 2007. May. Personal interview with author. Mamelodi, South Africa.

Magagula, Katherine. 2008, July. Personal interview with author. Mamelodi, South Africa.

Makope, Mabel. 1996, 30 April. Testimony before the Truth and Reconciliation Commission Human Rights Violations Committee, Johannesburg.

————. 2007, May. Personal interview with author. Mamelodi, South Africa.

Mandela, Nelson. 1995. *Long walk to freedom: The autobiography of Nelson Mandela*. Boston: Little, Brown.

Mashike, Lephophotho. 2008. Age of despair: The unintegrated forces of South Africa. *African Affairs* 107, no. 428:433–453.

Mashike, Lephophotho. 2007. "Some of us know nothing except military skills": South Africa's former guerrilla combatants. In *State of the Nation: South Africa 2007*, edited by Sakhela Buhlungu, John Daniel, Roger Southall, and Jessica Lutchman, 351–378. Cape Town: HSRC Press.

Mbembe, Achille. 2003. Necropolitics. *Public Culture* 15, no. 1:11–40.

Meli, Francis. 1988. *South Africa belongs to us: A history of the ANC*. Harare: Zimbabwe Publishing House.

Missing Persons Task Team. 2006. *Report for the Period 1 July 2005–30 June 2006*, edited by National Prosecuting Authority Priority Crimes Litigation Unit.

MKMVA. 2008, 9 October. Press Statement on the Mamelodi 10. www.cosatu.org.za/press/2008/oct/press22.htm [Accessed 30 March 2009].

MKMVA. 2008, 10 October. "Briefing on the Mamelodi 10." Available at: *groups.google.com/group/COSATU-press/msg/19865005138f6ff4*. [Accessed 30 March 2009].

Ntuli, Maria. 2008, July. Personal interview with author. Mamelodi, South Africa.

Ottaway, David. 1993. *Chained together. Mandela, De Klerk, and the struggle to remake South Africa*. New York: Times Books.

Pauw, Jacques. 1997. *Into the heart of darkness: Confessions of apartheid's assassins*. Johannesburg: Jonathan Ball.

Prinsloo, Hendrik Johannes. 1999, 19 October. Testimony before the Truth and Reconciliation Commission Amnesty Hearings, Pretoria.

Rademeyer, Julian. 2005. Digging up murder and lies. *Sunday Times* (South Africa), 4 April, 19.

Sampson, Anthony. 1999. *Mandela: The authorised biography*. London: HarperCollins.

Sanford, Victoria. 2003. *Buried secrets: Truth and human rights in Guatemala*. New York: Palgrave Macmillan.

Seekings, Jeremy. 2000. *The UDF: A story of the United Democratic Front in South Africa 1983–1991*. Cape Town: David Philip.

Sefolo, Lizzie Thandi. 1996, 30 April. Testimony before the Truth and Reconciliation Commission Human Rights Violations Committee, Johannesburg.

———. 2007, May. Personal interview with author. Mamelodi, South Africa.

———. 2008, July. Personal interview with author. Mamelodi, South Africa.

Sheehan, Helena. 2002. Interview with Jeremy Cronin. webpages.dcu.ie/~sheehanh/za/cronin02.html [Accessed March 25, 2009].

Southall, Roger. 2007. Introduction: The ANC state, more dysfunctional than developmental? In *State of the nation: South Africa 2007*, edited by Sakhela Buhlungu, John Daniel, Roger Southall, and Jessica Lutchman, 1–24. Cape Town: HSRC Press.

Sparks, Allister. 1995. *Tomorrow is another country: The inside story of South Africa's road to change*. New York: Hill and Wang.

Suttner, Raymond. 2002. Culture(s) of the African National Congress of South Africa [ANC]: Contribution of exile and prison experiences. In *WISER Seminar Series*. Witwatersrand University.

———. 2007. African National Congress (ANC): Attainment of power, post liberation phases, and current crisis. *Historia* 52, no. 2:1–46.

Thomspon, Leonard. 2000. *A history of South Africa*, 3rd edition. New Haven: Yale University Press.

van Vuuren, Paul. 1996, 21 October. Testimony before the Truth and Reconciliation Commission Amnesty Hearings, Johannesburg.

Wagner, Sarah. 2008. *To know where he lies: DNA technology and the search for Srebrenica's missing*. Berkeley: University of California Press.

Waldmeir, Patty. 1997. *Anatomy of a miracle: The end of apartheid and the birth of the New South Africa*. London: Viking.

Winter, Jay. 1999. Forms of kinship and remembrance in the aftermath of the Great War. In *War and remembrance in the twentieth century*, edited by Jay Winter and Emmanuel Sivan, 40–60. Cambridge: Cambridge University Press.

Zunes, Stephen. 1999. The role of non-violent action in the downfall of apartheid. *Journal of Modern African Studies* 37, no. 1:137–169.

Conclusions

The Unsettled Past

18

<hr />

Forbidden or Forsaken?

The (Mis)Use of a Forbidden Knowledge Argument in Research on Race, DNA, and Disease

REANNE FRANK

On June 16, 2006, an article appeared in the *Wall Street Journal* profiling the research of Dr. Bruce Lahn, a University of Chicago professor of human genetics (Regalado 2006). The article summarized two of Lahn's published research papers in which he and his co-authors identified two genes that they argued likely provided an adaptive advantage in the form of improved cognition (Evans et al. 2005; Mekel-Bobrov et al. 2005). An additional finding was that the favored alleles demonstrated a pronounced geographic pattern that made them the least common in sub-Saharan Africa.

Critics immediately challenged the paper's conclusions, arguing that there was no evidence that the genes were related to any brain-related phenotype and, additionally, that there was no evidence that the gene regions identified underwent selection (Currat et al. 2006). Lahn's research team eventually backed away from the claim that that there was an association between the genes and cognitive ability (Mekel-Bobrov et al. 2007). Nonetheless, the *Wall Street Journal* article on Lahn noted that he touched a "raw nerve in science." Dr. Lahn himself was quoted as saying that his work on potential racial differences in intelligence was "getting too controversial" and that the "intellectual police in the U.S. make such questions difficult to pursue." Responding to the failure to correlate the genes with differences in intelligence Lahn responded: "On a scientific level, I am a little bit disappointed. But in the context of the social and political controversy, I am a little bit relieved" (Balter 2006). The *Wall Street Journal* article ends with a reference to a student's recent inquiry to Dr. Lahn asking him, "whether some knowledge might not be worth having."

A profile of population geneticist David B. Goldstein in the *New York Times* made similar claims about how fear and politics stood in the path of true knowledge about race. Following a description of Goldstein's work on the possibility that many of the genes that bear the mark of natural selection tend to differ from one race to another, the reporter Nicholas Wade wrote: "[t]his newish finding has raised fears that other, more significant, differences might emerge among races."

For his part Goldstein remarks that, "there is a part of the scientific community which is trying to make this work off limits, and that I think is hugely counter-productive" (Wade 2008).

The cases of Dr. Lahn and Dr. Goldstein and the subsequent coverage in the *Wall Street Journal* and the *New York Times* are illustrative of an increasingly prevalent narrative characterizing the new genetic enterprise. I label the narrative "forbidden knowledge" and borrow from past research that has defined the concept of forbidden knowledge as the idea that there are certain things that we should not know, because the knowledge has been obtained by unacceptable means, the knowledge is perceived as too dangerous, or the knowledge is prohibited by religious, moral, or secular authority (Kempner et al. 2005). The claim that genetic explanations for racial difference represent forbidden knowledge is a common, yet often overlooked, narrative that has emerged in contemporary research. At its core, this powerful rhetorical argument misleadingly casts geneticists' writing on race as seeking objective truths, while portraying all skeptics as motivated by unscientific fears, passions, and politics.

The forbidden-knowledge argument is a powerful, yet flawed, one that reveals much about the ways in which claims about DNA, race, and history—however mistaken or specious—are crafted and rhetorically defended against criticism. As we have seen throughout this volume, the arguments about race and history originating from diverse genetics enterprises are themselves multifaceted and often conflicting. The applicability of these arguments—in criminal justice, in medical and pharmaceutical settings, in genealogy and other commercial enterprises, and at the level of politics and national building—are numerous. However, even as debate has raged about the validity and evidence supporting genetic claims about race and the past, many geneticists have sought to defend themselves against debate by resorting to a bold declaration: that any objections are rooted in fear.

A close look at examples of the forbidden knowledge argument used in the context of contemporary genetic research offers crucial insight into the genetics enterprise itself, and into some of its more troubling consequences. Perhaps most pressing is the fact that the forbidden knowledge argument functions to subvert the scientific process itself, by suggesting that critiques, such as those presented in this volume, come from a place of fear instead of representing legitimate scientific discourse.

Forbidden Knowledge in the Academic Literature

In the existing literature, the forbidden knowledge argument used in response to criticism of contemporary genetic research on racial difference follows a fairly consistent pattern. First, a genetic explanation is put forth as a causal agent in explaining a racial difference in health or a related outcome. Second, in response to a specific critique or in a related commentary, a forbidden knowledge argument is invoked, whereby the genetic explanation is depicted as "forbidden," that is, unwanted knowledge that is perceived as too dangerous or politically unpalatable to be accepted.

When scientists and others label genetic explanations for racial differences as "forbidden," it follows that those who support a genetic perspective are doing so in the face of societal pressure. For bringing to light what society has deemed forbidden knowledge, these scientists are seen as pioneers who ask the difficult questions that others are too fearful to ask. Fee (2006) has pointed out that they are often represented (and represent themselves) as "brave scientific martyr-pioneers" who are fighting against the repressive forces of political correctness to bring to light knowledge that other scientists consider taboo. Hammonds provides an example in her critique of Armand Marie Leroi's *New York Times* op-ed piece of March 2005, in which he asserts "the return of biological race," arguing that race is a "shorthand that allows us to speak sensibly, though with no great precision, about genetic rather than cultural or political differences" (Leroi 2005). In doing so, Hammonds argues that "he becomes the hero of his own tale for his obvious courage in going against the forces of political correctness in the service of addressing health disparities" (Hammonds 2006).

The flip side of this scenario is that those scientists who do *not* support a genetic explanation for a given racial difference are characterized as giving in to political constraints that restrain further investigation of biological factors. The forbidden knowledge argument provides little room for those who question genetic explanations because of concerns with the methodological quality of the research. Critics of contemporary genetic research on racial difference are labeled as "politically correct" or as too afraid to accept the evidence. This is a dynamic that has played out fairly consistently in the contemporary research that lies at the intersection of race and genetics.

Ancestry Testing

One of the more publicly recognized components of the new genetic enterprise is the practice of ancestry testing, that is, inferring "biogeographical" ancestries of individuals from predetermined genetic markers (Rosenberg et al. 2003; Shriver and Kittles 2004). A related practice involves distinguishing population groupings on the basis of individual genotypes, that is, clustering of individuals by genotype until a certain number of genetically distinct groups are defined (Bamshad et al. 2003; Bamshad et al. 2004; Rosenberg et al. 2002; Shriver et al. 2005). Both research areas have captured the public's imagination and have inevitably crossed over into debates concerning the genetic basis of race. In the popular press, research on genetic ancestry has been lauded as simultaneously "bringing us all a little closer together" and, at the same time showing that, "looked at the right way, genetic data show that races clearly do exist" (Leroi 2005; Wells 2007).

Critics of ancestry testing and related enterprises have been less enthusiastic about the promise of such claims. Several chapters in this volume raise concerns with the methodological practices underlying both ancestry testing and attempts to cluster individual genotypes into distinct population-based groupings that roughly correspond to popular notions of race. In the chapter "The Dilemma of Classification" Braun and Hammonds discuss how the sub-Saharan Working Group, one of the components of the Human Genome Diversity Project (HGDP), sampled groups using outmoded maps from the middle of last century. In doing so, the Working Group ignored the diffuse and changing nature of the populations sampled, instead converting them into fixed and unchanging databases that reify a biological concept of race. For example, the HGDP and other related databases have been used to argue that, "people's self-identified race/ethnicity is a nearly perfect indicator of their genetic background" (Risch 2005).

Concerns surrounding sampling methodology extend into the arena of ancestry testing. Although ancestry testing has become an increasing lucrative business that claims to allow "the general public to use the power of genomics to discover their genetic ancestry,"[1] others have questioned the authoritative nature of these results. In the chapter "A Biologist's Perspective of DNA and Race in the Genomics Era," Gabriel argues that the research area suffers from some basic technical problems. Essentially, ancestry identification relies on probabilistic tests, whose reliability depends completely on the sample size and the representativeness of the standard group analyzed for each population. Consequently, scientists engaged in the business of ancestry testing are forced to make many methodological decisions about how they are going to partition human population variation to determine a person's ancestry. These decisions involve issues of sample size, number of loci, number of clusters, assumptions about correlation in allele frequencies across populations, and the geographic dispersion of the sample (Rosenberg et al. 2005). The existence of such decisions calls attention to the fact that there is substantial disagreement as to how human genetic variation is structured as well as how to categorize this variation. While it is clear that there is human genetic and phenotypic variation across population groups that is geographically correlated, it is also true that this variation is not categorically distributed at the population level and, as a result, does not match up in any uniform way to supposed racial categories (Kittles and Weiss 2003).

Methodological critiques (such as the ones raised in this volume by such authors as Rajagopalan and Fujimura, Chow-White, and S. Lee regarding admixture, mapping, information databases, and forensics, respectively) have been cited as turning a promising area of research into a "contentious" debate (Bamshad 2005). Instead of viewing the critiques as raising legitimate methodological concerns, they are seen as denying the reality of clear genetic clusterings and questioning the reliability of ancestry tests. Dr. Neil Risch, a Stanford geneticist, has suggested that "*denying* the existence of racial or ethnic differences in gene frequencies . . . is unlikely to benefit minority populations" (Risch 2006). This lament is cited particularly when the subject matter moves from one involved in discerning ancestry towards the much more complicated task of disease identification and explaining racial disparities in disease. One such approach involves admixture mapping.

Admixture Mapping

Admixture mapping is a procedure that attempts to identify candidate disease genes. It follows in the tradition of genome-wide association studies, but differs in that it makes explicit use of race. By leveraging DNA markers whose frequencies differ significantly between populations, admixture mapping aims to reduce the work of narrowing down the location of disease genes. But as Rajagopalan and Fujimura argue, the admixture mapping research process deserves closer scrutiny. Their extensive work inside a laboratory that is currently using admixture mapping in research on prostate cancer suggests that the line between expert laboratory-generated knowledge and popular beliefs is blurry, and that American folk ideas of race figure prominently in many of the methodological decisions made. For example, many of the "ancestral" frequencies used in admixture mapping were assessed by genotyping contemporary samples (using European Americans as stand-ins for ancestral European populations and African Americans as stand-ins for ancestral West African or sub-Saharan African populations). Whereas the African American samples are conceived as African enough to approximate the corresponding frequencies in ancestral African groups, they are considered admixed with European ancestral contributions for the sake of the admixture analysis. In the process, the social history that made even the idea and possibilities for admixture possible is ignored.

What are we to do with the concerns raised by biologists themselves about the scope and character of genetic claims about race and history? In one of the earlier chapters of this volume, Abram Gabriel expresses surprise that "geneticists, known for their usual care in designing experiments, would be so willingly lax" in their use of socially constructed race variables in genetic studies. But instead of calls for more critical engagement of such research, a more frequent response to the criticism of admixture analysis, and the use of racial categories in genetic research more generally, is a forbidden knowledge argument.

A *New York Times* profile of geneticist Dr. Neil Risch states that: "in asserting that race is a valid concept for medical research, Dr. Risch has plunged into an arena where many *fear* to tread" (Wade 2002; emphasis added). A separate article argues that "it may be tempting to abandon the notion of race altogether" but this would be "detrimental to the very populations and persons that this approach allegedly seeks to protect" (Burchard et al. 2003). As reported in the *New York Times*: "[m]any people, including some African-Americans, have long been uneasy with the concept of race-based medicine, in part from *fear* that it may legitimize less benign ideas about race" (Wade 2004; emphasis added). Instead of a legitimate scientific discourse where issues about the construction of samples, the definition of populations, the probabilistic nature of results, and other methodological concerns are debated in an open forum, the invocation of the forbidden knowledge argument functions to silence critiques, taking away the basis for any informed scientific discourse on the matter.

The Slavery Hypothesis

Gabriel also expresses concern regarding the links being made between race and genetics for disease predisposition because "these links may become accepted without recognition of the limitations of the underlying science." Such a case is found in the development of "the slavery hypothesis," which was formulated as an explanation for the frequent and more severe hypertension found in African Americans. The slavery hypothesis refers to the possibility that, during the slave trade and transatlantic voyage, only those slaves who could retain salt survived, that is, did not die from heat stress and salt and water deprivation (Fryer 2005). As a result, New World Blacks are hypothesized to display an exaggerated hypertensive response to salt because of a genetic predisposition that originated in the slave trade. This idea has received considerable attention since it was first introduced ten years ago, including mention in most cardiology textbooks (Kaufman and Hall 2003). The slavery hypothesis was even showcased on an episode of the *Oprah Winfrey Show* with Dr. Mehmet Oz, her resident physician:

DR. OZ: "Do you know why African Americans have high blood pressure?"

OPRAH: "The reason why African Americans have higher blood pressure, Dr. Oz, is because during the Middle Passage [when Africans were taken as slaves to America], the African Americans who survived were those who could hold more salt into their body. And those who didn't survive were the ones who couldn't hold more salt into their body."

DR. OZ: "I'm off the show, you don't need me anymore—that's perfect!"

Despite Oprah's stamp of approval, epidemiologists Jay Kaufman and Susan Hall have argued that the slavery hypothesis is not supported by data (Kaufman and Hall 2003). While mention of the hypothesis is pervasive in both the popular and academic presses, a more thorough evaluation has shown that it lacks a base in either evolutionary theory or in empirical evidence. In particular, it suffers from an inaccurate estimation of the mortality rates that would have had to have occurred during the Middle Passage to make the slavery hypothesis tenable (Curtin 1992).

In response to Kaufman and Hall's critique, Clarence Grim, one of the two original formulators of the slavery hypothesis, accused his critics of forbidden knowledge and argued that: "Kaufman and Hall would have us stop all genetic research (hypothesis testing) for *fear* that we may discover information that 'marks a group as permanently distinct from other groups'" (Grim and Robinson 2003). Grim's remarks suggest that the slavery hypothesis is "forbidden" in the sense that it is not a socially acceptable explanation. In this rhetorical gambit, those who are unwilling to cow to the pressures of fear (as Grim casts himself) become the scientific heroes who are brave enough to raise and debate unpopular ideas. On the flip side, critics of genetic explanations are perceived as being too fearful of the knowledge that such a hypothesis would produce. But as we've seen in this volume, whether the focus is on the production of genetic knowledge in the laboratory, its use in courts and in clinics, or its utility in political discussions of national identity, a continuous theme promoted by those who would defend the enterprise is the claim that criticism is driven fundamentally by ignorance and fear. By invoking the forbidden knowledge argument, the methodological concerns raised by Kaufman and Hall cease to have scientific merit and instead become an issue of emotion, irrationality, and undue alarm.

The Future

The completion of the Human Genome Project in 2003 and the continued emergence of new genetic data repositories have revolutionized the fields of molecular biology and genetics and ushered in a new era of research. These developments hold great promise for our understanding of human history as well as for future discoveries in the field of human health. They also hold warnings from the past regarding the costs associated with the uncritical acceptance of genetic claims. These cautionary lessons take on an added urgency when race and DNA become conflated in the genetic enterprise.

The chapters included in this volume all, to some degree or another, remind us of the importance of monitoring research that occurs at the intersection of race and genetics, and of scrutinizing the methods, selective data sources, interpretive logic and illogic, and claims that can and cannot be supported by the evidence from genes. The work of the authors presented in these pages urge caution and skepticism, as well as engagement with the complexities of genetic research that uses racial categories. They urge greater attention to mistakes made in past research, awareness of assumptions made in current research, and thoughtful questioning of the methodological decisions underpinning genetics research; and above all, they provoke us to recognize the persistent and pervasive role that cultural assumptions play in these areas of science.

In contrast to the forbidden knowledge argument (which too often intends to close down debate and discussion), the goal of this volume is to facilitate a necessary and sustained dialogue on research that uses the concept of race (or more recently "biogeographic ancestry") in genetic research. For an optimal dialogue to take place, however, it will first be necessary to confront and move beyond the forbidden knowledge argument—the specious belief whether made by, or on behalf of, scientists and others, that all criticism of contemporary research on race and genetics originates out of a place of fear. Although the examples presented in this chapter involved biomedical or molecular genetics researchers, versions of the forbidden knowledge argument have also been used on behalf of social scientists, as illustrated in a special issue of the *American Sociological Review* on genetics and social science, where it was noted that sociologists often greet genetic research with "*fear* and loathing" (Bearman 2008; emphasis added). While it is likely true that many social scientists approach research that purports to demonstrate a genetic basis for human behavior with skepticism, it is counterproductive and fundamentally wrong to frame this skepticism as driven by irrational fear of the unknown.

Once a forbidden knowledge argument is invoked, rhetorical battle lines are drawn and the potential for meaningful scientific discourse is sharply curtailed. Critiques of racial genetic research are characterized as coming from a place of fear and not the result of legitimate concerns with the research itself. In this sense, claims of forbidden knowledge are unproductive at best and a form of scientific censorship at worst. They work to move research beyond critique and relegate those who argue alternative perspectives to the sidelines. Pigeonholed as cultural critics who are squelching potentially beneficial discoveries, voices of dissent are quickly silenced by a forbidden knowledge argument. Those who invoke the forbidden knowledge argument to defend their work also have something to lose. Scientists who think they are bravely employing race as an explanatory factor in the face of political correctness are not able to benefit from the critiques of their peers. If the only potential issue with the research is that it is not "politically correct," then the authors are less likely to be open to methodological critiques. As a result, the scientific research process (itself based on robust internal critique and the rejection of flawed ideas) is not able to run its due course.

Gabriel concludes his chapter in this volume with a list of recommendations for scientists who work at the intersection of molecular biology, genetics, health and race, arguing that they have a responsibility to: "inform the public about their work, explain their methods and their rigor, admit the limitations and areas of controversy and uncertainty, and examine its wider relevance." To his list I would add one additional recommendation: that the forbidden knowledge argument in response to critiques be eliminated. Only by forgoing references to fear, forbidden knowledge, or political correctness as a central motivating force in scientific and public debate can the research process move forward in a manner that ensures that future generations will truly benefit from the rise of a new genetics, and not look back on our century's research of race and genetics as a continuation of the eugenics work of early population geneticists from last century, with their own deeply flawed and politically noxious ideas about race, genes, and human history. This earlier history is also a reminder that science cannot settle the meaning of race.

NOTE

1. As quoted on the DNA Print website. January 2007. www.dnaprint.com/welcome/ corporate.

WORKS CITED

Balter, Michael. 2006. News focus. Bruce Lahn profile: Links between brain genes, evolution, and cognition challenged. *Science* 314 (5897):1872.

Bamshad, Michael J., Stephen Wooding, W. Scott Watkins, Christopher T. Ostler, Mark A. Batzer, and Lynn B. Jorde. 2003. Human population genetic structure and inference of group membership. *American Journal of Human Genetics* 72 (3):578.

Bamshad, Michael, Stephen Wooding, Benjamin A. Salisbury, and J. Claiborne Stephens. 2004. Deconstructing the relationship between genetics and race. *Nature Reviews Genetics* 5 (8):598.

Bearman, Peter. 2008. Exploring genetics and social structure. *American Journal of Sociology* 114 (suppl.):v–x.

Burchard, Esteban Gonzalez, Elad Ziv, Natasha Coyle, Scarlett Lin Gomez, Hua Tang, Andrew J. Karter, Joanna L. Mountain, Eliseo J. Perez-Stable, Dean Sheppard, and Neil Risch. 2003. The importance of race and ethnic background in biomedical research and clinical practice. *New England Journal of Medicine* 348 (12):1170.

Currat, Mathias, Laurent Excoffier, Wayne Maddison, Sarah P. Otto, Nicolas Ray, Michael C. Whitlock, and Sam Yeaman. 2006. Comment on "Ongoing adaptive evolution of ASPM, a brain size determinant in Homo sapiens" and "Microcephalin, a gene regulating brain size, continues to evolve adaptively in humans." *Science* 313 (5784): reply 172.

Curtin, P. D. 1992. The slavery hypothesis for hypertension among African-Americans: The historical evidence. *American Journal of Public Health* 82:1681–1686.

Evans, Patrick D., Sandra L. Gilbert, Nitzan Mekel-Bobrov, Eric J. Vallender, Jeffrey R. Anderson, Leila M. Vaez-Azizi, Sarah A. Tishkoff, Richard R. Hudson, and Bruce T. Lahn. 2005. Microcephalin, a gene regulating brain size, continues to evolve adaptively in humans." *Science* 309 (5741):1717–1720.

Fee, Margery. 2006. Racializing narratives: Obesity, diabetes and the Aboriginal thrifty genotype. *Social Science and Medicine* 62 (12):2988–2997.

Fryer, Roland. 2005. Racial differences in life expectancy: the impact of salt, slavery, and selection. Paper presented at the Malcolm Wiener Inequality and Social Policy Seminar Series.

Grim, Clarence, and Miguel Robinson. 2003. Commentary: Salt, slavery, and survival: Hypertension in the African diaspora. *Epidemiology* 14 (1):120–122.

Hammonds, Evelynn M. 2006. Straw men and their followers: The return of biological race. *Is Race Real?* A Web forum organized by the Social Science Research Council (SSRC). raceandgenomics.ssrc.org/.

Kaufman, J. S., and Susan A. Hall. 2003. The slavery hypertension hypothesis: Dissemination and appeal of a modern race theory. *Epidemiology* 14 (1):111–118.

Kempner, J., C. S. Perlis, and J. F. Merz. 2005. Forbidden knowledge. *Science* 307 (5711):854–854.

Kittles, Rick A., and Kenneth M. Weiss. 2003. Race, ancestry, and genes: Implications for defining disease risk. *Annual Review of Genomics and Human Genetics* 4 (1):33.

Leroi, Armand Marie. 2005. Op-Ed: A family tree in every gene. *New York Times,* March 14.

Mekel-Bobrov, Nitzan, Sandra L. Gilbert, Patrick D. Evans, Eric J. Vallender, Jeffrey R. Anderson, Richard R. Hudson, Sarah A. Tishkoff, and Bruce T. Lahn. 2005. Ongoing adaptive evolution of ASPM, a brain size determinant in *Homo sapiens. Science* 309 (5741): 1720–1722.

Mekel-Bobrov, Nitzan, Danielle Posthuma, Sandra L. Gilbert, Penelope Lind, M. Florencia Gosso, Michelle Luciano, Sarah E. Harris, Timothy C. Bates, Tinca J. C. Polderman, Lawrence J. Whalley, Helen Fox, John M. Starr, Patrick D. Evans, Grant W. Montgomery, Croydon Fernandes, Peter Heutink, Nicholas G. Martin, Dorret I. Boomsma, Ian J. Deary, Margaret J. Wright, Eco J. C. de Geus, and Bruce T. Lahn. 2007. The ongoing adaptive evolution of ASPM and Microcephalin is not explained by increased intelligence. *Human Molecular Genetics* 16 (6):600–608.

Regalado, Antonio. 2006. Scientist's study of brain genes sparks a backlash. *Wall Street Journal,* June 16.

Risch, Neil. 2005. Racial groupings match genetic profiles, Stanford study finds. Stanford School of Medicine news release, January 27, 2005.

———. 2006. Dissecting racial and ethnic differences. *New England Journal of Medicine* 408.

Rosenberg, Noah A., Lei M. Li, Ryk Ward, and Jonathan K. Ancestry. 2003. Informativeness of genetic markers for inference of ancestry. *American Journal of Human Genetics* 73 (6):1402.

Rosenberg, Noah A., Saurabh Mahajan, Sohini Ramachandran, Zhao Chengfeng, Jonathan K. Pritchard, and Marcus W. Feldman. 2005. Clines, clusters, and the effect of study design on the inference of human population structure. *PLoS Genetics* 1 (6):e70.

Rosenberg, Noah A., Jonathan K. Pritchard, James L. Weber, Howard M. Cann, Kenneth K. Kidd, Lev A. Zhivotovsky, and Marcus W. Feldman. 2002. Genetic structure of human populations. *Science* 298 (5602):2381.

Shriver, Mark D., and Rick A. Kittles. 2004. Opinion: Genetic ancestry and the search for personalized genetic histories. *Nature Reviews Genetics* 5 (8):611–618.

Shriver, Mark, Rui Mei, Esteban J. Parra, Vibhor Sonpar, Indrani Halder, Sarah A. Tishkoff, Theodore Schurr, Sergev Zhadanov, Ludmila P. Osipova, et al. 2005. Large-scale SNP analysis reveals clustered and continuous patterns of human genetic variation. *Human Genomics* 2 (2):81–89.

Wade, Nicholas. 2002. Race is seen as real guide to track roots of disease. *New York Times,* July 30.

———. 2004. Race-based medicine continued . . . *New York Times,* November 14.

———. 2008. A dissenting voice as the genome is sifted to fight disease." *New York Times,* September 16.

Wells, Spencer. 2007. Building a family tree for all humanity. in *Ideas worth spreading,* edited by TED. www.ted.com/index.php/talks/spencer_wells_is_building_a_family_tree_for_all_humanity.html.

19

Genetic Claims and Credibility

Revisiting History and Remaking Race

KEITH WAILOO, CATHERINE LEE, AND ALONDRA NELSON

We may think we know who we are and where we come from, but we live in an age when science and business compete for our attention—telling us in the media, in courtrooms, in clinical settings, and in political contexts that they possess the secrets to our identities. Observing the multiple clashes in law, medicine, and politics, we may rightly ask: What degree of authority should we grant to the claims that geneticists have unlocked the past and uncovered the truth about racial or ethnic or national identities? Does the evidence support the sweeping claims that we have solved historical mysteries of racial origin and lineage once and for all, or settled other contentious disputes from the past with genetic analysis?

Many geneticists and some social scientists answer, yes—the genetic view of race and history has opened the doorway to a future where true differences can be identified, irrefutable historical knowledge obtained, and better, scientifically informed social policies developed. Although our questions about identity and origin may be at once political and scientific, science apparently holds a stronger hand on the truth. The myriad applications of DNA analysis have not merely focused on predicting a future that is "written in our genes,"[1] but also made fundamental, if problematic, claims about who we are in the present, who we have been in the distant past, and what will become of us in the years ahead. Yet, these assertions of scientific truth remain contentious, and the essays above highlight the care with which we must approach genetic claims about identity and the past. Caution is warranted because of geneticists' own conflicted history with the race concept. Many of today's assertions echo the field's noxious claims about race and heredity from the eugenics age of the early twentieth century—claims, which can now be seen as warnings about how a myopic science legitimated the era's racism and racial politics. While the picture of genetics, race, and history today cannot be reduced to such easy caricatures, what is particularly notable is the way in which genetics ventures enact still-unfolding "racial projects" in diverse national contexts.[2]

These new ideas about race and the past can offer both liberating and limiting possibilities. Genetic testing and analysis in these arenas can expand a sense of connection among social groups, foster an individual's sense of reconciliation and belonging to the nation, or even—in the case of the well-known Innocence Project—support actual liberation in the form of release from unjust imprisonment. However, genetic analysis is also a constraining vehicle (for example, by promoting racial reification, supporting scientifically-sanctioned social exclusion, or fostering essentialism around dangerous notions about the primacy of biological kinship). Clearly, questions of race and genetics must be answered with insights drawn from many cases and contexts. As the essays in this volume highlight, the uses of DNA in the United States, Canada, across Europe, or in South Africa cannot be understood apart from the politics of race in these diverse locales; nor can search for an "Irish genome," a French-Canadian genetic identity, or a Native-American genetic past be separated from the politics of citizenship and nation.

Genetic Claims and Credibility

Genetic claims about the knowable past engender a modern collision between identity and identification, on the one hand, and scientific credibility, on the other. The essays here illustrate the contingent nature of credibility as science intersects with business and commercial interests; as science is deployed in courtroom and policing settings; and as the science of race comes into play in political arenas. The question of credibility, as sociologist Howard Becker wrote four decades ago, illuminates the fundamentally social character of belief and knowledge. He invoked "the notion of a hierarchy of credibility" to describe situations in which in "any system of ranked groups, participants take it as given that members of the highest group have the right to define the way things really are." To be sure, this social negotiation is evident wherever DNA-based insights are invoked in courtrooms, in genetic genealogy, or in other settings, to override or supplant popular beliefs about the past. In Becker's classic view of the hierarchy of credibility, "members of lower groups will have incomplete information, and their view of reality will be partial and distorted in consequence."[3] In works that followed Becker, however, historians and sociologists of science have suggested a more complex interaction of expert, lay, and political knowledge in the maintenance of credibility by scientists as they struggle for public relevance and authority. In these accounts, contests over professional authority are commonplace in the sciences.[4] Drawing on such insights, the essays in this volume trace how genetic analysis becomes credible and is, in turn, linked to various kinds of authoritative political (that is, group and governance) claims.

One should be careful about painting all genetic claims about race and history with one brush, because genetic evidence never speaks for itself; it must be interpreted and spoken for. With this in mind, the chapters above illustrate convergences, divergences, and diverse pathways by which authoritative claims about DNA, race, and history develop. The forensic credibility of DNA claims in the courtroom highlights the ways in which legal standards of evidence and proof are used to evaluate assertions about DNA in relationship to innocence, guilt, liability, and family, backed by the power of the state. In the context of civics and governance, however, political credibility has another standard of evidence—one group's claims about genetic identity are weighed in relation to other groups' claims. In this context, science becomes more credible when it affirms already-existing ideas about the group, its history, and its political agenda. The commercial credibility of genetic genealogy is a different affair—for it depends on the existence, for example, of enough customers who believe that the match between their DNA sample and the company's records can transport them into the past to meet imagined ancestors. Thus, commercial or financial credibility relies too on the reliability of profits. The essays above illuminate the ways in which genetic credibility is an ongoing process, operating at these and many other levels of society.

While lawyers, politicians, and entrepreneurs, along with geneticists do much of the work of translating the complex scientific findings into information and products that are credible to jurors, aggrieved groups, or stockholders, the news media play a powerfully important role in conveying the legitimacy and significance of new genetic findings and disseminating these in the public sphere. Thus, the media is yet another site where scientific credibility is constructed, with recurring stories in which small, even inconsequential, research studies based on limited evidence are woven into grand narratives about what genes mean for identity. Consider, for example, press coverage of a December 2009 genome-wide association study (GWAS) of the genetic relationship between Africans and African Americans. Reporting on the findings, a *Science Daily* story noted that the research team (led by geneticists and computational biologists) had revised what it means to be African American: "People who identify as African-American may be as little as 1 percent West African or as much as 99 percent."[5] When *Science Daily* expounded on the finding, noting that "the data . . . point to the ability of geneticists to *reliably discern* ancestry using such data [emphasis added]," a potential discrepancy between perceived racial identity, lived identity, and scientifically-validated identity emerged. As the news account continued, "Scientists found . . . that they could distinguish African and European ancestry at each region of the genome of self-identified African Americans."[6] In such accounts, genetics is presumed to simultaneously reveal the speciousness of phenotypic views of monolithic races and validate and affirm true historical origins and social identity. Furthermore, the scientists were presented as having a precise tool for revealing an African American identity. Drawing from a press release that had been circulated by the University of Pennsylvania where some of the research was done, the article concluded that the GWAS tool could have "implications for personalized ancestry reconstructions, personalized medicine and more effective drug treatments," not to mention the mapping of genetic risk factors for diseases common to African Americans.[7]

The GWAS study suggests that genetic analyses take on resonance in contexts in which issues of identity and belonging remain unresolved. In the United States, where racial segregation was legally and socially codified but where the intermixing of groups regularly occurred nevertheless, the contested nature of genetic identity takes its meaning from the nation's vexing and still-unresolved ethnoracial ambivalences. In this context, questions of origins and identity have been central to an American cultural imagination," as Jennifer Hamilton notes, and it is perhaps not surprising that the marriage of colonial settler origins, a coerced and volitional migration history, ethnic uncertainty, and capitalism have allowed this brand of genetic genealogy to spread widely from the commercial realm to other social arenas. Thus, context matters enormously to both the production of that genetic evidence and its particular applications and to racial and historical debates. Surveying the map from South Africa to the United States and Canada, we see in the pages above precisely how the locating of genetic ancestors and the meaning associated with one's genetic history play out from one nation to the next. In many instances, the turn toward genetic analysis for resolution is no resolution at all, but rather a step in the evolving cultural process of adjudicating and negotiating identity and national belonging.

Ambiguities and Contradictions

What role should genetic knowledge and analysis play, for example, in ancestry analysis, in the promise of personalized medicine, or in criminal justice—where the pressures to solve a crime or settle an old case are urgent ones? At stake in these settings is the question of the relative credibility of privileged scientific knowledge and lay knowledge about people and the past. Even as national origins stories have become the domain of geneticists, there is an evolving tension between the supposed absolute nature of genetic tests and the seemingly contingent nature of personal accounts. Describing this tension and situating it in particular contexts—as evident in the laboratory, the clinic, the courtroom, the media, and public debates and public policy—has been the topic of the preceding pages. And even with genetic information commanding our attention in these settings, the answers to life's fundamental questions of origin and identity are still necessarily uncertain and contingent. In the end, "the genetic ancestors" are not figures discovered by genomic science who really existed in the past, but they are, rather, assemblages materialized at the intersection of legal and scientific practice, spawned in laboratories, conjured into being by breathless and imaginative reporters, and generated at the intersection of entrepreneurial genealogy businesses and consumer desire.

Close examination of the ambiguities of how race is made and unmade via genetic analysis should lead to greater caution at all levels of society—among scientists, policymakers, and consumers. The process of making convincing and credible links between race and ancestry from genes has involved several levels of deft rhetorical sleights of hand. The essays above track the diverse pathways by which the credibility of genetic claims about race and history are established, including discursive claims to the scientific purity and integrity of earlier historical and political racial categories; scientists' control and use of specialized methods and data; and general boundary control over the scientific enterprise by both scientists and business leaders. Geneticists, for example, today are quick to note that they are not concerned with "races" in the classic sense but with gene pools that are clustered by continents. However, as Lundy Braun and Evelyn Hammonds point out, these continental clusters are often only thinly disguised surrogates for race. Moreover, one important yet unheralded problem in genetic thinking about these originary continental clusters is how (when looking at what were in fact mixed and diverse populations in the past) scientists see them as pure—thereby producing "purity out of mixture, something of great importance to Europeans." The past's continental clusters that are imagined by geneticists, in other words, are ones in which pure groups prevailed and little mixing occurred—defying the historical reality. (Such assumptions of purity are indeed being undermined by genetic scientists themselves. Recent analysis of a 2,000-year-old Italian skeleton suggested maternal Asian ancestry.)[8]

In addition to these curious and historically flawed presumptions of genetic fixity, there is another contradiction in genetic typologies of race today—the science both depends upon nation-specific political categories of race, ethnicity, and identity to characterize populations (Irish, English, Native-American, and French Canadian genomes) and support its claims, while also criticizing those political identities as inferior to scientific views of difference. The genetics of human difference, in other words, is itself caught in the paradox of race. As Hinterberger explains above, although terms such as *ethnic stock* may have fallen into disuse, geneticists still must depend on population classification given to them by the census which continues to shape the identification, monitoring, and inclusion of the kinds of people that make up the nation. Through this process, the evidence of difference that originates in the political process of ethnic identification feeds into the collection of genetic materials for people of the same *ethnic stock*, and thus genetics (for example, in Canada) is caught up in the classification logic of institutionalized multiculturalism, where the "the category *visible minority* is an exemplar of the political logic of multicultural classification."

What are we to make of the fact that, in one context after another, genetic claims relate so intimately and almost seamlessly to site-specific debates about culture, difference, heritage, and diversity? These rhetorical similarities are not coincidental. Marianne Sommer suggests, for example, that we live in a time when public awareness of issues surrounding cultural heritage is heightened and when initiatives like the Human Genome Diversity Project seek to speak to those cultural needs by analogizing the human gene pool to human languages and archeological and historical legacies. The cultural politics of genetic genealogy in Canada is but one instance in which authority is built around, and rests on, the claims to scientific credibility. Nina Kohli-Laven observes above that the affinities between the ways people in the world of medicine and genetics draw population boundaries and the way Quebec nationalists have used those boundaries to forward their historiographic and ideological agendas are striking. Indeed, "the tendency to represent French-Canadians as homogenous and endogamous, whether in science or society at large, is a symptom of the dominance of the nationalist mood, even though those characterizations of a homogeneous French-Canadian past flies in the face of archival work, which suggests a highly mixed society of French and native interaction. The credibility of genetic analysis in this instance, then, overrides historical evidence while reinforcing the political tendencies of the moment. In this and many other instances, the work of constructing scientific, genetic categories is deeply intertwined with the political and social agendas of the classifiers and classified. In this context, the notion that any racial science can also be an apolitical science is deeply flawed. What emerges from these essays is a view of genetic analysis that, owing to an array of processes, has the appearance of a science that stands separate from politics, but where scientific legitimacy depends intimately upon political logic to locate each of us in the social world.

To demonstrate this point, many of our essayists peer into the black box of how genetic data are turned into racial evidence and observe how troubling assumptions about race are intrinsic to the science of techniques such as admixture mapping. "First, admixture mapping methods assume a particular form of relatedness and unrelatedness among and between the individuals they study," observe Ramya Rajagopolan and Joan Fujimura. That is, they use socioculturally defined categories of race to infer a higher level of relatedness among people in one race category and a lower level of relatedness between people in different categories, and so the associations they find between race and biology cannot be seen in nature. These associations are technical and epistemological products. As Rajagopolan and Fujimura conclude, "the link between disease and group is a product of the scientists' assumptions about relatedness within race groups."

Building Credibility

Nationalists, genetic scientists, and business entrepreneurs build credibility around problematic claims regarding historical events and identities with a complex system of signification in which the manipulation of a database (the larger the better) lends authority to the findings. As Peter Chow-White observes, whatever the limitations of genetic thinking, its power is derived from the operation of massive databases of information, and from the fact that "at all levels of society, from institutions to individual identities, information has become the material that social and political meaning is constructed from, new companies profit from, and states use to govern." By looking into the manipulation of information we see how data translate into power, influence, and credible knowledge. And then, when this system is tied to the raw commercial marketing and popular consumer appeal of genetic claims about race, genes, and history and linked to specific consumer products, the circular logic of genes and identity is buttressed further. But as Marianne Sommer writes, the "sex appeal of the new technologies is more likely to be due to the aura of old myths." That is, for many individuals, these new genetic technologies are appealing, because they suggest the possibility of the imprimatur of science on origin stories passed down over generations. And in the process, the line between genetics' role in public memory as a science, and as a business enterprise becomes increasingly blurred.

Technological advances in computing have enabled these manipulations of data. Since the beginning of the recombinant DNA technology in the mid 1970s, commercial goals have infiltrated the fields of genetics and molecular biology. The promise of genetics as a business enterprise, aided by the high-throughput technological abilities of supercomputers and micro-chip storage capacities, has shifted the terminology of the field from "pharmacogen-etics" to "pharmacogen-omics." Whereas the former focused on investigations of single gene-to-gene interactions, the latter relies on technological advances to make possible instantaneous comparisons of multiple genes. Genetic scientists and entrepreneurs tout these advances as laying the foundations for "genetic recipes," which will link genes to identity and products and yield the holy grail of genomic medical research—individualized medicine. It remains to be seen how these pharmacogenomic drugs (if and when they are ever produced) will support, undermine, or intersect with existing notions of identity and difference. In the meantime, commercial claims about the potential for genetic science to identify and ameliorate diverse problems, especially medical ones, outpace actual discoveries. And, potential consumers—patients and physicians—wait for a time when genetic science will lead to medical cures (despite the fact that some leading geneticists are cautious about when, if ever, these advances will materialize).[9]

In contrast to medicine, the courtroom has been one important realm in which the power of genetic information to validate ancestral claims has been actually deployed, tested, and challenged. But even here, ultimately the logic and appeal of these innovative linkages between race, genetics, and history (from North America, through Europe and Africa) are political in character—that is, these linkages are fundamentally concerned with public governance and the power to manage and organize people and their interactions in a society. The complexities of DNA's links to race and the past are as numerous as those of the political terrain itself. In post-apartheid South Africa, for example, Jay Aronson observes that DNA is not so much being used to define the boundaries of race, or to trace the origins of a particular group of people, but rather to ameliorate past injustices to a historically marginalized group defined entirely by race. The success or failure of this effort depends not on the logic of the evidence, but on the shifting politics of reconciliation, blame, and retribution.

In this legal arena, Jonathan Kahn finds a complex interplay between old and new racial concepts. The legal credibility of a genetic race hinges upon our everyday understanding and acceptance that there are indeed different races—a fundamental feature of racialist thinking in American society. In practical terms, the criminal justice system's use of racially identified population databases may improve only slightly the odds of implicating a matched defendant in a criminal case. Nevertheless, there is "an inertial power" to racial thinking that propels its continued use long after any original rationale for its introduction may have passed away. The powerful valence of racial thinking in the courtroom explains how, in one locale, tools like Forensic DNA Phenotyping (FDP), despite its numerous flaws, has succeeded in effectively redirecting investigations, by shifting police attention from suspects in one racial grouping to those in another. In another setting, Native Americans and other groups might turn to genetic information to try to validate their claims to land, restitution, and belonging. This variability in legal uses of genetics and biological evidence indicates the highly charged nature of claims that cry out for a political denouement. The diversity also illuminates the fact that science cannot provide the final blueprint for resolving these essentially political, legal, and social tensions.

Often, scholars championing the next discovery in the genetics of race are quick to dismiss any critics as politically correct naysayers. Reanne Frank rightly observes that defenders of the science "are often represented (and represent themselves) as 'brave scientific martyr-pioneers' who are fighting against the repressive forces of political correctness to bring to light knowledge that other scientists consider taboo." These authors see a stark division between the world of politics and the world of science—a simple, dichotomous view that we do not share. For these martyr-pioneers, politics is not a constituent part of science; rather, science becomes mired in politics only when those who do not fully understand its complexity, constraints and limitations misuse or misinterpret it. As opposed to these views, the preceding chapters have illustrated that the genetic science at the heart of this book is constituted from these complexities, constraints and limitations. All efforts to connect to the past are bound to be speculative, fraught with supposition, and troubled by problems of evidence. Just as selective editing and interpretation is common in the way we each fashion ourselves and our historical identities, so too genetic analysis is shown to be highly selective and politicized from its very inception. If the essays above demonstrate anything, it is that the line between the political and the scientific is blurry and ever-shifting—particularly when geneticists, savvy politicians, and enterprising business leaders wander into the realms of race and history and push us all to revise our ideas about who we are, to what family and community we belong, and what nation we should call home.

NOTES

1.   Adam Geller, "Consumers Turn to Their DNA for Answers," *Boston Globe,* March 28, 2006; www.boston.com/business/personalfinance/articles/2006/03/28/consumers_turn _to_their_dna_for_answers/ [Accessed March 19, 2010].

2. Michael Omi and Howard Winant, *Racial Formations in the United States: From the 1960s to the 1990s*, 2nd ed. (New York: Routledge, 1994), 56–58.

3. Howard S. Becker, "Whose Side Are We On?" *Social Problems* 14 (Winter 1967):241.

4. Abby J. Kinchy and Daniel Lee Kleinman, "Organizing Credibility: Discursive and Organizational Orthodoxy on the Borders of Ecology and Politics," *Social Studies of Science* 33 (December 2003):869–896; Steven Epstein, *Impure Science: AIDS, Activism and the Politics of Knowledge* (Berkeley: University of California Press); Tomas F. Gieryn, *Cultural Boundaries of Science: Credibility on the Line* (Chicago: University of Chicago Press, 1999); Sheila S. Jasanoff, "Contested Boundaries in Policy-Relevant Science," *Social Studies of Science* 17 (1987):195–230; Bruno Latour and Steve Woolgar, "The Cycle of Credibility," in *Science in Context: Readings in the Sociology of Science*, ed. Barry Barnes and David Edge (1979; rpt. Milton Keynes: Open University Press, 1982), 35–43.

5. Katarzyna Bryc, Adam Auton, Matthew R. Nelson, Jorge R. Oksenberg, Stephen L. Hauser, Scott Williams, Alain Froment, Jean-Marie Bodo, Charles Wambebe, Sarah A. Tishkoffh, and Carlos D. Bustamante, "Genome-Wide Patterns of Population Structure and Admixture in West Africans and African Americans," *Proceedings of the National Academy of Sciences* 107 (December 22, 2009), www.pnas.org/content/107/2/786.full.pdf+html?sid=1dee1ff6–68b9–40bc-96bd-a1ad7806cbe7.

6. "Genetic Study Clarifies African-American Ancestry," *Science Daily* (December 24, 2009): www.sciencedaily.com/releases/2009/12/091221212823.htm [emphasis added].

7. Ibid.

8. "DNA Testing of 2,000-Year-Old Bones in Italy Reveal East Asian Ancestry," *Science Daily* (February 2, 2010): *www.sciencedaily.com/releases/2010/02/100201171756.htm*. In this same year, there were also reports, based on so-called "ancient DNA" analyses, that Native Americans had traveled to the Americas 500 years prior to Columbus and that a woman of Native American or East Asian ancestry had lived among the Vikings. See Giles Tremlett, "First Americans 'Reached Europe Five Centuries before Columbus Discoveries'" *Guardian*, 16 November 2010, www.guardian.co.uk/science/2010/nov/16/first-americans-europe-research?CMP=twt_gu; and "Vikings Brought Amerindian to Iceland 1,000 Years Ago: Study," *The Independent* (November 21, 2010), www.independent.co.uk/life-style/ health-and-families/vikings-brought-amerindian-to-iceland-1000-years-ago-study-2140130.html.

9. The tenth anniversary of the decoding of a draft of the human genome in July 2010 brought with it cautious appraisals of the genomics era and medical genetics from unlikely quarters. The *New York Times* reporter Nicholas Wade, typically an enthusiatic booster of developments in genetic science, wrote that the "primary goal" of the Human Genome Project—medical applications—"remains largely elusive." More strikingly, maverick geneticist Craig Venter declared in the press that we "have learned nothing from the genome other than probabilities." In late 2011, there was news of a successful instance in which whole genome sequencing resulted in treatement for symptoms of a genetic condition called dopa-responsive dystonia. At present, however, such developments continue to be quite rare, and personalized medicine, indeed, remains elusive. See Nicholas Wade, "A Decade Later, Genetic Map Yields Few Cures," *New York Times*, June 10, 2010, www.nytimes.com/2010/06/13/health/research/13genome.html; "Spiegel Interview with Craig Venter: 'We Have Learned Nothing from the Genome,'" *Der Spiegel*, July 29, 2010, www.spiegel.de/international/world/0,1518,709174–2,00.html; and Ericka Check Hayden, "Genome Study Solves Twins' Mystery Condition," *Nature* (June 15, 2011), www.nature.com/news/2011/110615/full/news.2011.368.html.

CONTRIBUTORS

Jay D. Aronson is an associate professor of Science, Technology, and Society at Carnegie Mellon University. His work focuses is on the interactions of science, technology, law, and human rights, in a variety of contexts. He is currently engaged in a long-term study of the ethical, political, and social dimensions of post-conflict and post-disaster DNA identification of the missing and disappeared. He is the founder and director of the Center for Human Rights Science at Carnegie Mellon. He received his Ph.D. in History of Science and Technology from the University of Minnesota and was both a pre- and post-doctoral fellow at Harvard University's John F. Kennedy School of Government.

Lundy Braun is Royce Family Professor in Teaching Excellence and Professor of Medical Science and Africana Studies and a member of the Faculty Committee on Science and Technology Studies at Brown University. She received her Ph.D. from Johns Hopkins University School of Hygiene and Public Health in 1982. Her current research focuses on the history of race, technology, and science and the burden of asbestos-related diseases in South Africa. She has published several articles on the contemporary debate over race, genomics, and health disparities. She is currently writing a monograph, tentatively titled *Race, Difference, and Vital Capacity Measurements: Historical Perspectives.*

Peter A. Chow-White is an assistant professor in the School of Communication at Simon Fraser University in Vancouver, Canada. He is coauthor, with Lisa Nakamura, of the edited book *Race after the Internet.* He has published on race, gender, technology, and genomics in *Science, Technology & Human Values*, *Media, Culture & Society*, and the *International Journal of Communication and Communication Theory.* Currently, he is working on two research projects. In the first project, he is collaborating with medical scientists who are developing a molecular diagnostic technology for cancer to research the management of personal genetic information in healthcare settings. In his second project, he is writing a scholarly monograph that draws from his research on social media and data mining.

Reanne Frank is an associate professor of sociology at The Ohio State University. Her research focuses on the sociology of immigration and race/ethnic inequality with a focus on health and mortality. Her primary research area concerns the role of migration in shaping demographic and health outcomes in both sending and receiving countries and communities. Her work in this area has centered primarily on the case of Mexico and Mexican immigration to the United States. A secondary research interest concerns the intersection of genetics and racial differences in health.

Joan H. Fujimura is a professor of sociology, and Science and Technology Studies, at the University of Wisconsin, Madison. She has written on the sociology of genetics, molecular biology, biotechnology, biomedicine, and systems biology. She is currently writing a book on her interdisciplinary study of the use of notions of population, race, and ancestry in biomedical and human variation studies. Her current field research project examines interdisciplinarity and collaboration in systems biology and epigenetics research.

Abram Gabriel is an associate professor of molecular biology and biochemistry at Rutgers, The State University of New Jersey. His research focuses on the study of mechanisms and consequences of retrotransposon reverse transcription, those parts of the genome knows as "jumping genes" or "mobile DNA." He was a member of the Geneticist-Educator Network of Alliances Project, an initiative aimed at developing methods for the improvement of high school science curricula. He holds an M.D. from the Johns Hopkins University School of Medicine.

Jennifer A. Hamilton is an assistant professor of Legal Studies and anthropology and the director of the Law Program at Hampshire College. She is a cultural anthropologist who is centrally interested in how ideas of difference shape institutional forms, and how they influence individual and social subjectivities. She is the author of *Indigeneity in the Courtroom: Law, Culture, and the Production of Difference of North American Courts* and is currently working on a project about legal standing and the life sciences.

Evelynn Hammonds is the dean of Harvard College and Barbara Gutmann Rosenkranz Professor of the History of Science and of African and African American Studies at Harvard University. She served previously as Harvard's first senior vice provost for Faculty Development and Diversity. Prior to joining Harvard, she was the founding director of the Center for the Study of Diversity in Science, Technology, and Medicine at the Massachusetts Institute of Technology. Her scholarly interests include the history of scientific, medical, and sociopolitical concepts of race, the history of disease and public health, gender in science and medicine, and African-American history. Her most recent book is *The Nature of Difference: Sciences of Race in the United States from Jefferson to Genomics* (2009). In 2010, she was appointed to President Barack Obama's Board of Advisors on Historically Black Colleges and Universities.

Amy Hinterberger is a research fellow at the Institute for Science, Innovation, and Society, University of Oxford. She received her Ph.D. in sociology from the BIOS

Centre at the London School of Economics and Political Science. She recently completed a postdoctoral fellowship at the Institute for the Study of the Americas in the School of Advanced Study, University of London. Her research explores the intersections among the state, science, and commerce in contemporary human genome science.

Michelle M. Jacob (Yakama) is an associate professor of Ethnic Studies at the University of San Diego. She holds a Ph.D. in sociology from the University of California at Santa Barbara. Her interests include racial and ethnic identity, American Indian studies, gender in Native America, American Indian health and education issues, social justice movements, and indigenous grassroots activism. Her research has been published in many venues, including *American Behavioral Scientist*, *Social Justice*, *International Feminist Journal of Politics*, *Wicazo Sa Review*, and several edited volumes. She is currently completing a book on cultural revitalization activism on the Yakama Reservation.

Jonathan Kahn is a professor of law at Hamline University School of Law. He holds a Ph.D. in U.S. history from Cornell University and a J.D. from the Boalt Hall School of Law, University of California, Berkeley. His current research focuses on the intersections of law, race, and genetics, with particular attention to how regulatory mandates intersect with scientific, clinical, and commercial practice in producing and classifying genetic information in relation to racial categories. He is currently working on a book titled *Race in a Bottle: Law, Commerce, and the Rise of Ethnic Medicine in a Post-Genomic Age* (2012).

Nina Kohli-Laven is currently a postdoctoral fellow in the Department of Social Studies of Medicine at McGill University and at the Institute for Health Policy Studies at the University of California, San Francisco. Her research explores the production of emergent health technologies, combining anthropology, history, and science and technology studies. She has published on the social production of biomedical evidence in cancer clinical trials. Her present work investigates the politics of breast cancer screening in the purview of new genomic technologies, looking at how regulatory and bioclinical infrastructures shape styles of reasoning about risk and therapy.

Catherine Lee is an assistant professor in sociology and a faculty associate at the Institute for Health, Health Care Policy, and Aging Research at Rutgers University. Her areas of research include race and ethnicity, immigration, law, and science and medicine. Her work on race and science has focused on the construction of race in biomedical research and government regulation of race in health policy. She is completing a book titled *Fictive Kin: Family Reunification and the Meaning of Race in Immigration Policy*, which explores the varying ideas about family and their centrality for constructing race and legislating American immigration policy from the mid-nineteenth century to today.

Sandra Soo-Jin Lee is a senior research scholar at the Stanford University Center for Biomedical Ethics. Her work as a medical anthropologist probes the social and cultural contexts of emerging genetic technologies and their application in biomedicine as well as the social and ethical implications of human genetic variation research. She is currently working on a book entitled *American DNA: Race, Justice, and the New Genetic Sciences.*

Alondra Nelson is an associate professor of sociology at Columbia University, where she also holds an appointment in the Institute for Research on Women and Gender. She is the author of *Body and Soul: The Black Panther Party and the Fight Against Medical Discrimination* (2011) and coeditor of *Technicolor: Race, Technology, and Everyday Life* (2001). She is currently at work on a book entitled *Reconciliation Projects*, which explores how claims about race, ethnicity, and ancestry are marshaled together with genetic analysis in a range of social and political ventures.

Ramya Rajagopalan is a postdoctoral research associate in the Department of Sociology and the Holtz Center for Science and Technology Studies at the University of Wisconsin, Madison. Her current research (jointly with Joan Fujimura) investigates contemporary developments in the life sciences, including human genetic variation research, and interdisciplinary collaboration in systems biology and epigenetics research. Her publications include "Different Differences: The Use of 'Genetic Ancestry' versus Race in Biomedical Human Genetic Research" (with J. H. Fujimura). Rajagopalan received her Ph.D. in genomics and molecular biology from the Massachusetts Institute of Technology.

Pamela Sankar is an associate professor of bioethics in the Department of Medical Ethics at the University of Pennsylvania. Her degrees are in history of ideas, anthropology, and communications, and she has completed postdoctoral training in health services research. Dr. Sankar's research and teaching interests include research ethics, genetics and race, and the history of privacy. Her current research concerns the use of genetics in law enforcement and public understanding of evolution.

Marianne Sommer is a professor of cultural studies at the University of Lucerne in Switzerland. Her research focuses on the cultural history of the life sciences, particularly the human origins sciences. Her latest monograph represents a (pre)history of paleoanthropology and related disciplines—including the genetic approach—from ca. 1800 to the present (*Bones and Ochre*, 2007). She has recently published "DNA and Cultures of Remembrance: Anthropological Genetics, Biohistories, and Biosocialities" (*BioSocieties*, 2010). She is director of the SNSF-Project "History Within: The Phylogenetic Memory of Bones, Organisms, and Molecules" (see www.phylogenetic-memory.uzh.ch).

Keith Wailoo, formerly Martin Luther King Jr. Professor of History at Rutgers University, is Townsend Martin Professor of History and Public Affairs at Princeton

University. He is author of *How Cancer Crossed the Color Line* (2011), *The Troubled Dream of Genetic Medicine: Ethnicity and Innovation in Tay-Sachs, Cystic Fibrosis, and Sickle Cell Disease* (2007) (coauthored with Stephen Pemberton), *Dying in the City of the Blues: Sickle Cell Anemia and the Politics of Race and Health* (2001), and *Drawing Blood: Technology and Disease Identity in Twentieth-Century America* (1997). He is also editor of *Three Shots at Prevention: The HPV Vaccine and the Politics of Medicine's Simple Solutions* (2010) (coedited with Julie Livingston, Steven Epstein, and Robert Aronowitz) and *Katrina's Imprint: Race and Vulnerability in America* (2010) (coedited with Karen O'Neil, Jeffrey Dowd, and Roland Anglin).

Priscilla Wald is a professor of English at Duke University, where she is a member of the Institute for Genome Sciences and Policy and an affiliate of the Trent Center for Bioethics and Medical Humanities and the Institute for Global Health. She teaches and works on U.S. literature and culture, particularly literature of the late-eighteenth to mid-twentieth centuries and the intersections among the law, literature, science, and medicine. Her most recent book is *Contagious: Cultures, Carriers, and the Outbreak Narrative.* She is also author of *Constituting Americans: Cultural Anxiety and Narrative Form* and is currently at work on *Human Being after Genocide,* a book-length study of changing ideas of the human that emerged from scientific and technological innovation in the wake of the Second World War.

INDEX

Aboriginal people: in Canada, 205, 214–216; Canadian classification of, 212, 221n1; identification of, 215

aboriginal population, defining, 184

admixture: "recent," 146, 147; use of term, 146, 194

admixture mapping, 51–53, 143; American identification in, 160; ancestral frequencies used in, 319; and assumptions about race, 330; compared with family linkage studies, 145; construction of populations, 148; continental and racial labels used in, 154; deconstructing admixture in, 145–149; explained, 145; goal of, 319–320; vs. GWAS, 159; limitations of, 147; maps, 150–151, 152; of populations and diseases, 159; practices of, 153–154; researchers' definition and categories used in, 146, 148, 150; study design for, 145

Adulthood Rites (Butler), 258, 260

adverse drug reactions (ADRs), reducing, 166–168

Africa: codification of languages of, 70; colonial interventions in, 78; before colonial penetration, 74; delimiting tribes in, 69–72; genetic diversity of, 152; importance for researchers of, 67; shaping image of, 67. *See also* Africans; South Africa

African American Heart Failure Trial (A-HeFT), 172, 173

African American Lives (documentary), 57, 267

African Americans: admixture mapping for, 51, 151; drug designed exclusively for, 171–176; end-stage renal disease in, 51; frequencies calculated in contemporary, 152; FyO allele among, 53; genetic makeup of, 59, 61; genetic relationship with Africans, 327; heart failure in, 172; health disparities in, 173–174; hypertension in, 320; label of, 170; multiple ancestries of, 147; in New World, 59; prostate cancer in, 155; risk factors for diseases, 327; self-identification as, 147; sickle cell anemia in, 60–61, 135, 144, 157

African Ancestry, Inc., 21, 22–23, 23, 24, 267, 271, 273; operations of, 29n8, 30n9

African Ancestry Project, 231

African Burial Ground Memorial, of U.S. National Parks Service, 24

"African chromosome," 154, 155

Africandna, 57–58

African Eve theory, 232

African Lineage Database (ALD), 24

African National Congress (ANC): African centers of, 300–301; elite of, 303–304; in exile, 301–302; history of, 300–301; and identification of missing, 302; military strategy of, 301; and reburials, 309; shift in modus operandi of, 302; unbanned, 302

"African risk allele," 157

Africans: databases for, 97; DNA analysis of, 59; FyO allele among, 53; genetic relationship with African Americans, 327; producing knowledge about, 69

African societies: categorizing of languages of, 70; classification of, 76; descent as organizing principle of, 73; ethnographies of, 77; internal dynamics of, 74; precontact, 74; reduced to static forms, 76

Afrofuturists, 85

Agamben, Giorgio, 274

Ahmed, Sara, 212

AIMs. *See* ancestry informative markers

Alcoff, Linda, 212, 213

allele frequencies: in ancestry testing, 318; in forensic analysis, 129; race-specific, 132

alleles, 46; in evolutionary science, 252; and geographic region, 107–108

allele specific primer extension (ASPE), in forensic analysis, 128–129

American Indian high school students, tutors and mentors for, 283–284. *See also* Native youth education program

American Indian Recruitment (AIR) Program, 280, 292; indigenous and scientific perspectives in, 291–292; NAGPRA introduced in, 283. *See also* Native youth education program

American Society of Human Genetics, 156, 267

ancestral groups, in making of AIMs, 151

ancestral origins: locating genetic, 328; role of DNA in, 43

ancestral populations: definitions of, 148; local histories in, 152